CLUSTER RANDOMISED TRIALS

CHAPMAN & HALL/CRC
Interdisciplinary Statistics Series

Series editors: N. Keiding, B.J.T. Morgan, C.K. Wikle, P. van der Heijden

Published titles

Published titles

Chapman & Hall/CRC
Interdisciplinary Statistics Series

CLUSTER RANDOMISED TRIALS

Richard J. Hayes

Lawrence H. Moulton

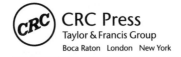

CRC Press
Taylor & Francis Group
Boca Raton London New York

CRC Press is an imprint of the
Taylor & Francis Group, an **informa** business

A CHAPMAN & HALL BOOK

Chapman & Hall/CRC
Taylor & Francis Group
6000 Broken Sound Parkway NW, Suite 300
Boca Raton, FL 33487-2742

© 2009 by Taylor & Francis Group, LLC
Chapman & Hall/CRC is an imprint of Taylor & Francis Group, an Informa business

Library of Congress Cataloging-in-Publication Data

Hayes, Richard J., DSc.
    Cluster randomised trials / authors, Richard J. Hayes and Lawrence H. Moulton.
       p. ; cm. -- (Interdisciplinary statistics)
    "A CRC title."
    Includes bibliographical references and index.
    ISBN 978-1-58488-816-1 (hardcover : alk. paper)
    1. Clinical trials. 2. Cluster analysis. I. Moulton, Lawrence H. II. Title. III. Series.
    [DNLM: 1. Cluster Analysis. 2. Randomized Controlled Trials as Topic--methods. 3.
Data Interpretation, Statistical. WA 950 H418c 2009]

R853.C55H39 2009
615.5072'4--dc22
                                                                             2008035804

Visit the Taylor & Francis Web site at
http://www.taylorandfrancis.com

and the CRC Press Web site at
http://www.crcpress.com

To our families:

Anne, Clare and Emma; Ann, Carine and Tyler.

Contents

Part C: Analytical Methods

Preface

Randomised controlled trials are the accepted gold standard for evaluating the effects of interventions to improve health, and the advantages of this study design are widely recognised. In the great majority of such trials, individual patients or participants are randomly allocated to the experimental conditions under study, for example to treatment and control groups. Sometimes, however, it is more appropriate to randomise *groups* of individuals to the different treatment arms. Trials of this kind are known as *cluster randomised trials*, and this book aims to discuss the design, conduct and analysis of such trials.

Few cluster randomised trials were carried out before the 1980s, but since then the design has become more widely known and many such trials are carried out and reported every year. In the early years, the special design and analysis requirements of these trials were not always understood, and there were many examples of trials that were designed, analysed or reported inappropriately. Over the past two decades, much work has been done on methods for cluster randomised trials, and the quality of reported trials has gradually improved.

This is still a relatively new study design, and methods for such trials are an active area of statistical research. A large number of alternative methods have been proposed and published, and their relative merits have not always been definitively established. We have reached the stage, however, where it is possible to present a set of core methods of design and analysis. In this book, we have not attempted to provide a comprehensive review of all possible methods. Rather we have aimed to select a more limited range of methods that are simple to understand, easy to apply with readily available statistical software and perform well under the conditions experienced in most cluster randomised trials.

The book has grown out of the personal involvement of the authors in a wide range of cluster randomised trials, mostly in the field of international public health. We hope it will provide a useful practical resource for investigators carrying out such trials. Toward this end, we have provided more material on study design options than is usually found in statistical texts.

While some equations are needed to describe and present the methods adequately, we have tried to avoid unnecessary mathematical detail. We have also worked hard to use consistent notation throughout the book, and this is set out in the Glossary of Notation.

We were particularly keen that readers should be able to apply the methods to their own trials. There is therefore a heavy emphasis on practical examples, many of them based on our own research. We have tried to include examples from a wide variety of settings, including both developing and industrialised countries. Cluster randomisation may confer particular advantages when evaluating the effects of interventions against *infectious diseases*. We feel that this aspect of the design has received insufficient emphasis in the literature, and have ensured that our examples cover such applications as well as studies of non-communicable diseases. To illustrate the application of analytical methods, we have provided several datasets from actual trials. These datasets can be downloaded from the "Downloads & Updates" section of the publisher's website at http://www.crcpress.com/e_products/downloads/. Computer output is displayed in text boxes to show how these data can be analysed using the *Stata®* statistical package. The reader is encouraged to reproduce these analyses and to explore alternative approaches. Equivalent analyses can usually be carried out using other packages such as *SAS®*.

While our examples focus on medical applications, the cluster randomised trial design is of equal relevance for the evaluation of other types of intervention, for example in the fields of education or social welfare. We hope that the book will be of value to practitioners working in these and other fields. We think that the rigorous evidence of intervention effects provided by cluster randomised trials has the potential to inform public policy in a wide range of areas.

This book could not have been written without the help of many friends, colleagues and collaborators. We have benefited from valuable discussions on methodology and applications with many colleagues. We are particularly grateful to Simon Cousens, Steve Bennett and Andrew Thomson for sharing their insights, and to the many statisticians and other colleagues who have worked with us on specific trials over the years. We would like to thank Fred Binka, John Changalucha, Heiner Grosskurth, Linda Morison, Kate O'Brien, Gillian Raab, Ray Reid, David Ross, Mathuram Santosham, Helen Weiss and Danny Wight for making available datasets from their studies. The first author was able to work on the first draft of this book during a sabbatical from his work as head of the Tropical Epidemiology Group, and wishes to thank Helen Weiss and Paul Milligan for looking after the group in his absence. The support and inspiration provided by the Consortium to Respond Effectively to the AIDS-TB Epidemic (CREATE), funded by the Bill and Melinda Gates Foundation, have been important factors in this book's conception and completion. We are grateful to Rebecca Hardy who reviewed the first draft of the manuscript and provided many useful comments and suggestions. Her input has considerably improved the book. We would also like to thank Natasha Larke and Liz Turner who checked and commented on various drafts of the material. Natasha Larke also worked with the first author on the adaptation of some of the material for use in a study module offered as part of the MSc distance learning course in Clinical Trials at the London School of Hygiene and Tropical Medicine. Finally, we are grateful for the constant love and support of our families, to whom this book is dedicated.

Authors

Richard Hayes is professor of epidemiology and international health at the London School of Hygiene & Tropical Medicine and Head of the MRC Tropical Epidemiology Group. He is a statistical epidemiologist whose main research interest is in the epidemiology of infectious diseases of public health importance in developing countries. He has a particular interest in the epidemiology and control of HIV and other sexually transmitted diseases, tuberculosis and malaria. He is one of the principal investigators of a collaborative programme of research in Mwanza, Tanzania, whose aim is to develop and evaluate effective preventive interventions against the HIV epidemic. He is also involved in collaborative research on HIV and related infections in other parts of Africa, including Uganda, Zimbabwe, Zambia and South Africa. Richard also conducts research on statistical and epidemiological methods, and is involved in work on the design and analysis of cluster-randomised trials, and on transmission models of HIV and other STDs.

Lawrence Moulton is professor of the departments of international health and biostatistics, at the Johns Hopkins Bloomberg School of Public Health. He has been the principal statistician on several large cluster randomised field trials of infectious disease interventions. His expertise is in correlated data analysis, study design, and statistical epidemiology. His substantive areas of interest include safety and effectiveness of childhood vaccines, and the prevention of HIV and tuberculosis transmission. At Johns Hopkins University, he directs the PhD program in global disease epidemiology and control and the Peace Corps/Masters International Program, and is co-director of the Institute for Vaccine Safety.

Glossary of Notation

Statistics and Parameters

d = observed number of events or number of subjects with the event
x = quantitative outcome
n = total number of individuals
m = number of individuals per cluster
y = person-years of observation
c = number of clusters
z = covariate
e = expected number of events or number of subjects with the event
$\bar{e}$ = expected mean of quantitative outcome
μ = population mean
π = population proportion
λ = population rate
σ = population standard deviation
σ_W = within-cluster standard deviation
$\bar{x}$ = sample mean
p = sample proportion
r = sample rate
l = log sample rate
h = difference in log sample rate between treatment arms
s = sample standard deviation
RR = risk ratio or rate ratio
OR = odds ratio
R_r = ratio-residual
R_d = difference-residual

Note: Greek characters are generally used for true (population) values and Latin characters for observed (sample) values.

Subscripts

i = treatment arm ($i=1$: intervention; $i=0$: control)
j = cluster ($j=1,..., c$)
k = individual ($k=1, ..., m$)
l = covariate ($l=1, ..., L$)
s = stratum ($s=1, ..., S$)

e.g., d_{ijk} = number of observed events in kth individual in jth cluster in ith treatment arm.

Measures of between-cluster Variability

k = coefficient of variation
k_m = coefficient of variation within matched pairs or strata
ρ = intracluster correlation coefficient
σ_B = between-cluster standard deviation

Expectation and Variance

$E()$ = expected value of a random variable
$Var()$ = variance of a random variable

Regression Coefficients

α = intercept parameter
β = regression parameter representing intervention effect
γ = regression parameter representing effect of covariate
u = random effect representing between-cluster variability

Standard Normal Distribution

$z_{\alpha/2}$ = standard normal distribution value corresponding to upper tail probability of $\alpha/2$
z_β = standard normal distribution value corresponding to upper tail probability of β
α = probability of Type I error
β = probability of Type II error

Note: z is used to denote both covariates and standard normal deviates. The meaning should be clear from the context.

Part A

Basic Concepts

1

Introduction

1.1 Randomised Trials

The past two decades have seen increasing acceptance that decisions regarding major public health interventions or clinical treatments should be based on careful review of the evidence from rigorously conducted studies to analyse the benefits and adverse effects of the proposed interventions. Resources for health care are limited even in the industrialised countries and may be severely limited in developing countries. Rational policy making requires that the limited resources available should be used to provide interventions that have been proven to be effective and cost-effective. This book focuses on the collection of evidence of effectiveness and in particular the use of cluster randomised trials to measure the population-level effects of interventions delivered to groups of individuals.

Randomised controlled trials have come to play a central role in evidence-based medicine because they are regarded as the "gold standard" for evaluating the effectiveness of interventions. This rests on three key features of the randomised controlled design. First, the interventions or treatment conditions are allocated to participants by the investigator. This means that it is possible to assemble treatment groups that are comparable in every respect other than the treatment condition, thus coming close to the principles of laboratory experimentation where the aim is to vary one factor while keeping other factors constant. Observational studies can also be used to provide information about the effects of interventions by comparing outcomes in individuals in a study population who happen to access a given intervention with those who do not. However, these groups of individuals are likely to vary with regard to many other characteristics that may be risk factors for the outcome of interest, and it may be difficult to control adequately for these differences.

Second, a key feature of the randomised controlled trial is that there should be a control group that is followed up in parallel to the intervention group using similar methods, so that outcomes can be compared between these groups over the same time period. Many health-related outcomes show substantial variations over time, referred to as *secular trends*. In a randomised controlled trial, any secular trends should affect the treatment groups equally and so comparisons between groups should not be distorted by these trends. In contrast, alternative study designs using *historical controls* or control groups from a different population may be seriously affected by secular trends.

Third, randomisation is used to allocate participants to the treatment conditions under comparison. This is not only an objective, fair and transparent procedure but, if implemented correctly and with an adequate sample size, should virtually ensure that the treatment groups are comparable with respect to all characteristics apart from the treatment conditions under study. Importantly, this includes potential confounding factors, even those that are unknown or unmeasurable. This is a very significant strength of the randomised study design.

In addition, there are a number of accepted procedures for the implementation of randomised controlled trials that further enhance their rigour, including allocation concealment, blinding, trial monitoring and intention-to-treat analysis.

Because of these methodological advantages, systematic reviews of the evidence regarding the effects of interventions—such as those carried out within the framework of the Cochrane Collaboration—are usually based primarily on data from randomised controlled trials. Moreover, the regulatory procedures for licensing of new products such as drugs and vaccines require the conduct of well-conducted randomised controlled trials. In addition to such "clinical trials", randomised trials may also be used to evaluate the effects of public health interventions, such as health education programmes, community-based vitamin A supplementation or provision of insecticide-treated bednets to reduce mortality from malaria.

1.1.1 Randomising Clusters

In most randomised controlled trials, individual participants are randomly allocated to treatment arms. We shall refer to such trials as "individually randomised trials". Methods for the design and analysis of such trials are well known.

In some trials, however, *groups* of individuals may be randomly allocated to treatment arms. These groups are referred to as *clusters*, and such trials are known as *cluster randomised trials*. Examples of clusters include schools, communities, factories, hospitals or medical practices, but there are many other possible choices. Depending on the definition of a cluster, there are a number of alternative terms for such trials, the most common of which are *group randomised trials* and *community randomised trials*. The term *community trial* is sometimes used, but is ambiguous since it does not distinguish between individually randomised trials carried out in the community and trials in which communities are randomised to treatment arms. We shall use the abbreviation CRT for cluster randomised trials throughout this book.

The reasons for adopting a cluster randomised design are discussed in more detail in Chapter 3, but the main reasons are as follows:

- The intervention by its nature has to be applied to entire communities or other groupings of individuals, or it is more convenient or acceptable to apply it in this way.
- We wish to avoid the *contamination* that might result if individuals in the same community were to be randomised to different treatment arms.
- We wish to capture the population-level effects of an intervention applied to a large proportion of a population, for example an intervention designed to reduce the transmission of an infectious agent.

There are two key features of CRTs which mean that special methods of design and analysis are needed for such trials. First, observations on individuals in the same cluster are usually correlated. Standard methods for designing and analysing randomised trials, including sample size calculations, assume that the observations on all individuals in the trial are statistically independent but this assumption is violated when clusters are randomised. Special methods are therefore needed for the design and analysis of CRTs that take these correlations into account.

Second, because the clusters are often large, it is usually not possible to randomise a large number of clusters to each treatment arm. With small numbers of clusters, we cannot rely on randomisation to ensure adequate balance between arms. A number of design strategies are used to address this problem, including the use of matching, stratification and restricted randomisation, and these will be discussed in later chapters.

The randomised controlled trial design was first used for medical trials in the 1930s and 1940s, but it was not until the 1980s that a significant number of studies were carried out using cluster randomisation. Practical experience with this design is therefore much more limited than for standard individually randomised trials, and a number of reviews have been carried out pointing to the poor methodological quality of many CRTs published during the past two decades (Donner, Birkett, and Buck 1990; Simpson, Klar, and Donner 1995).

Despite this, some CRTs have been carried out to a high standard and have had a major effect on global health policy. An important example is a linked set of four CRTs that were carried out in sub-Saharan Africa to determine the effect of insecticide-treated bednets on child mortality (Binka et al. 1996; D'Alessandro et al. 1995; Habluetzel et al. 1997; Nevill et al. 1996). The results of the trials, showing a 20% reduction in all-cause child mortality across four disparate study populations, have provided definitive evidence of the value of this important intervention which remains a cornerstone of malaria control efforts in Africa.

1.1.2 Some Case Studies

To illustrate the range of possible applications, we briefly introduce three case studies. Each of these will be discussed in more detail in later chapters.

Example 1.1

A number of large CRTs have been carried out in developing countries to measure the effects of a range of public health interventions. Most commonly in these trials, the cluster is an entire community, for example a village, district or other type of geographical zone. Because the clusters are typically large, it is usual for the number of clusters to be quite small. Many of these trials are of interventions against infectious diseases and, as noted above, the CRT design allows us to measure the population-level effects of interventions and thus to capture indirect effects of an intervention, acting through a reduction in transmission of an infectious agent, as well as direct effects.

We illustrate this with a CRT carried out in the Mwanza region, Tanzania in the early 1990s (Grosskurth et al. 1995). The sexual transmission of HIV between infected and uninfected partners is known to be enhanced in the presence of other sexually transmitted diseases (STDs) in either partner. Improved treatment of STDs has therefore been proposed as an indirect strategy to prevent HIV infection in populations where STDs are highly prevalent and existing treatment services are inadequate.

The trial was carried out in 12 rural communities, where each community was defined as the catchment population of a health centre and its satellite dispensaries. These 12 communities were arranged in six pairs that were matched on geographical location, type of community (roadside, lakeshore, island or rural villages) and prior STD rates recorded at the health centre. Based on previous data from the region, HIV incidence rates were expected to be similar in the two communities in each pair as a result of the matching. Within each pair, one community was randomly chosen to receive the intervention immediately, the other acting as a control community. The intervention was extended to all comparison communities at the end of the trial.

The intervention consisted of training of staff at government health centres and dispensaries to deliver improved treatment services for STDs using the approach of syndromic management. To evaluate the population-level impact of the intervention, a random sample of approximately 1000 adults was selected from the general population in each of the 12 communities, and followed up over a two-year period to measure the incidence of HIV infection. A total of 12,537 adults were recruited and 8845 (71%) were seen at follow-up. The trial reported a 40% reduction in HIV incidence in the intervention arm compared with the control arm.

Note that cluster randomisation was chosen because the intervention had to be delivered at community level since it involved the training of health unit staff, but the CRT design also allowed population-level effects of the intervention to be captured. Given the small number of clusters randomised, the matched pairs design was adopted in an effort to improve the balance between treatment arms and to reduce between-cluster variability.

Example 1.2

In both industrialised and developing countries, the CRT design is often selected to examine the effects of interventions in institutions, such as schools, factories or other workplaces.

Project SHARE was a CRT carried out in Scotland to measure the impact of a school-based sexual health education programme (Wight et al. 2002). In this trial, 25 secondary schools in Scotland were randomly allocated to the intervention and control arms. The intervention consisted of a teacher-delivered programme of 20 classroom sessions on sexual health, 10 sessions in the third year and 10 in the fourth year of secondary school. The control schools continued with their existing sex education programmes.

To evaluate the effects of the SHARE intervention, two successive cohorts of third year students were recruited and followed to the start of their fifth year, approximately 6 months after the end of the intervention sessions. A total of 8430 students were enrolled in the cohort (around 340 per school) and 5854 (67%) were successfully followed up 2 years later. No differences were seen in sexual activity or risk taking at follow-up, although students in the intervention arm reported less regret of first sexual intercourse with their most recent partner.

Note that the CRT design was chosen for this study because the SHARE intervention programme was designed for application to groups of school students. If the intervention were effective in changing attitudes or behaviours, its impact might be further enhanced if delivered across all third and fourth year students in a school, through effects on peer norms. Randomisation of schools allowed for any such population-level effects to be captured.

Example 1.3

CRTs are sometimes carried out to examine the effects of interventions at the level of medical practices. This design is particularly suited to the UK where most residents are registered with a general practice that forms part of the National Health Service. Randomisation of practices has allowed the effects of different strategies of treatment, diagnosis or prevention to be investigated.

In the POST trial, 52 general practices in the London Borough of Hackney were randomised to test the effects of an intervention to improve secondary prevention of coronary heart disease (Feder et al. 1999). The intervention involved the sending of postal prompts to patients 2 weeks and 3 months after discharge from hospital following admission for myocardial infarction or unstable angina, providing recommendations on methods of lowering the risk of a coronary event and encouraging patients to make an appointment with their GP for further discussion; letters were also sent to the GP for each recruited patient, with a summary of effective prevention measures.

To evaluate the effects of the POST intervention, the 52 practices were randomly allocated to intervention (25 clusters) and control (27 clusters) arms. A total of 328 patients from the study practices were recruited at the time of discharge from hospital and allocated to the intervention or control arms according to the allocation of their general practice. Six months after discharge, each patient was sent a questionnaire and information was extracted from medical records to determine the proportions of patients who had a consultation with their GP, received advice on risk factors and prevention, had tests to record levels of risk factors such as serum cholesterol and were prescribed beta-blockers or other medication.

GP consultation for coronary prevention was significantly increased in the intervention arm, and more patients in intervention practices had their serum cholesterol measured. Disappointingly, there were no significant effects on the prescription of effective drugs for secondary prevention or on self-reported changes in lifestyle.

Note that postal prompts to patients might potentially have been allocated at individual level, but since the intervention also included interventions at the level of the general practice it was decided to randomise at this level.

Also note that the CRTs described in Example 1.2 and Example 1.3 were essentially *unmatched*, in contrast to the *pair-matched* trial in Example 1.1, although in each case special methods of randomisation were used to improve the balance between arms.

1.1.3 Overview of Book

The book is divided into four parts. Part A introduces the reader to *basic concepts* underlying the use of cluster randomisation. As we have already noted, a key feature of CRTs is that observations on individuals from the same cluster tend to be correlated, as a result of variation between clusters in the outcomes of interest. In Chapter 2, we discuss some alternative measures of between-cluster variability and the relationships between them. Chapter 3 discusses the circumstances when cluster randomisation should be used. The design is sometimes used to capture the indirect effects of interventions against infectious diseases when applied to entire populations, and we define and explain the terms *direct*, *indirect* and *total effects*.

In Part B, we consider a range of specific issues in the *design* of CRTs. Chapter 4 considers the choice and definition of the clusters to be randomised and discusses strategies for minimising *contamination* effects in CRTs. Chapter 5 discusses the use of *matching* and *stratification* to improve the balance between treatment arms and to reduce between-cluster variability, and provides guidelines on when these strategies should be adopted. Chapter 6 discusses randomisation procedures in CRTs, including the use of *restricted randomisation* to improve balance between treatment arms. Special methods for sample size calculation are needed for CRTs, and these are set out in detail in Chapter 7. In Chapter 8, we discuss some alternatives to the simplest two-arm CRT, including trials with more than two arms, factorial designs and stepped wedge trials.

Part C considers analytical methods for CRTs. Basic principles of analysis are discussed in Chapter 9. The next two chapters consider the analysis of simple unmatched CRTs, starting with methods based on cluster-level summaries in Chapter 10 and proceeding to regression methods based on individual-level data in Chapter 11. The analysis of CRTs with matched, stratified or other study designs is discussed in Chapter 12.

Part D covers miscellaneous topics in the conduct of CRTs. Ethical issues of special relevance to CRTs are discussed in Chapter 13, while trial monitoring and interim analyses are explored in Chapter 14. Finally, the reporting and interpretation of CRTs are discussed in Chapter 15.

2

Variability between Clusters

2.1 Introduction

In a conventional clinical trial, in which individual subjects are randomly allocated to the different treatment arms, we can generally assume that observations on all individuals are statistically independent. In a CRT, in which groups or clusters of individuals are randomly allocated to treatment arms, the assumption of independence is usually invalid because observations on individuals in the same cluster are *correlated*. Much of this book is devoted to describing statistical methods of design and analysis that take such correlations into account.

Observations on individuals in the same cluster will be correlated, in the statistical sense, if and only if knowledge of one individual's outcome confers more information about the outcome of another individual in that same cluster than it provides about the outcome of an individual in a separate cluster. Note that within-cluster correlation depends on the existence of other clusters, and has no meaning if there is just one study population under consideration.

As an example, suppose we consider as a response variable the beverage of choice of residents of Paris and Dublin. Suppose we randomly select one resident of Dublin and find that he or she drinks Guinness, a popular Irish beer. If we then randomly select a Parisian, and guess that he or she also drinks Guinness, our guess is less likely to be correct than if we make the same guess for another randomly selected resident of Dublin. This is an example of positive within-city correlation. If, however, our sample consists only of residents of Dublin, the issue of within-city correlation becomes moot as it is the only city remaining under consideration. If Dublin is broken down into its constituent neighbourhoods, of course, the outcome may show within-neighbourhood correlation. We shall see later that the extent of intracluster correlation often depends on the nature and size of the clusters.

In CRTs, there will almost always be positive within-cluster correlation due to variability in the underlying, or *true*, means of outcomes between clusters. If clusters have different mean response levels, it follows that persons in the same cluster will tend to have responses that are more similar to each other than responses of persons in different clusters. As we shall see, the variance of observed cluster means will be the sum of the within-cluster sampling variance and the between-cluster variance in the underlying means.

Negative within-cluster correlation, on the other hand, is rarely encountered in practice. It can arise in situations where there is minimal variability between cluster means, coupled with a competition for resources that renders cluster means less variable than they would be if observations were independent. Consider a CRT of a pneumococcal vaccine in a rural population where the outcome is hospitalisation due to pneumonia. Suppose that each study community is a 3-day drive from the hospital and that there is only one vehicle in any given community. Then, even if residents need hospitalisation at the rate of one every 2 days, or 15 per month, only four to five patients per month will actually arrive at the hospital. Thus, the observed rate will be a relatively constant value of four or five every month. In contrast, if there were several vehicles available, there would be much greater month-to-month variability, perhaps modelled by a Poisson random variable, generally varying from 5 to 25. The *underdispersion* induced by the availability of only one vehicle would be reflected as negative within-community correlation. Admittedly, this is a highly contrived situation, and in practice we would not wish to proceed with the trial if the outcome variable were constrained in this way; but it is only in such extreme situations that we will be faced with cluster means varying less than would be expected if individual responses were uncorrelated. A more natural example is that of the size of wildlife populations in designated regions with limited food supplies.

As we shall see, between-cluster variability and within-cluster correlation provide two different perspectives on the same underlying phenomenon, and we shall use both approaches during the chapters that follow. It is therefore important to understand the relationship between them.

We begin in Section 2.2 with some simple examples to illustrate the importance of between-cluster variability in making inferences from a CRT. In Section 2.3, we then define and discuss two alternative measures of between-cluster variability, the *coefficient of variation between clusters* (k) and the *intra-cluster correlation coefficient* (ρ), and go on to explain the relation between the two measures. We also explore, in Section 2.4, how they are related to the *design effect*. Finally, Section 2.5 presents some practical examples of how correlations may arise in CRTs.

2.2 The Implications of Between-cluster Variability: Some Examples

We present two simple examples to demonstrate why between-cluster variability cannot be ignored when designing and analysing a CRT.

Example 2.1

First, consider the two hypothetical CRTs shown in Figure 2.1. In each trial, 10 villages have been randomly allocated to two treatment arms, five villages receiving a community-wide health education programme designed to improve hygiene behaviour and the other five villages forming a control group. The primary outcome is the prevalence of diarrhoea in children aged under 5 years at the end of follow-up, and Figure 2.1 and Table 2.1 show the observed prevalences in the 10 villages in each trial.

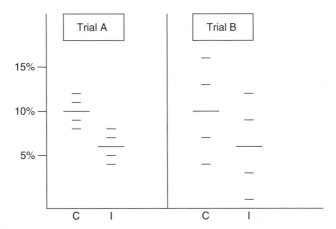

FIGURE 2.1
Prevalence of diarrhoea in children in ten villages in two hypothetical CRTs (C: Control arm, I: Intervention arm).

TABLE 2.1

Prevalence of Diarrhoea in Children in Ten Villages in Two Hypothetical CRTs

Trial A		Trial B	
Control	**Intervention**	**Control**	**Intervention**
8/100 (8%)	4/100 (4%)	4/100 (4%)	0/100 (0%)
9/100 (9%)	5/100 (5%)	7/100 (7%)	3/100 (3%)
10/100 (10%)	6/100 (6%)	10/100 (10%)	6/100 (6%)
11/100 (11%)	7/100 (7%)	13/100 (13%)	9/100 (9%)
12/100 (12%)	8/100 (8%)	16/100 (16%)	12/100 (12%)
50/500 (10%)	30/500 (6%)	50/500 (10%)	30/500 (6%)

With equal numbers of children in each village, the overall prevalence of diarrhoea in each treatment arm is simply the mean of the village-level prevalences. In each trial, the overall prevalences in the intervention and control arms were 6 and 10%, respectively, implying that the intervention was associated with a 40% reduction in prevalence.

If we analysed these two trials using standard methods, ignoring the cluster-randomised design, we would simply compare the overall prevalences in the intervention and control arms. This yields an identical chi-squared statistic of $\chi^2 = 5.43$ (1 degree of freedom) for both trials, giving a *P*-value of 0.02 in each case.

It is clear from Figure 2.1, however, that Trial A provides much stronger evidence than Trial B of an intervention effect. In Trial A, all five villages given the intervention had equal or lower prevalences of diarrhoea than all of the five control villages, whereas in Trial B there was substantial overlap in the prevalences observed in the two arms. Using an appropriate method of analysis that takes account of the cluster-randomised design (see Chapter 10), the P-values were 0.004 for Trial A and 0.22 for Trial B, showing clearly how the inferences that can be made from a CRT depend on the degree of between-cluster variability in the outcome of interest.

Example 2.2

Now consider a CRT carried out to measure the effect of a training programme for general practitioners (GPs) to improve their treatment of a specific type of back pain. A total of 50 GPs are selected for the study and 25 are randomly allocated to receive the new training programme, the other 25 serving as a control group.

To assess the effects of the training programme on the quality of diagnosis and treatment, medical records are collected and analysed for a random sample of five patients with back pain seen by each GP during a 1-year period, giving a total sample of 125 patients in each arm of the study. Based on review of the records, an algorithm is used to derive a GP performance score for each patient. Mean scores are then compared for the patients in each arm of the trial.

In this example, the scores for patients of the same GP are likely to be correlated, since it is probable that the GP will use similar diagnostic and treatment procedures for patients presenting with the same condition. In a conventional individually randomised trial, doubling the sample size provides twice the information so that, for example, the variances of estimates are halved. In the CRT in this example, however, doubling the number of patients sampled in each practice would *not* provide twice the information. In the extreme case in which GPs are entirely consistent in their practices, so that all scores within each practice are identical, it is clear that only one patient needs to be sampled to provide complete information on the performance of each GP. The (identical) data for the other four patients are redundant in this case.

A consequence of this is that if we decide to increase the power of the trial by doubling the sample size from 125 to 250 per arm, the amount of additional information provided will depend on how the increased sample size is achieved. Doubling the number of GPs to 50 per arm while continuing to sample five patients per GP will provide more information (and possibly much more information, depending on the strength of correlation) than continuing to study 25 GPs per arm but doubling the patients per GP from 5 to 10.

Clearly the application of standard statistical methods based on an assumption of independent data to such CRTs would lead to invalid inferences, since these methods take no account of the structure of the data or of the correlations between observations.

Note that, in this example, the scores for the patients of each GP will only be correlated if there are differences in the performance of different GPs. If the performance of all GPs was similar, then two patients of the same GPs would be no more likely to have similar scores than two patients of different GPs, and the within-cluster correlation would be zero. This reiterates the point that within-cluster correlation and between-cluster variability are merely two ways of viewing the same phenomenon. We explore this point in more detail in Section 2.3.

2.3 Measures of Between-cluster Variability

2.3.1 Introduction

In order to take account of between-cluster variability in the design and analysis of a CRT, we need to define an appropriate measure of variability. In this section, we define two alternative measures of variability and explain the relationship between them.

We begin by considering data on an outcome of interest from a single set of clusters. These could represent baseline data from the set of clusters that are to be enrolled in a CRT, prior to randomisation and intervention. Alternatively, they could represent follow-up data from the clusters in one arm of a CRT. The point is that at this stage we are not considering any effects of intervention. Intervention effects will be considered in detail in later chapters.

In this book, we shall focus mainly on three types of outcome that are of interest in most medical and epidemiological studies:

2.3.1.1 Binary Outcomes and Proportions

Each individual subject either does or does not satisfy a certain condition. The parameter of interest is the *proportion* of individuals satisfying the condition, or equivalently the *probability* that a randomly chosen individual satisfies the condition. We use data from the finite sample of individuals studied in the trial to estimate π, the *true value* of the proportion in a notional wider population from which the trial subjects are assumed to be randomly sampled. Examples would be the *point prevalence* of some medical condition (e.g., proportion obese at end of study) or the *cumulative incidence* of a disease during a fixed follow-up period (e.g., proportion developing clinical malaria during 3 months' follow-up).

2.3.1.2 Event Data and Person-years Rates

Individuals are followed up over time, and the number of occurrences of a defined event recorded together with the person-years of follow-up. The parameter of interest is the *rate*. We use data from a finite sample of follow-up time to estimate λ, the *true value* of the rate in a notional wider population from which the trial follow-up time is assumed to be randomly sampled. An example is the *incidence rate* of a disease, sometimes referred to as the *hazard* or *force of morbidity* (e.g., incidence of tuberculosis expressed per 100 person-years in a TB vaccine trial).

An alternative way to handle event data is to model the intervals between events. Such *time-to-event* data are the subject of *survival analysis*, which aims to explain why some intervals are longer than others. Analysing the time until a person is diagnosed with TB, rather than just whether or not he or she is diagnosed, can result in a more powerful analysis. In most CRTs, however, the occurrence of disease is of greater interest than the timing of the occurrence.

2.3.1.3 Quantitative Outcomes and Means

A quantitative variable, which may be either discrete or continuous, is measured on each individual. We will generally assume that the parameter of interest is the *mean*, although other measures are possible (e.g., median, geometric mean). We use data from the finite sample of individuals studied in the trial to estimate μ, the *true value* of the mean in a notional wider population from which the trial subjects are assumed to be randomly sampled. Examples might include mean blood pressure in a treatment trial for hypertension, or mean number of sexual partners in an HIV prevention trial.

Note that by *true value* we refer to a parameter with a fixed but unknown value. Thus, we are working in a frequentist rather than Bayesian framework, and assume that our observations refer to a random sample from a notional infinite population.

2.3.2 Coefficient of Variation, k

Suppose there are c clusters, and that the *true value* of the parameter of interest in the jth cluster ($j=1, \ldots, c$) is given by μ_j. In general, μ_j will be a proportion, rate or mean, as discussed above.

We assume that the μ_j are randomly sampled from a probability distribution with mean $E(\mu_j)=\mu$ and variance $Var(\mu_j)=\sigma_B^2$, where σ_B^2 represents the *between-cluster variance*. Then the *coefficient of variation* is defined as:

$$k=\sigma_B/\mu \tag{2.1}$$

This definition is quite general, and applies whether the parameter of interest is a proportion, rate or mean. If it is a proportion or rate, μ in Equation 2.1 is replaced by π or λ, respectively.

It is important to recognise that the μ_j in this definition represents the *true value* of the parameter in each of the c clusters. The μ_j are not directly observable, since we collect data only on a finite sample of individuals (or person-time) in each cluster. However, as we shall see later, it is possible to use the *observed values* of the proportion, rate or mean in each cluster to obtain valid estimates of σ_B, μ and hence k.

Example 2.3

Suppose we are planning a CRT to investigate the effect of providing insecticide-treated bednets on the prevalence of malaria parasitaemia in village children aged under 5 years. We plan to randomly allocate entire villages to the intervention and control arms, and need an estimate of between-village variability to assist with the study design.

Malaria parasitaemia is a binary outcome, and we are interested in making inferences about the *proportion*, π, with this outcome. Malariologists who are familiar with the area tell us that the prevalence of malaria parasitaemia averages around 30% but could easily vary between 15 and 45% in individual villages. If we are prepared to assume that the village prevalences are approximately normally distributed, this would imply a σ_B of around 0.075, since roughly 95% of prevalences would fall within two standard deviations of the mean ($30\% \pm 2 \times 7.5\%$ gives the interval $15-45\%$). Thus we could obtain an estimate of k as:

$$k = \sigma_B/\pi = 0.075/0.30 = 0.25$$

Note that this should be treated as a rough estimate of k for at least two reasons. First, it is unlikely that the village-level prevalences exactly follow a normal distribution. Second, we are assuming that the statement "could easily vary between" translates roughly to a 95% range.

We are sometimes in the fortunate position of having observed data on cluster-level proportions. We shall see how to use these to obtain an unbiased estimate of k in Chapter 8.

2.3.3 Intracluster Correlation Coefficient, ρ

We have already seen that between-cluster variability and within-cluster correlation are two ways of viewing the same phenomenon. The degree of within-cluster correlation can be measured by the *intracluster correlation coefficient*, ρ. This represents how much more similar are measurements of individuals from the same cluster than those from different clusters.

Let x_{jk} be the observed outcome for the kth individual in the jth cluster ($j = 1, \ldots, c$). We assume here that x is either a binary or quantitative outcome, as ρ is not defined for event data based on person-years rates. Then the *intracluster correlation coefficient*, ρ, is defined as:

$$\rho = \frac{E(x_{jk} - \mu)(x_{jk'} - \mu)}{E(x_{ik} - \mu)^2} \tag{2.2}$$

In this equation, the expectation in the numerator is over all distinct pairs of individuals ($k \neq k'$) taken from the same cluster and over all clusters; the expectation in the denominator is over all individuals and all clusters; and μ is the true mean over the entire population.

In general, ρ will fall between zero and one. A ρ of zero implies that there is no clustering so that individuals within the same cluster are no more similar than individuals from different clusters, in other words there is no between-cluster variability. A ρ of one implies that individuals in the same cluster are perfectly correlated, in other words they all have the same outcome.

It is technically possible to have a ρ of less than zero. This occurs if each cluster is more heterogeneous than a randomly selected sample from the population. However, this is very uncommon in practice as we have seen in Section 2.1, and we do not consider this possibility further.

2.3.3.1 Quantitative Outcomes

If x is a quantitative outcome, Equation 2.2 reduces to:

$$\rho = \frac{\sigma_B^2}{\sigma^2} = \frac{\sigma_B^2}{\sigma_B^2 + \sigma_W^2} \tag{2.3}$$

where σ_B^2 is the between-cluster variance, or $Var(\mu_j)$ in the notation of Section 2.3.2; σ_W^2 is the within-cluster variance $Var(y_{jk}/\mu_j)$; and σ^2 is the overall variance for a randomly selected individual. Note that $\rho=0$ if $\sigma_B^2=0$ (no between-cluster variability) while $\rho=1$ if $\sigma_W^2=0$ (no within-cluster variability).

2.3.3.2 Binary Outcomes

For a binary outcome, the denominator σ^2 is replaced by the variance $Var(x_{jk})$ of the outcome in a randomly selected individual from the entire population. This random variable is typically assumed to follow the Bernoulli distribution with probability π, where π is the true proportion for the entire population, and we therefore obtain $Var(x_{jk})=\pi(1-\pi)$, so that:

$$\rho = \frac{\sigma_B^2}{\pi(1-\pi)} \tag{2.4}$$

where σ_B^2 is $Var(\pi_j)$, the variance of the cluster-specific true proportions.

2.3.3.3 Estimation of ρ

While the intracluster correlation coefficient is perhaps less intuitive to use than the coefficient of variation, we can obtain estimates of ρ by using Equation 2.3 and Equation 2.4. With quantitative data, we need estimates of σ_B and σ_W, and these may be obtained either by informed judgement or, if there are empirical data available on the outcome of interest, by one-way analysis of variance of between and within cluster variation. With binary data, we need estimates of σ_B and π, and note that these are the same estimates needed to obtain $k=\sigma_B/\pi$.

2.3.4 Relationship between k and ρ

For binary outcomes, a simple relationship exists between k and ρ. From Equation 2.4 we have:

$$\sigma_B^2 = \rho\pi(1-\pi)$$

while from Equation 2.1, we note that:

$$\sigma_B^2 = k^2\pi^2$$

It follows that:

$$\rho = \frac{k^2\pi^2}{\pi(1-\pi)} = \frac{k^2\pi}{1-\pi} \tag{2.5}$$

Note from Equation 2.5 that $\rho=0$ when $k=0$, as we would expect. Note also that, since $\rho<1$, it follows that:

$$k < \sqrt{\frac{1-\pi}{\pi}}$$

This provides a useful upper bound for k.

For quantitative outcomes, there is no simple relationship between ρ and k, although Equation 2.1 and Equation 2.3 confirm that $\rho=0$ when $k=0$, as for binary outcomes. For event data we recall that the intracluster correlation coefficient is undefined, and this is a disadvantage of methods that rely on this measure of between-cluster variability.

2.4 The Design Effect

When we carry out a CRT, we can consider this as equivalent to collecting data from a *cluster sample* of individuals in each treatment arm, rather than a *simple random sample* as in a conventional individually randomised clinical trial. It is well known that, in general, cluster sampling provides less precise estimates of parameters of interest than simple random sampling, and the *design effect (DEff)* (Kish 1965) is used to measure the increase in variance resulting from the use of this sampling design:

$$\text{Design effect} = \frac{\text{Variance for cluster sampling}}{\text{Variance for simple random sampling}}$$

Since the variance for a simple random sample is inversely proportional to the sample size, the design effect also gives the *effective sample size* for the cluster sampling design:

$$\text{Effective sample size} = \text{Actual sample size}/DEff$$

For example, if $DEff=2$, this means that the cluster sample will provide the same precision as a simple random sample of half the size.

To see how the design effect relates to k and ρ, we first derive an equation for the variance of the parameter estimate of interest based on our cluster sample, and see how this relates to the variance under simple random sampling. We consider only the simplest design, with a random sample of c clusters each of size m.

2.4.1 Binary Outcomes

Assume that the outcome in each individual is labelled a *success* or a *failure*, and let d_j be the number of "successes" in the jth cluster. Then the *observed proportion* in that cluster is given by $p_j=d_j/m$.

Since the number of successes in the jth cluster follows the binomial distribution, we note that the variance of p_j conditional on the true proportion π_j in that cluster is:

$$Var(p_j \mid \pi_j) = \frac{\pi_j(1-\pi_j)}{m}$$

Based on this expression, it may be shown that the unconditional variance of p_j is given by:

$$Var(p_j) = \frac{\pi(1-\pi)}{m} + \frac{m-1}{m}\sigma_B^2$$

Our overall estimate of the proportion, based on c clusters, will be:

$$\bar{p} = \frac{1}{c}\sum_{j=1}^{c} p_j$$

and so:

$$Var(\bar{p}) = \frac{\pi(1-\pi)}{mc} + \frac{(m-1)\sigma_B^2}{mc} \qquad (2.6)$$

Note that this variance has two components. The first is the binomial variance implicit in estimating a proportion π based on a finite sample of size mc. The second is the additional variability due to the between-cluster variation, as measured by σ_B^2.

Using Equation 2.4 and rearranging, we can show that:

$$Var(\bar{p}) = \frac{\pi(1-\pi)}{mc}[1+(m-1)\rho]$$

and since $\pi(1-\pi)/mc$ is the variance of an estimate based on a simple random sample, it follows that the design effect in this case is:

$$DEff = 1+(m-1)\rho$$

The corresponding formula for k follows from the relationship between ρ and k:

$$DEff = 1+(m-1)\frac{k^2\pi}{1-\pi}$$

2.4.2 Quantitative Outcomes

With a quantitative outcome x_{jk} measured on each individual, we now obtain the observed mean $\bar{x}_j$ for each cluster. The variance of $\bar{x}_j$ conditional on the true mean μ_j in that cluster is given by:

$$Var(\bar{x}_j \mid \mu_j) = \frac{\sigma_W^2}{m}$$

Based on this expression, it may be shown that the unconditional variance of $\bar{x}_j$ is given by:

$$Var(\bar{x}_j) = \frac{\sigma_W^2}{m} + \sigma_B^2$$

Our overall estimate of the mean π, based on c clusters will be:

$$\bar{x} = \frac{1}{c} \sum_{j=1}^{c} \bar{x}_j$$

and so:

$$Var(\bar{x}) = \frac{\sigma_W^2}{mc} + \frac{\sigma_B^2}{c}$$

Using Equation 2.3 and recalling that the overall variance $\sigma^2 = \sigma_B^2 + \sigma_W^2$ this simplifies to:

$$Var(\bar{x}) = \frac{\sigma^2}{mc}[1 + (m-1)\rho]$$

and since σ^2/mc is the variance of an estimate based on a simple random sample, it again follows that the design effect is:

$$DEff = 1 + (m-1)\rho$$

The corresponding formula for k is:

$$DEff = 1 + (m-1)\frac{k^2\mu^2}{\sigma^2}$$

We see that, when using the intracluster correlation coefficient, the formula for the design effect takes the same simple form for both types of outcome. We note that the design effect increases with the intracluster correlation coefficient, ρ, but also with the cluster size, m. This means that the design effect may be substantial when we have large clusters, even if the intracluster correlation is small.

Since the design effect for a CRT is generally greater than one, the required sample size when clusters are randomised is greater than for an individually randomised trial addressing the same study question. Increased sample size clearly has cost and logistical implications and we shall be returning to this point in more detail in Chapter 7 and Chapter 15.

2.5 Sources of Within-cluster Correlation

Within-cluster correlation, or equivalently between-cluster variability, can occur in CRTs for three main reasons.

2.5.1 Clustering of Population Characteristics

The first reason is the most obvious, which is that health conditions tend to exhibit geographical variations or variations between the different institutions, such as schools or medical practices, that may form the basis of the cluster randomised design. These variations may be due to differences in the characteristics of the *individuals* that make up each cluster, including demographic, socioeconomic, behavioural and other factors. They may also be due to differences in *cluster-level* variables. For example, rates of infectious diseases may vary according to the environmental characteristics of the cluster, including climate, soil, breeding sites of vectors and other variables. And the outcome of interest may also be influenced by the performance or behaviour of key players operating at cluster level such as teachers, community leaders or medical practitioners. Regardless of their source, clustering of population characteristics will lead to within-cluster correlation even in the absence of any intervention.

2.5.2 Variations in Response to Intervention

A perhaps less obvious point is that different clusters may respond differently to the intervention so that, even in the absence of any prior between-cluster variation in the outcome of interest, following the intervention there is variation in outcomes between clusters. Such within-cluster correlation in intervention response may occur either because individual responses are correlated, due to interaction between the intervention and geographically clustered population characteristics as described above, or because the intervention is implemented by one or a small number of individuals (e.g., the staff of a medical practice) who may be responsible for varying responses across the clusters.

2.5.3 Correlation Due to Interaction between Individuals

As we shall discuss in Chapter 3, cluster randomisation may be particularly appropriate in trials of interventions against infectious diseases, since effects of the intervention on the acquisition or natural history of infection in one individual may have subsequent effects on transmission to other individuals in the same community. The transmission of infections from one person to another, either directly or through vectors or intermediate hosts, implies that the assumption of statistical independence of outcomes between individuals is not strictly correct, and is an additional and important cause of within-cluster correlation. Other types of interaction between individuals can also lead to such correlations. For example, community members may discuss their opinions of health education messages, leading to similarities in risk behaviour between members of the same community.

Example 2.4

In the *MEMA kwa Vijana* trial in Tanzania, 20 rural communities were randomly allocated to an intervention arm receiving an integrated adolescent sexual health programme or a control arm (Hayes et al. 2005; Ross et al. 2007). The main component of the intervention was a school-based sexual health education programme delivered by teachers in all the primary schools in each community.

All of the above sources of within-cluster correlation may have been important in this trial. First, there were substantial variations between communities in social, economic and demographic factors. Some communities were remote rural villages, others were trading settlements on main roads and two communities were located close to gold mining areas where higher risk sexual behaviour may be more common. Second, the delivery of the intervention was largely dependent on the skill and commitment of teaching staff, so that the response in each community was influenced by the performance of a small number of individuals. For example, poor implementation of the programme by teachers in a community could significantly influence the response in that community. Finally, the sexual behaviour of one individual clearly has effects on other individuals in the same community, while the incidence rates of sexually transmitted infections that were the primary outcomes of this trial are influenced by population-level transmission dynamics as well as individual risk behaviour.

3

Choosing Whether to Randomise by Cluster

3.1 Introduction

We have seen in Chapter 2 that correlations between observations on individuals within the same cluster lead to estimates that are less precise than those based on simple random samples. In a CRT, we collect data on a sample of clusters in each treatment arm, and our estimates of treatment effect are based on comparison of the results from these cluster samples. It follows from this that, in general, a CRT will provide less precise estimates than an individually randomised trial with the same total number of individuals.

Because of the loss of statistical efficiency implicit in the CRT design, individual randomisation is usually the method of choice unless there are cogent reasons for adopting cluster randomisation. In this chapter, we discuss the main reasons for using the CRT design. Ultimately, the choice of a design is driven by the nature of the intervention, the logistics of implementing the intervention and the particular scientific question of interest.

We begin in Section 3.2 with reasons for adopting the CRT design that may apply to any kind of intervention. There are a number of additional reasons for randomising by cluster that apply to interventions against *infectious diseases*, and these are considered in Section 3.3. In particular, we see how a CRT may capture the *indirect effects* of an intervention on the transmission of infection when it is applied to a large proportion of a population, in addition to the *direct effects* that are captured by individually randomised trials. Indirect effects may also be of importance in studies of non-infectious diseases. Finally, in Section 3.4, we discuss some of the disadvantages and limitations of cluster randomisation.

3.2 Rationale for Cluster Randomisation

3.2.1 Type of Intervention

In a conventional clinical trial, we are generally interested in measuring the efficacy of a treatment or other medical intervention delivered to an individual patient. Individual randomisation is the natural choice in these circumstances. Sometimes, however, we wish to measure the effects of interventions which *by their nature* are applied to entire communities or other groupings of individuals.

Example 3.1

A new programme of peer-led sex education has been developed for implementation in secondary schools. This involves training older students to act as peer-educators and to work with classes of younger students during scheduled classroom sessions. It would not be possible to randomise individuals to receive this intervention, as it is designed for delivery to entire classes. We might therefore choose to randomise classes. Alternatively, for logistical convenience and to avoid contamination (children in intervention classes sharing information with those in control classes), we might decide to randomise entire schools.

Example 3.2

A programme to provide improved water supplies to villages in a rural area of a developing country is to be evaluated to measure its effect on childhood diarrhoea. Since the programme is implemented at village level, and involves provision of clean water through boreholes and hand-pumps that are shared by all the villagers, it would not be possible to randomise individuals to receive or not receive the intervention. Instead it would be more appropriate to randomise at the village level. In the case of a programme which is to be rolled out throughout a region, it may be decided to use a "stepped wedge" design whereby all villages receive the intervention but it is introduced in random order so that a valid measure of its effects can be obtained (see Chapter 9).

Example 3.3

The UK National Health Service wishes to evaluate a new health promotion intervention which involves the provision in general practice waiting rooms of information leaflets on healthy eating. Since the intervention is based on leaving the leaflets in the waiting room for patients to pick up, it would not be possible to randomise individual patients to receive the intervention. It is therefore decided to randomise general practices to receive the leaflets or to act as control practices.

3.2.2 Logistical Convenience and Acceptability

In Section 3.2.1, we considered interventions which, by their nature, could not be evaluated in an individually randomised trial. If we wish to obtain evidence from a randomised trial for these interventions, we have no choice but to adopt cluster randomisation. Sometimes, however, we wish to evaluate an intervention which could in principle be delivered at the individual level, but where cluster randomisation would offer greater logistical convenience.

Example 3.4

A placebo-controlled trial was carried out in northern Ghana to measure the effect of regular vitamin A supplements on childhood mortality (Ghana VAST

Study Team 1993). Because this is a rare outcome, even in high mortality countries, a large sample size was needed to detect a clinically significant reduction in mortality. More than 20,000 children were enrolled in this trial. Vitamin A or placebo was delivered by field workers through household visits at four-monthly intervals. It would, in principle, be possible to randomise individual children to receive vitamin A or placebo. However, it was decided that this would be practically difficult to organise, as field workers would then have to take with them lists of the allocations for all children in the trial and identify them individually at each visit. Instead, the study area was divided into 185 geographical clusters, averaging just over 100 children per cluster. These clusters were randomly allocated to the intervention (92) or control (93) arms. This was much more convenient as field workers only needed to take the appropriate medication (vitamin A or placebo) with them on their visit to each cluster.

Cluster randomisation may also be more acceptable to the community than a design whereby different individuals in the same community receive different treatments, especially if blinding is not possible. This may be particularly the case in rural communities in some less industrialised countries, where key decisions are often made communally. Individual allocation of neighbours to receive or not receive an intervention in such a setting might cause resentment, and might be unacceptable to village leaders who may be looked to by the community to ensure that externally provided resources are distributed equitably.

Example 3.5

In a rural area of Bangladesh, a study is conducted to look at the effects of enhanced micro-credit services on utilisation of health services. Enabling women to have greater access to funds to run small enterprises may provide them with higher disposable incomes and empower them to take their children to health facilities. Although the lending process is carried out at an individual level, it would not seem fair for one woman to have access to credit while her neighbour does not. Thus, the investigator decides to randomise at the village level, allowing all women in a selected intervention village to participate in the programme.

3.2.3 Contamination

In an individually randomised trial, the term *contamination* usually refers to a situation where individuals in one treatment arm actually receive part or all of the intervention allocated to another treatment arm. The term *crossover* may also be used for this situation, but is usually reserved for trials in which the change in intervention status is part of the study design. The result of contamination is that outcome differences between the treatment arms will be diluted, biasing the trial toward smaller effect estimates. Contamination can occur in many ways:

Example 3.6

Patients undergoing cataract surgery are individually randomised to two groups. The first is given a new solution to apply following surgery to aid healing, the second group receiving usual standard of care. Participants given the new solution may share it with friends and neighbours undergoing cataract surgery.

Example 3.7

Secondary school students who are smokers are randomly allocated to receive individual counselling using cognitive behavioural therapy (CBT) to help them give up smoking, or to a control group. Smoking quit rates are compared in the two arms of the trial. It is likely that students in the CBT group will talk to friends in the control group about the counselling they have received. This may have some influence on the behaviour of control group participants, leading to dilution of the measured intervention effect.

Contamination is also an issue in trials carried out in general practice. If individual patients treated by the same doctor are randomised to different treatment groups, it is likely that treatment methods in the intervention arm will spill over to the control arm.

Contamination is particularly likely in non-blinded studies, where participants are aware which treatment arm they are in. Participants who know they are in the control arm may take steps to obtain the intervention. In a trial of male circumcision to reduce HIV transmission in South Africa, for example, 10.3% of men who were randomised to the control arm had been circumcised by other providers by the 21 month follow-up visit (Auvert et al. 2005). Contamination may also occur in blinded studies, although probably to a lesser extent as participants should be unaware of whether they are in the active or placebo arm.

Example 3.8

There is considerable evidence that the sexual transmission of HIV is enhanced in the presence of genital herpes. In a trial of suppressive therapy for herpes as an HIV prevention measure in Africa, women were individually randomised to receive twice daily treatment with acyclovir or placebo. On random urine testing, a small proportion of women in the placebo arm had metabolites of acyclovir detected in their urine. The investigators postulated that some of the women shared the same residences or workplaces, and that there may have been some sharing of product, either inadvertently or deliberately—for example, if one woman had forgotten to bring her medication to work.

Contamination is one of the most common reasons for adopting cluster randomisation. However, contamination may still present an important problem in CRTs and this issue is discussed further in Chapter 5. Furthermore, as we shall see, the CRT design has its own disadvantages and limitations. In some instances, investigators may decide that it is worth accepting a certain level of contamination in order to benefit from the advantages of an individually randomised trial.

3.3 Using Cluster Randomisation to Capture Indirect Effects of Intervention

3.3.1 Introduction

Conventional individually randomised trials are designed to measure the direct effect of the intervention on the individuals that receive it. Sometimes, however, individuals may benefit from an intervention provided to *other members of the community.* Such effects are referred to as *indirect effects* of an intervention.

Indirect effects are particularly important when we consider interventions against *infectious diseases*, since these may influence the *transmission* of infection within the community. This may lead to benefits in those not receiving the intervention, and also to additional benefits in those receiving the intervention, over and above the direct effect. As we shall see, indirect effects may also be of importance outside the field of infectious diseases.

In this section, we shall explore the various ways in which indirect effects may occur, and discuss how cluster randomisation can be used to capture both the direct and indirect effects of intervention, providing a measure of the overall effect of implementing an intervention throughout a population.

3.3.2 Effects of an Intervention on Infectiousness

We focus here on interventions designed to impact on the incidence or severity of *infectious diseases.* In a conventional trial, individuals are randomised to receive or not receive an intervention (or to receive different interventions) and followed up over time to record the *direct effects* of the intervention on the disease outcomes of interest in those same individuals.

The main outcome of interest might be the *incidence of the infectious disease* under study, by which we mean the occurrence of clinical disease due to the infection of interest satisfying a specified *case definition.* Alternatively, it may be the *incidence of infection* as detected by a diagnostic test. In either case, comparison of incidence in the intervention and control arms of the trial provides a measure of the direct effect of the intervention on *acquisition* of disease or infection. We define the *protective effectiveness* of the intervention on *susceptibility* to acquisition of disease or infection as:

$$PE_S = 1 - \frac{I_1}{I_0}$$

where I_1 and I_0 are appropriate incidence rate measures in the intervention and control arms, respectively.

Conventional trials are well placed to measure the direct effects of intervention on acquisition, since individual randomisation of large numbers of participants helps to ensure, across the study arms, similar *exposure* to the infection as well as similar *susceptibility* apart from any effects of the intervention. Individually randomised trials have therefore been the usual method of choice for Phase III trials of vaccine efficacy.

If an intervention has an effect on *acquisition of infection*, it is likely to have an effect on the transmission of infection to other members of the community, since there will be fewer infected individuals in the population. We consider this effect further in Section 3.3.3. Whether or not they have an effect on acquisition, however, some interventions may influence the *infectiousness* or *infectivity* of recipients who do become infected or who are already infected on enrolment. We consider two examples:

Example 3.9

Malaria remains a serious public health problem in many parts of the world, and the search for effective malaria vaccines continues. While present in a human host, the malaria parasite passes through several stages. Some vaccines are designed to act against the liver and pre-erythrocytic stages of the parasite. These vaccines aim to prevent the occurrence of a febrile episode of clinical malaria, or to ameliorate the severity of a clinical episode, in the vaccine recipient. Other vaccines are designed to act against the gametocyte stage of the parasite. These vaccines would have no direct effect on infection or disease expression in the recipient, but would block or reduce transmission of the parasite, via the mosquito vector, to other members of the community. They are therefore known as *transmission blocking vaccines*. The effects of such a vaccine on infection rates in the community cannot be measured directly in a conventional individually randomised trial, but would be captured by randomising communities to the vaccinated and control arms.

Example 3.10

The sexual transmission of HIV between an infected and uninfected partner is known to be enhanced in the presence of other sexually transmitted infections (STIs) in either partner. Improved treatment of STIs has therefore been proposed as an HIV prevention strategy in populations where STIs are highly prevalent. Cluster randomisation has been used to measure the effects of this strategy for two main reasons. First, improved treatment services are by their nature delivered through health facilities, and so individual randomisation is inappropriate (see Section 3.2.1). Second, part of the postulated effect of the intervention would be to reduce the *infectiousness* of HIV-infected individuals to their sexual partners. Such an effect could not readily be measured in an individually randomised trial.

Corresponding to PE_S which measures the direct protective effect of an intervention on acquisition of infection or disease, we can also define the *protective effectiveness* of an intervention on *infectiousness* as:

$$PE_I = 1 - \frac{T_1}{T_0}$$

where T_1 and T_0 are appropriate measures of transmissibility or infectiousness in the intervention and comparison arms, respectively.

In both the above examples, it may be possible to obtain some measure of the effect on infectiousness within a conventional individually randomised trial. In the malaria example, this could be done by comparing gametocyte rates in blood films taken from vaccinated and unvaccinated individuals. Alternatively, mosquito vectors can be fed on individuals in each arm of the trial, and the mosquitoes collected and examined for malaria parasites. In each case, this provides only a *proxy* measure of infectiousness, and it may be difficult to deduce how any such effects would translate into effects on the transmission of malaria in a natural setting.

Proxy measures may also be possible within individually randomised trials of STI treatment for HIV prevention. For example, trials have been undertaken to measure the effect of suppressive therapy for genital herpes, involving daily treatment with antiviral drugs such as acyclovir, on HIV infectiousness. In one such trial in Burkina Faso, HIV-infected women were enrolled and randomised to receive twice-daily valacyclovir or placebo, and followed up for 3 months (Nagot et al. 2007). Genital specimens were collected to quantify the shedding of HIV in the genital tract. This is assumed to be a proxy for HIV *infectiousness* to sexual partners although, as in the malaria example, the exact relationship between genital shedding data and risk of transmission is not known.

A further trial looking at this question provides an example of how individually randomised trials can be augmented to collect direct evidence of intervention effects on infectiousness. In this trial, HIV-serodiscordant couples are being enrolled, that is, couples in which one partner is HIV-infected and the other is HIV-uninfected. The infected partner is randomised to herpes suppressive therapy or placebo, and the couple is followed up to record HIV seroconversions among the uninfected partners. The intention is to recruit monogamous partnerships, so that any seroconversions can be assumed to result from transmission of infection from the index case. Alternatively, it is now possible to use molecular techniques to confirm whether the virus is identical, providing strong evidence for transmission within the couple.

The above examples illustrate how we can obtain some information on intervention effects on infectiousness from individually randomised trials. However, the difficulties in interpreting proxy measures of infectiousness and the logistical complexities in carrying out trials of discordant partners impose limitations on the ability of this design to evaluate such effects. We shall see that cluster randomisation allows the effects of interventions on infectiousness, as well as other indirect effects, to be captured although it may be difficult to separate out these effects.

3.3.3 Mass Effects of Intervention

We have seen that indirect effects may accrue when an intervention leads to a reduction in infectiousness even if it has no direct effect on the incidence of infection or disease in recipients. However, this is not the only way in which indirect effects may occur.

By the *mass effect* of an intervention, we mean the additional effect achieved when a substantial proportion of the population receive the intervention. Consider an intervention which reduces the incidence of infection in recipients, but has no other biological effect; for example, it has no effect on the infectiousness of those who become infected. A prophylactic vaccine against a respiratory infection would be a good example. Suppose that a substantial proportion of the (susceptible) population (say 70%) is vaccinated and that the protective efficacy of the vaccine is high (say 90%). Then, as a direct result of vaccination, the incidence of infection in the population will be reduced by 63%. We now recognise that, as an indirect result of this, incidence in unvaccinated individuals will also fall since their exposure to infected (and infectious) individuals will be substantially reduced. Furthermore, in due course, the incidence in vaccinated individuals will fall by more than the 90% protection afforded by the vaccine, since their exposure too will now be reduced due to the overall fall in incidence in the population. The *overall reduction* achieved by vaccinating 70% of the population may therefore substantially exceed the 63% reduction corresponding to the *direct protective effect* of the vaccine.

In fact, under certain conditions, vaccination at this level may lead to complete elimination of the infection from the population. We recall that R_0, the basic reproduction number of an infection, is defined as the number of secondary infections resulting from one primary infection in a completely susceptible population (Anderson and May 1991). If a proportion p of the population is given a vaccine with efficacy e, the number of secondary infections is reduced to $R_0 \times (1 - pe)$ and, if this falls below one, then the infection cannot be sustained in the population. It follows that the infection will be eliminated if $p > (R_0 - 1)/eR_0$. For example, if $R_0 = 4$ and $e = 0.90$ (vaccine with 90% efficacy), elimination will occur if $p > 0.83$. This type of mass effect is well known, and referred to in the infectious disease literature as *herd immunity*.

These calculations are based on a number of simplifying assumptions related to homogeneity of the population and random mixing, but nevertheless illustrate how the population-level effect of the widespread application of an intervention can exceed the efficacy of the intervention against acquisition in individual subjects. A distinction is often made between *explanatory trials*, which aim to measure the *efficacy* of an intervention when applied under optimal conditions; and *pragmatic trials*, which aim to measure the *effectiveness* of an intervention when applied routinely in a population. Effectiveness is generally assumed to be lower than efficacy due to imperfect compliance and other deficiencies in delivery of the intervention. We have seen above, however, that for interventions against infectious diseases it is possible for population-level effectiveness to *exceed* individual-level efficacy when there are important mass effects of the intervention.

Example 3.11

A slightly different type of mass effect is illustrated by a trial of insecticide-impregnated bednets to reduce child mortality from malaria. The mosquito vectors that transmit malaria are killed if they come into contact with these nets. It was postulated that if a substantial enough proportion of villagers were sleeping under impregnated bednets, this would have a *mass killing* effect on the vectors, leading to an overall reduction in the transmission of malaria. As before this would result in an indirect benefit to those not receiving the intervention, in this case individuals who did not sleep under an impregnated bednet.While we have emphasised infectious disease applications, there are other examples of mass effects not related to infectious diseases:

Example 3.12

Health education interventions may be more effective when delivered to a substantial proportion of the population, even if they are delivered at individual level. Consider a national health promotion initiative involving an interview with a nurse about the importance of taking adequate exercise, delivered to patients following routine visits to the doctor. If a large proportion of the population go to the doctor at least once a year, we can assume that many people will take part in these interviews and discuss them with their relatives, friends and colleagues. This process of repeated discussion may reinforce the effects of the interview and lead to enhanced effectiveness. Similarly, mass media campaigns may have greater effect if their coverage of the population is high, since even individuals who do not see or hear the media messages may hear about them from friends and colleagues.

Example 3.13

It has been argued that individual behaviours and other characteristics are often influenced by the distribution of those characteristics in the population at large (Rose 1992). For example, epidemiologists working on risk factors for cardiovascular disease have argued the importance of interventions designed to *shift the entire distribution* of blood pressure rather than just targeting the small proportion of "hypertensive" individuals in the upper tail of the distribution. This is partly because, despite a high relative risk in the upper tail, the majority of cases of cardiovascular disease occur among the much larger group of people with moderately increased risk in the main body of the distribution. However, it is also because it may be *easier to achieve* changes in the tail if the entire distribution is shifted. For example, it may be easier for hypertensives to change their dietary habits if societal norms have changed, there is strong peer-pressure to modify food intake and there is a general change in the nutrient content of restaurant and shop-bought food products.

Where population-wide implementation is being considered and important mass effects are expected, the most important information for health policy makers is the overall effectiveness of the intervention given community-wide application. Individually randomised trials are unlikely to provide this evidence and cluster randomisation is a useful alternative to consider.

3.3.4 Direct, Indirect, Total and Overall Effects

When considering the design of a CRT to capture the indirect as well as direct effects of an intervention, it is helpful to distinguish clearly between the different effects of interest that we may wish to measure. To define appropriate measures of protective effectiveness (Halloran, Longini, and Struchiner 1999; Halloran and Struchiner 1991), we consider an idealised CRT with two arms (Figure 3.1). In intervention clusters, we assume that the intervention is delivered to a randomly sampled fraction f of the population, the remaining fraction $(1-f)$ not receiving the intervention.

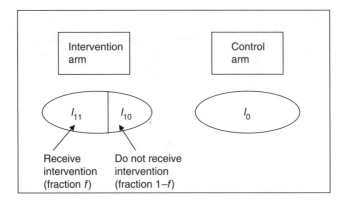

FIGURE 3.1
Schematic diagram showing incidence rates in intervention and control arms used to define measures of direct, indirect, total and overall effects.

We first note that the *direct effect* is simply the protective effectiveness for susceptibility defined in Section 3.3.2, and can be estimated by comparing the incidence rates of the outcome of interest in those receiving and not receiving the intervention *within the intervention clusters*, denoted I_{11} and I_{10}, respectively:

$$PE_{\text{direct}} = PE_S = 1 - \frac{I_{11}}{I_{10}}$$

The *indirect effect* is assessed by comparing the incidence rate in individuals *not* receiving the intervention in the intervention clusters with the overall incidence rate in the control clusters, denoted I_{10} and I_0, respectively:

$$PE_{\text{indirect}} = 1 - \frac{I_{10}}{I_0}$$

Note that this effect may be due to effects of the intervention on infectiousness, as measured by PE_I, or the *mass* effects of the intervention on exposure to infection or both.

We next define the *total effect* of the intervention as:

$$PE_{\text{total}} = 1 - \frac{I_{11}}{I_0}$$

where the incidence rate in those receiving the intervention in the intervention clusters is compared with the overall incidence rate in the control clusters. Note that those receiving the intervention benefit from both the direct effect of the intervention on susceptibility as well as an indirect effect due to the reduction in exposure resulting from effects on infectiousness and/or mass effects.

Finally, the *overall effect* of intervention is obtained by comparing the overall incidence in the intervention and control arms as:

$$PE_{\text{overall}} = 1 - \frac{I_1}{I_0} = 1 - \frac{f \times I_{11} + (1-f) \times I_{10}}{I_0}$$

where the numerator is a weighted average of incidence in the fractions of the population with and without the intervention in the intervention clusters.

Note that the incidence rates in the above equations are assumed to be *true* parameter values, so that they represent the theoretical incidence that would be measured with an infinite number of clusters and individuals in each arm.

We recall that the above formulation assumes that, in the intervention clusters, those receiving the intervention are a random sample of all individuals in those clusters and hence are comparable to those not receiving the intervention. In practice, the aim is usually to provide the intervention to as large a proportion of the population as possible, but some do not receive the intervention because of refusal, temporary absence from the community or other reasons. In this case, our estimates of PE_{direct}, PE_{indirect} and PE_{total} will all be subject to selection bias since those receiving and not receiving the intervention in the intervention clusters may differ with respect to other characteristics that affect risk. The estimate of PE_{overall} should be valid if the trial is well designed, however, as it compares overall rates in the two arms.

In some CRTs, the control clusters may receive a placebo intervention, an example being the vitamin A supplementation trial in Ghana described in Example 3.4 (Ghana VAST Study Team 1993). This design is shown in Figure 3.2. If the placebo is effective in achieving perfect blinding, it may be reasonable to assume that the selection effects in the two arms of the trial are identical. This means that those receiving the intervention in the

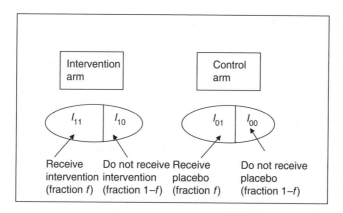

FIGURE 3.2
Alternative schematic diagram showing incidence rates in intervention and control arms when a placebo is delivered in the control arm.

intervention clusters can be assumed to be comparable to those receiving the placebo in the control clusters, apart from any effects of the intervention.

In this scenario, we can now obtain unbiased estimates of $PE_{indirect}$ and PE_{total} as follows:

$$PE_{indirect} = 1 - \frac{I_{10}}{I_{00}}$$

$$PE_{total} = 1 - \frac{I_{11}}{I_{01}}$$

where I_{01} and I_{00} now denote the incidence rates in those receiving and not receiving the placebo intervention in the control clusters. Note that our estimate of PE_{direct} will still be subject to selection bias, however.

We observe that the indirect, total and overall effects of an intervention will generally vary according to the coverage of the intervention. For example, the indirect effect of a vaccine due to herd immunity will generally increase with vaccine coverage. Thus, the generalisability of results from a trial will depend on the uptake of the intervention that can be achieved when the intervention is implemented in practice. This may be either higher or lower than in the trial. Usually, uptake during a trial is higher because of the additional resources and intensive follow-up that are often available during a research study. However, in a study of an unlicensed vaccine against a rare disease, in a population that may be suspicious of vaccines, uptake during the trial may be less than when the vaccine is licensed and recommended for universal use.

To explore the effects of coverage on indirect effects, trial designs have been suggested in which different clusters are randomised to different coverage levels, the intervention being allocated randomly to individuals within clusters (Longini et al. 1998). An alternative approach when using a simple two-arm CRT design is to take advantage of variations across clusters in achieved levels of coverage and to model the risk of disease among those who did not receive the intervention as a function of the proportion in their cluster that did (Moulton et al. 2006). This method can provide a determination of the coverage level at which indirect effects become manifested in a given population.

A less well-recognised fact is that, in some circumstances, the *direct* effect of an intervention may also vary according to coverage. For example, the efficacy of a vaccine may vary according to the infectious challenge which may be influenced by the mass effects of vaccination on the population-level burden of infection.

While the concepts of direct, indirect, total and overall effects are useful in discussing the rationale and objectives of a trial, it may be difficult in practice to separate out these effects in any specific CRT. Additionally, because of the selection biases discussed above and dependence of effects on coverage levels, our inferences will in general be made conditional on the coverage levels observed in a given study. These points are discussed further in later chapters.

3.4 Disadvantages and Limitations of Cluster Randomisation

In Section 3.2 and Section 3.3, we have focused on situations where cluster randomisation offers important advantages because of the nature of the intervention to be studied, the logistical feasibility of individual randomisation, concerns over contamination or the need to capture the indirect effects of an intervention. These advantages need to be weighed against a number of important limitations and disadvantages of this study design, and we now discuss these.

3.4.1 Efficiency

As a result of between-cluster variability, the power and precision of a CRT will generally be lower than for an individually randomised trial of the same overall size. We have already seen in Section 2.4 that the *design effect* associated with cluster sampling is given by:

$$DEff = 1 + (m - 1)\rho$$

and increases with the sample size in each cluster and with the intracluster correlation coefficient. Where we have large clusters (for example extensive geographical communities) or where there is substantial variability between clusters, the design effect may be considerable, so that a CRT design is much more costly. Even where the design effect is moderate, and the overall sample size is not increased substantially, a CRT may still be much more expensive and complex to implement due to the logistical aspects of working in several different communities. This may necessitate separate mobilisation and community liaison activities in each cluster, increased travel costs if clusters are widely distributed and sometimes a need to establish separate study offices and field teams in each cluster. In addition, considerable effort may be required to establish the exact location of cluster boundaries and to track the residential status of participants.

The statistical and cost efficiency of a CRT may therefore be much lower than for an individually randomised trial, and this needs to be carefully considered when choosing between alternative study designs. Sample size requirements for CRTs are discussed in more detail in Chapter 8.

3.4.2 Selection Bias

In a sample survey, designed to obtain valid estimates of disease rates or other characteristics in a well-defined population of interest, *selection bias* refers to any effect causing the sample estimates to deviate *systematically* from the true population values. In a randomised trial, designed to obtain rigorous evidence on the effects of an intervention, it is usual to deliberately choose a *study population* that is more restricted than the intended *target population* for the intervention. For example, we will typically choose a population that is likely to comply with the intervention and in which it is easy to achieve high follow-up rates. This raises issues of *generalisability* that are discussed in Section 3.4.4. However it does not, in itself, lead to biased estimates of intervention effect so long as the individuals allocated to the two arms of the trial are comparable. The trial will then show *internal validity* even if its *external validity* may be open to question.

Randomisation is the principal method used to help ensure comparability between study arms, on both known and unknown confounding factors, and thus to ensure internal validity. If random allocation is used, selection bias can only occur if there is selective drop-out from the study arms subsequent to randomisation. Such drop-outs can occur either immediately (before intervention) or subsequently during the follow-up period. The importance of the latter and of the need for rigorous measures to ensure high follow-up rates, are well known. Immediate drop-out may occur, for example, if participants decide not to continue in the trial after learning the study arm to which they have been allocated. Such losses could be differential between study arms and thus lead to selection bias. Investigators usually attempt to avoid this type of selection bias by requiring subjects to consent to participate on the basis that they will accept the results of the subsequent randomisation. However, it is difficult in practice to avoid some withdrawal following randomisation, so that the possibility of selection bias remains.

Selection bias at the enrolment stage may be a particularly serious concern for some types of CRT. Consider a CRT in which medical practices are randomly allocated to implement two alternative strategies for treating patients with a specific condition. Having been informed of the study arm they have been allocated to, doctors in each practice are then asked to enrol a given number of patients with the condition of interest and to implement the appropriate treatment strategy. Because the study arm is already known, both doctors and patients will be aware of the treatment that will be given if the patient is enrolled. Depending on prior opinions of the different treatment strategies and beliefs about their efficacy for different types of patient, either the doctor or patient may be influenced in their decisions regarding enrolment, and this may lead to significant selection bias.

While this is potentially a serious disadvantage of the CRT design for such applications, it is worth considering how such effects could be minimised:

- In conventional trials, *randomisation concealment* is one of the important methods used to avoid selection bias at the enrolment stage. This means that both participants and study staff (including those responsible for recruitment and enrolment) are kept blind to the study arm a participant is allocated to until after their enrolment is agreed and registered. Some version of this approach may be possible in some CRTs. For example, in a trial based on medical practices, doctors may be asked to prepare and submit a list of potentially eligible patients satisfying specified enrolment criteria *prior* to the random allocation of practices to study arms. This should reduce selection bias resulting from prior opinions of medical practitioners, although patients in the two study arms may still show a differential tendency to opt out of the trial.

- Prior selection of patients is only likely to be feasible if the trial is looking at the treatment of *prevalent cases* of a relatively chronic condition. For trials of treatment for acute conditions, requiring the enrolment of *incident cases* of the disease at the time they first present to their medical practice, prior selection is not possible. Selection bias may be reduced in these circumstances if there are *transparent* and *objective* criteria for patient enrollment that are agreed by all participating practices prior to randomisation. This should be combined with regular visits by trial monitors to check medical records at each practice to ensure that all patients meeting the agreed criteria have been invited to enrol.

When such strategies are expected to be ineffective, investigators should consider whether it would be preferable to adopt an individually randomised trial design, even if this is at the cost of some contamination (Torgerson 2001). In this case, it is important to collect data to measure the extent of contamination to assist with the interpretation of the trial results.

Another option for reducing selection bias is to perform a two-stage randomisation that first assigns clusters to either high- or low-intervention study arms, and then randomises individuals within clusters to the intervention or control status with either a high (80%, say) or low (20%) probability. Borm et al. refer to this approach as *pseudo randomisation* (Borm et al. 2005). This can avoid selection bias that occurs when participants are recruited individually into a cluster of known treatment status. For example, someone may be unwilling to enrol in a study if, given their place of residence, receipt of the standard treatment is a certainty. Pseudo randomisation is not possible, however, when treatments are applied at the cluster level.

Practical experience suggests that selection bias is much less of a problem in CRTs in which *entire communities* or *institutions* are randomised, and where the intervention is applied at the cluster level. For example, trials in which entire geographical communities are covered by experimental or control interventions; or in which schools are randomised to different health education strategies. Of course, refusal to participate in the surveys carried out to measure intervention impact in these trials may still lead to selection bias. It is thus important to implement measures to maximise participation and to monitor coverage rates during the trial so that remedial steps can be taken if they are too low.

3.4.3 Imbalances between Study Arms

As we have seen in Chapter 1, one of the major advantages of randomised controlled trials is that, if large numbers of individuals are randomly allocated to the different study arms, we can rely on the randomisation process to provide study arms that are similar with respect to all potential confounding factors, both known and unknown.

As a result of practical and financial constraints, the number of clusters randomised in a CRT is often quite small. In many trials of public health interventions, for example, only 20 or 30 communities are randomised. With such a small number of randomisation units, it is quite likely that there will be some imbalance on one or more potential confounding factors. While there are analytical methods than can be used to adjust for these factors (see Chapters 10 through 12), there is no question that the credibility of the trial results may be weakened in the presence of such imbalances. In Chapter 5 and Chapter 6, we shall review design strategies that can be used in an attempt to avoid imbalances.

3.4.4 Generalisability

As discussed in Section 3.4.2, the main emphasis in randomised trials is on achieving *internal validity* so that unbiased estimates of efficacy can be obtained *within the study population*. To achieve this, the chosen study population is usually more restricted than the potential *target population* in which the intervention would be applied. For example, the study population is likely to be chosen with regard to the likelihood of achieving high compliance with the intervention and with the study schedule to minimise losses to follow-up and hence reduce selection bias. There may also be additional exclusion criteria, perhaps relating to pre-existing medical conditions or the values of clinical laboratory parameters, which would not be applied if the intervention were provided in the general population.

For this reason, when trial results are reported, it is usually necessary to consider to what extent their results are *generalisable* to a wider target population, or to populations in different geographical settings. This is an important issue for regulatory agencies when they review evidence from trial data in order to agree on the *indications* for use of new products at the stage of licensing.

While the effects of drug treatments and vaccines on individual patients may show some variation between populations, community-level interventions may show much more variation for several reasons:

- Many community-level interventions are less clearly defined than patient-based interventions, and are likely to differ in their *implementation* in different settings. For example, peer-assisted health education for sex workers to prevent HIV transmission may depend in its implementation and effectiveness on the local structure and organisation of the sex-work industry in any given location. And the impact of village-based provision of mosquito nets to prevent malaria may depend on the availability and skills of village health aides or the coverage of local health centres.

- The *response* to complex interventions may also show considerable variation between populations, particularly where they involve behaviour change. For example, the effectiveness of a sexual health education programme in schools might vary depending on (i) the training and skills of teachers delivering the programme; (ii) the educational level and social skills of the children; (iii) local community norms that might influence the support of parents and community members for the adoption of changed behaviours.

- The *indirect* effects of interventions, particularly those against infectious diseases, may vary substantially between populations. For example, the indirect and overall effects of a community-wide vaccination programme will depend not only on vaccine coverage but also on the basic reproduction number R_0. If R_0 is close to 1, even moderate coverage with a vaccine with limited efficacy may reduce transmission below the epidemic threshold and lead to elimination of the infection; while if R_0 is large the indirect effect of the same vaccine may be negligible. R_0 may, for a given disease, differ across populations because of differences in population density, congregration patterns, age distribution and many other factors.

Example 3.14

A good example is provided by three trials of STI control for HIV prevention carried out in East Africa (Figure 3.3). These CRTs were based on the premise that the sexual transmission of HIV is enhanced in the presence of other STIs, and that improved STI treatment should reduce the population prevalence of STIs and hence decrease HIV incidence. The design and results of the three trials are summarised in Table 3.1 (Grosskurth et al. 1995; Kamali et al. 2003; Wawer et al. 1999).

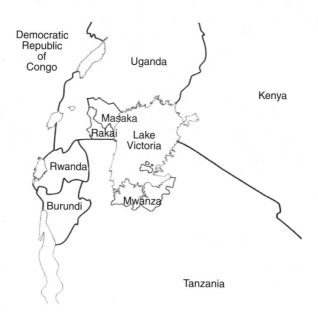

FIGURE 3.3
Locations of three STD treatment trials in East Africa. (From Grosskurth, H., Gray, R., Hayes, R., Maybey, D., and Wawer, M. Control of sexually transmitted diseases for HIV-1 prevention: Understanding the implications of the Mwanza and Rakai trials. *Lancet* 2000, 355, 1981–87. With permission.)

TABLE 3.1

Summary of Designs and Results of Three STD Treatment Trials in East Africa

	Mwanza	Rakai	Masaka	
Design	CRT with six matched pairs of communities	CRT with five matched pairs of communities	CRT with six matched triplets of communities (three arm trial)	
Intervention	Syndromic STI management	Mass STI treatment	IEC campaign	IEC campaign + syndromic STI management
Impact on HIV incidence (*RR* with 95% CI)	0.62 (0.45–0.85)	0.97 (0.81–1.16)	0.94 (0.60–1.45)	1.00 (0.63–1.58)

All three trials recorded some effect of the interventions on STI prevalence or incidence. However, the effects on the primary outcome of HIV incidence differed considerably. In Mwanza, Tanzania, improved syndromic treatment of STIs led to a 40% reduction in HIV incidence, which was statistically highly significant, while little effect on HIV incidence was observed for mass treatment or improved syndromic treatment of STIs in Rakai, Uganda and Masaka, Uganda, respectively.

Several hypotheses have been suggested for these apparently conflicting findings (Korenromp et al. 2005; Orroth et al. 2003). It has been suggested that the results could be due to (i) differences between the STI treatment strategies; (ii) differences in rates of curable STIs between the study populations; (iii) differences in the maturity of the HIV epidemic; or (iv) bias or random error in the trials. Subsequent re-analysis of trial data combined with mathematical modelling suggested that *differences between the study populations* provided the main explanation for the different effects measured in the three trials:

- At the time that the trials were conducted, there was more risky sexual behaviour and higher rates of curable STIs in Mwanza than in Masaka and Rakai.
- The HIV epidemic was more mature in the two Ugandan study sites than in Tanzania, with a much higher prevalence in the general population and most HIV transmission occurring between spouses and stable sexual partners rather than in groups at high risk, who are more likely to have STIs.

These two factors together imply a much higher prevalence of curable STIs in discordant couples (one partner HIV-positive and the other HIV-negative) in Mwanza than in the Ugandan sites, and mathematical modelling provided supporting evidence that this could result in HIV impact results similar to those observed in the three trials (White et al. 2004).

There is increasing recognition that considerable care is needed in generalising the results of CRTs, particularly those evaluating interventions against infectious diseases, from the study populations where they are conducted to populations elsewhere with different characteristics. We return to this issue in Chapter 15.

Part B

Design Issues

4

Choice of Clusters

4.1 Introduction

One of the first decisions to be taken when designing a CRT relates to the choice and definition of the *clusters* that are to be randomised during the trial. In practice, published trials have used a wide variety of types and sizes of clusters. These have ranged from CRTs of families or households, with only a few individuals in each cluster, to CRTs of large geographic regions in which each cluster may include millions of individuals. While the general principles of CRT design may be similar for these widely varying situations, the practical aspects of implementing such trials are clearly very different.

In Section 4.2, we consider the different *types* of study cluster, including those which are geographically demarcated, those based on different kinds of institution or organisation and those based on small groups such as households. Having decided on the basic type of unit, the investigator sometimes has a choice to make concerning the exact *size* of the clusters that are to be randomised. In Section 4.3, we discuss some of the key issues to be considered in choosing cluster size, including statistical considerations, logistical factors and contamination. For infectious disease studies, the concept of the *transmission zone* of an infectious agent may also be of relevance. Finally, in Section 4.4, we consider what design strategies are available to reduce the degree of *contamination* in a CRT.

4.2 Types of Cluster

4.2.1 Geographical Clusters

Geographically demarcated clusters are the most common choice for trials of interventions directed at entire populations or subgroups of the population. They are also appropriate when we wish to measure the population-level impact of an intervention, including any *indirect effects* as well as *direct effects* (see Section 3.3). Examples include:

- Trials of health education initiatives delivered through the *mass media*. By their nature, these are delivered to entire populations.
- Trials of treatment programmes for infectious diseases, where the outcome of interest is the prevalence or incidence of disease or infection in the population as a whole, and not just those accessing health services.
- Vaccine trials where the aim is to measure the overall effect of introducing a vaccine taking into account the indirect effects operating through herd immunity or effects on infectiousness (see Section 3.3).
- Trials of water and sanitation programmes which are delivered to entire villages or districts.

Geographical clusters have also been used quite widely for trials of individual-level interventions which could in principle be studied through individually randomised trials, but where considerations of practical convenience and acceptability favour cluster randomisation. Examples are given in Section 3.2.2.

4.2.1.1 Communities

In many cases, geographical clusters are based on well-defined communities, such as villages or towns, which are clearly separated from other communities. Problems of contamination tend to be less severe where there is clear separation of this kind, although we shall discuss this further in Section 4.3 and Section 4.4.

Example 4.1

A CRT was carried out in The Gambia to evaluate the effects of the National Impregnated Bednet Programme (D'Alessandro et al. 1995). In this trial, 104 large villages were randomly allocated to the intervention arm, in which villagers were provided with insecticide-impregnated bednets through the national programme, or to the control arm. Villages in The Gambia are clearly defined settlements which are well separated from neighbouring villages.

Example 4.2

A CRT has been carried out in Peru to evaluate the effect of an STD prevention intervention (Hughes 2005). In this trial, 20 medium-to-large cities, each with a population of 50,000 or greater, have been randomly allocated to the intervention or control arms. The intervention consisted of training seminars for pharmacy staff in the treatment of STDs as well as outreach services for commercial sex workers and their clients. The primary outcome was the prevalence of STDs in random samples of adults in each city.

4.2.1.2 Administrative Units

Sometimes, clusters are based on *administrative units* such as districts or regions. This has some clear advantages. First, it is likely that maps will be available which clearly show the boundaries between neighbouring units. Second, such units may facilitate arrangements for obtaining approval for trial participation from political authorities. Such units also tend to be quite large, and this reduces concerns over contamination and may decrease between-cluster variability (see Section 4.3). One disadvantage is that administrators may be reluctant to participate in a trial where the whole of the administrative unit they are responsible for may be allocated to the control arm. Another is that implementation of trials with such large randomisation units can be logistically complex and involve high transport costs. A further concern is that boundaries between administrative units sometimes pass through communities or populated areas. While this carries a risk of contamination across these boundaries, if the areas are sufficiently large this may affect only a small proportion of the study population and have a negligible effect on the measured outcomes.

Example 4.3

A trial was carried out in France to evaluate the impact of an STD prevention campaign on STD cases seen at GP surgeries. Six *départements* (large geographical units with an average population of around half a million) were grouped into three matched pairs, and randomly allocated to the intervention and control arms. Such large randomisation units considerably reduce the risk of contamination, although with only six clusters it is unclear whether this trial was adequately powered.

Example 4.4

In a CRT to measure the effectiveness of a pneumococcal vaccine in infants, it was initially intended to take the clusters to be large administrative units in a Native American population in the Southwest United States. Four Indian Health Service administrative units were to be randomised to receive the pneumococcal vaccine and four others to receive the control vaccine. Contamination would have been minimal with this design, but it was decided that the study power might be inadequate, depending on the level of between-cluster variation in incidence rates, and that a larger number of randomisation units would be desirable. It was therefore decided to use a local administrative area known as a "chapter", of which there were 110 on the reservation, and to group them into approximate communities of two to four chapters each, resulting in 38 clusters. A meeting with tribal demographers and fieldworkers was held to identify clusters that were as "independent" as possible, so that children from one cluster would not attend the same school as children from another cluster. The locations of shops, government services, roads and other topographical features were also considered in defining the clusters.

4.2.1.3 Arbitrary Geographical Zones

Some CRTs have been carried out in areas where the population is widely scattered and not divided up into clearly defined and well separated communities. Other strategies need to be used to define clusters in this type of setting. One option is to arbitrarily divide the area into zones, for example using grid squares on a map. While it is easy to draw straight lines on a map, the grid squares may not produce clusters that make geographical sense on the ground. An alternative in this case is to use the map combined with local geographical knowledge, and perhaps aerial photographs if these are available, to construct zones that take account of logistical factors and seek to minimise contamination; for example, by drawing boundaries along natural barriers such as hills or rivers and ensuring that any denser population aggregations do not cross zone boundaries.

Example 4.5

A CRT was carried out in a rural area of Northern Ghana to measure the effect of impregnated bednets on child mortality (Binka et al. 1996). This area consists of widely scattered households rather than clearly defined villages. Prior to the trial, the study area was mapped and a census was carried out. Using this information, the study area was divided into 96 clusters of geographically contiguous households, with an average of about 1400 persons per cluster (Figure 4.1). Impregnated bednets were provided to households in 48 randomly selected intervention clusters, and were also provided in the 48 control clusters at the end of the trial.

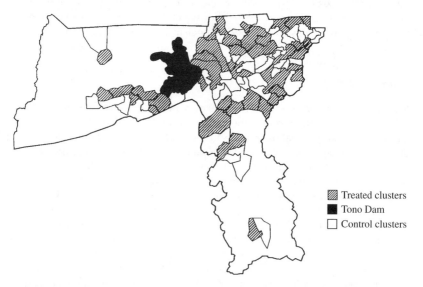

FIGURE 4.1
Map of study area of Ghana bednet trial showing intervention areas (shaded) and control areas (unshaded). Black area is the Tono Dam irrigation project. (From Binka, F.N., Kubaje, A., Adjuik, M., et al. Impact of permethrin impregnated bednets on child mortality in Kassena-Nankana district, Ghana: A randomized controlled trial. *Tropical Medicine and International Health* 1996, 1, 147–54. With permission.)

4.2.2 Institutional Clusters

Many CRTs aim to measure the effectiveness of interventions that are to be implemented by specific institutions or organisations, such as schools, health units or workplaces. Randomisation of institutions is the usual choice for such trials.

4.2.2.1 Schools

There are many examples of CRTs in which schools have been randomised to measure the effects of educational or health interventions. This is the natural choice for interventions, such as health education programmes, that are to be implemented through schools. While randomisation of individual classes within each school to different treatment arms is an option, this is usually avoided because of the substantial risk of contamination due to social contact between siblings and friends who are in different classes.

Two major advantages of schools as settings for trials are worth noting. First, for interventions aimed at children and adolescents they provide a simple way of recruiting a study population that is representative of the intended target population, at least in countries in which school attendance rates are high. In some developing countries, only a small minority of children attend school, particularly at post-primary level, and the generalisability of data from trials based on schools would need to be considered carefully in such settings. Second, schools offer considerable logistical advantages in carrying out trials. Because students are generally at school every day, recruitment and survey procedures are greatly facilitated. For example, it may be possible to arrange for trial activities to be incorporated into the school timetable. Because students generally attend the same school for several years, high follow-up rates can often be achieved. This advantage is less clear-cut for interventions aimed at older students, since this may require follow-up after they have left school.

Because of the logistical advantages of school-based trials, schools are sometimes used as convenient settings for trials of individual-level interventions. Individual randomisation is likely to be the method of choice for such trials, unless *indirect effects* of the intervention need to be captured or there are concerns over contamination.

Example 4.6

Project SHARE was a CRT carried out in Scotland to measure the impact of a school-based sexual health education programme (Wight et al. 2002). As previously discussed in Example 1.2, the intervention consisted of a programme of classroom sessions on sexual health delivered by teachers to students in the third and fourth years of secondary school. A total of 25 secondary schools in the east of Scotland were randomised to the intervention and control arms and a cohort of 8430 students aged 13–15 years was followed up for 2 years to measure the effects of the intervention.

4.2.2.2 Health Units

Health units that have been randomised in CRTs include hospitals, clinics, general practices and individual practitioners. The clusters in these trials generally consist of the patients attending these health units.

New drugs and vaccines are usually tested for *efficacy* in individually randomised trials, while capturing the *indirect effects* of interventions against infectious diseases generally requires randomisation of geographical clusters so that population-wide impact can be measured. Randomisation of health units is therefore most often used to evaluate the *effectiveness* of new *strategies* for the diagnosis and management of medical conditions. These often require the training of medical staff in new approaches, and a common reason for choosing cluster randomisation is a concern that contamination may occur if individual patients are randomised. A similar concern may argue against randomising practitioners in the same health units to different treatment arms.

Example 4.7

The POST trial was previously discussed in Example 1.3, and was carried out to measure the effectiveness of an intervention to improve the secondary prevention of coronary heart disease (Feder et al. 1999). In this trial, 52 general practices in the London Borough of Hackney were randomised to intervention or control arms. The intervention consisted of postal prompts to patients after discharge from hospital following admission for heart disease, providing recommendations for prevention of coronary events and encouraging patients to make an appointment with their GP, and letters were also sent to the GP with a summary of preventive measures. As noted in Example 1.3, the main outcomes were measured by following up patients 6 months after discharge. The groups of patients discharged with heart disease at the 52 practices therefore constitute the clusters in this trial.

Example 4.8

The directly observed therapy, short-course (DOTS) approach to case finding and treatment for tuberculosis (TB) has become the mainstay of TB control programmes all over the world and is strongly promoted by WHO. However, there are still many settings where this strategy has not been implemented effectively and where adherence to treatment is inadequate. In a CRT in Senegal, 16 government district health centres in different parts of the country were randomised to an intervention aimed at improving adherence (eight centres) or to usual standard of care (eight centres) (Thiam et al. 2007). The intervention involved training of health personnel to provide improved patient counselling, decentralisation of treatment, patient choice of a directly observed therapy (DOT) supporter and reinforced supervision. A total of 1522 TB patients at these centres were followed up to record successful completion of the course of treatment as well as the proportion of patients defaulting from treatment.

4.2.2.3 Workplaces

Workplaces may offer the same advantages for adult populations as schools do for younger age groups. They may be chosen for study in CRTs either to evaluate interventions specifically designed for implementation in occupational settings, or simply because of their convenience for recruiting and following up substantial numbers of adults. In the latter case, issues of generalisability need to be carefully considered. The *healthy worker effect* is well recognised in occupational epidemiology, meaning that occupational cohorts often differ in their health status from the general population, and the socioeconomic and demographic characteristics of different occupational groups can clearly show substantial variation.

Example 4.9

In populations with a high prevalence of HIV infection, rates of TB have increased substantially due to the effects of HIV-related immune deficiency. Standard approaches to TB control based on case finding and management do not seem sufficient to bring the disease under control in such settings, and more intensive control strategies are therefore under consideration. In a CRT in South Africa, the effects of mass isoniazid treatment are being investigated among gold miners, who have some of the highest TB rates anywhere in the world. After case finding to exclude active cases of TB, miners are asked to take isoniazid for 6 months. By eliminating latent TB infection, this intervention is known to be effective at the individual level in reducing the incidence of active TB. Through use of cluster randomisation, however, the investigators aim to capture the *overall* effects of the intervention on TB. Since active cases of TB are the source of new infections with *Mycobacterium tuberculosis*, the intervention is designed to reduce TB transmission at population-level, leading to *indirect effects* of the intervention in both miners who take isoniazid and those who decline it. In this CRT, the randomisation units are 15 mineshafts operated by three different mining companies. The primary outcome will be the incidence of TB during a 1 year period following completion of the intervention.

4.2.3 Smaller Clusters

The main focus of this book is on CRTs with large or moderately sized clusters. There are, however, numerous examples of CRTs with small clusters and we consider some examples here.

We have seen in Section 2.4 that the *design effect* of a CRT based on clusters of equal size m is given by:

$$DEff = 1 + (m-1)\rho$$

where ρ is the intracluster correlation coefficient. If both m and ρ are small, it follows that the design effect may be very close to 1, and in some cases the effect of the cluster design may be negligible. While sample size formulae and analytical methods designed for individually randomised trials can often be applied to such trials with little error, it is generally safer to use methods designed for CRTs.

4.2.3.1 Households and Other Small Groups

Randomisation of households or families may be considered for two main reasons: first, for logistical convenience and to avoid the contamination that may occur if different members of the same family were to be randomised to different treatment arms; and second, for the study of interventions which are designed to be delivered to households.

Example 4.10

Intermittent preventive therapy (IPT) is a malaria control strategy whereby infants or children in endemic areas are given antimalarial treatment at specified time intervals, irrespective of symptoms, with the aim of reducing the incidence of clinical malaria. Consider an individually randomised trial in which young children living in a defined area are randomised to IPT or placebo arms. To avoid the contamination that could occur if children living in the same household were allocated to different treatment arms, for example due to sharing of drugs, it may be stated in the protocol that children from the same household will always be allocated to the same arm. Even though many households may only have one child participating in the trial, this means in principle that the trial should be considered as a CRT.

While we have indicated that the design effect for such trials may be close to one, this will only be the case if ρ is small, and this assumption needs to be examined for any given study. For example, some genetically acquired diseases show strong familial clustering and some lifestyle outcomes such as diet and exercise are also likely to show strong within-household correlation. The design effect may substantially exceed one in such cases.

4.2.3.2 Individuals as Clusters

In most CRTs, the clusters comprise groups of individuals. In some trials, however, individual people may themselves be considered as clusters.

Example 4.11

Consider a trial in dental medicine where individual patients are randomised to different approaches to preventive dentistry. For example, they might be randomised between six-monthly or annual dental check-ups. The patients are followed up for 2 years, and the condition of their teeth examined at the end of this period. It is likely that there will be quite a strong correlation in the outcomes for the teeth of any given patient. This is an example of *intracluster correlation* where the patient is regarded as the cluster and the teeth as the individuals.

Similar examples can be found in ophthalmology where measures on patients' eyes may be strongly correlated, and in other fields of medicine. Although investigators may see trials in these disciplines as standard individually randomised trials, statistically they share many of the features of CRTs with small clusters. One difference in the case of dental trials is that the different teeth are not all equivalent, so that measures on molars might be quite different from canines, for example. Thus, our usual assumption that measures for individuals *within* a cluster are independently and identically distributed may not be tenable.

More generally, when measurements are carried out repeatedly over time on the same individual, the observations for each individual can be regarded as a "cluster". The analysis of longitudinal data is concerned with such situations and takes account of the time sequence of the observations. We shall not be concerned with such situations explicitly in this book, but note that many of the statistical methods designed for longitudinal data are appropriate for the clustered data that arise from randomising groups of individuals. Such methods will be discussed in later chapters.

4.3 Size of Clusters

4.3.1 Introduction

Having decided on the *type* of cluster that will be randomised in a CRT, the investigator may still have some latitude in choosing the *size* of each cluster. This is particularly the case with geographical clusters, where arbitrary boundaries are to be drawn, or where there are administrative units at different levels. Even when we have institutional clusters, however, there may be some flexibility—for example to group neighbouring schools or medical practices into one cluster. We briefly discuss the issues that need to be considered when choosing cluster size in such circumstances.

In some CRTs, a *sample* of individuals is selected from each cluster to measure the outcomes of interest, rather than measuring these on the entire cluster. In this section, we focus on the size of the entire cluster. Sampling within clusters is discussed further in Chapter 7.

4.3.2 Statistical Considerations

We consider again the formula for the *design effect* of a CRT relative to an individually randomised trial:

$$DEff = 1 + (m-1)\rho \qquad (4.1)$$

This formula shows that, for a given total sample size, precision is maximised with a cluster size of $m = 1$, corresponding to individual randomisation. If ρ, the intracluster correlation coefficient, remains constant, the design effect increases with cluster size. This implies that a large number of small clusters is statistically more efficient than a small number of large clusters.

While this is a useful general result, the condition of constant ρ may often be violated. In practice, ρ often decreases with the size of the cluster. An example shows why.

Example 4.12

Suppose we are considering carrying out a CRT in 20 large towns. Each town comprises several neighbourhoods, and there are a total of 100 neighbourhoods. The choice is between randomising towns or neighbourhoods. Assuming that ρ is 0.005 for both choices of cluster and that the total sample size is 10,000, this would imply m of 500 and 100 for randomisation of towns and neighbourhoods, giving design effects of 3.5 and 1.5, respectively.

However, suppose now that the neighbourhoods in each town are a mix of communities with higher and lower socioeconomic status. This may mean that there are substantial variations in health outcomes *between neighbourhoods*, but that these average out so that overall there is little difference in outcomes *between towns*. This would imply that ρ is much higher for neighbourhoods than for towns.

For example, if $\rho = 0.005$ as before for neighbourhoods, but is reduced to $\rho = 0.001$ for towns, both the design effects would be about 1.5.

This hypothetical example illustrates the importance, when estimating sample size requirements for CRTs, of obtaining ρ or k estimates which relate to the actual types and sizes of cluster that are under consideration.

Sample size requirements for CRTs are discussed in more detail in Chapter 7.

4.3.3 Logistical Issues

Statistical issues are not the only consideration when deciding on an appropriate choice of cluster size. Issues of cost and logistical feasibility are also very important.

The relative cost and feasibility of designs based on alternative cluster sizes will depend critically on the particular type of cluster and geographical setting. We give two examples to illustrate this.

Example 4.13

Consider a CRT with geographical clusters based on arbitrary zones as in the bednet trial in Ghana (see Example 4.4). In this trial, boundaries were drawn across the study area to define 96 clusters, with an average of around 170 young children in each cluster. Now suppose that larger zones had been constructed, so that there were instead 48 clusters each comprising around 340 children. In terms of statistical efficiency, the design effect would depend on the extent to which ρ changes as the cluster size increases, and whether any reduction in ρ would be sufficient to compensate for the increase in m (see Section 4.3.2). In logistical terms, it is unlikely that in this case the cost or feasibility of the trial would be significantly altered by the choice of cluster size. Since the entire study area was included in the trial, all compounds in the area had to be visited at regular intervals, and the costs of fieldwork would be very similar irrespective of the zone boundaries.

Example 4.14

Now consider a CRT in which the clusters are well-defined and separated communities. Suppose the choice is between a design in which 20 towns are randomised with 100 subjects studied in each town, and an alternative design in which 50 villages are randomised with 40 individuals studied in each village. The total sample size is 2000 in each case. However, the cost and logistical complexity of carrying out fieldwork in 50 communities may be considerably higher than for 20 communities. This may depend, however, on the geographical spread of the communities. If the 50 villages are all located in a relatively limited area, transport and supervision costs may be much lower than for the towns if they are spread over a much larger area.

These examples should be sufficient to demonstrate that it is difficult to make general statements about the relative cost efficiency of different cluster sizes. The investigator is therefore advised to cost alternative designs, taking into account statistical requirements as well as the logistical and budgetary implications of different cluster sizes.

4.3.4 Contamination

As we have seen in Chapter 3, avoidance of *contamination* is one of the primary reasons for using cluster randomisation rather than individual randomisation. However, contamination may still be a significant problem in some CRTs.

Contamination occurs in a CRT when responses in one cluster are distorted because of contacts with individuals from outside the cluster. This can happen in several ways.

4.3.4.1 Contacts between Intervention and Control Clusters

This may occur when members of an intervention cluster have friends, relatives or neighbours who are members of a control cluster, or through travel or migration between intervention and control clusters. For example, in a CRT of a school-based health education campaign, if there are intervention and control schools in the same geographical area, social mixing between students from the two treatment arms may influence trial outcomes in both arms. The usual effect of contamination in this situation will be *dilution* of the differences between treatment arms. Control subjects may gain some benefit from hearing second-hand the health education messages received by the intervention subjects. Conversely, the effects of health education among intervention subjects may be reduced if they are undermined by the differing beliefs of those not receiving the intervention.

Similarly in a CRT based on randomisation of medical practices to different treatment strategies, contamination may occur if some patients attend more than one practitioner, or through social or professional contact between practitioners in different treatment arms. In either case, these contacts may influence the treatment strategy adopted and hence the outcomes of the trial.

4.3.4.2 Contacts between Intervention Clusters and the Wider Population

Similar effects can occur because of social and other contacts between members of intervention clusters and individuals who are members of *neither* intervention nor control clusters. This may happen because of movements across cluster boundaries. For example, intervention participants may travel outside the cluster; individuals from outside may migrate or travel into the cluster; or there may be contacts between neighbours living close to the *boundaries* of the cluster, so-called *edge effects*.

These population movements may influence trial outcomes in different ways. In the case of health education messages, the arrival of new community members who have not received the messages may undermine the effects of the intervention. In the case of infectious disease interventions, new members may bring with them the infection of interest, leading to reinfection of study participants and a higher infection rate than if the cluster were hermetically sealed.

It could be argued that population movements are a reality and that any intervention will have to contend with the results of such movements. The effectiveness observed in a CRT may therefore be viewed as giving a valid measure of the actual effect if the intervention were to be routinely introduced into communities of similar size and characteristics as the trial clusters. We note however that, if shown to be effective, the intention would often be for the intervention to be introduced on a much wider scale, and possibly nationally. Under these circumstances, new entrants to a community would generally have received the intervention in their previous home community, so that the same dilution effect would not occur. In the presence of contamination, CRT results may therefore underestimate the true effects of interventions if introduced on a wide scale.

4.3.4.3 Contacts between Control Clusters and the Wider Population

While such contacts may occur as for intervention clusters, they are unlikely to have an appreciable effect on trial outcomes unless the control clusters receive some alternative intervention that distinguishes them from the wider population.

4.3.4.4 Effects of Cluster Size on Contamination

In general, contamination is likely to decrease as cluster size increases. Rates of travel and migration across area boundaries generally decrease as the size of the area increases. For example, villagers are likely to travel outside their village much more frequently than across the district boundary. Edge effects are also likely to diminish with the size of the cluster, since the proportion of the population living close to the boundary of an area decreases as the area is increased.

In Section 4.4, we consider a number of strategies to reduce the effects of contamination in CRTs.

4.3.5 Transmission Zones of Infectious Diseases

We have seen in Chapter 3 that CRTs are of particular value for the study of interventions against infectious diseases, because they capture the *indirect effects* as well as *direct effects* of an intervention. The aim here is usually to measure the *overall effect* of an intervention if implemented throughout a population with a certain level of coverage. Clearly, this effect will be under-estimated if the clusters are chosen in such a way that there is considerable transmission across cluster boundaries.

To avoid this special type of contamination, investigators may seek to select clusters that are as far as possible equivalent to *transmission zones* for the infection of interest. Some examples will illustrate this idea.

Example 4.15

In a trial of an intervention against a sexually transmitted infection such as HIV, it would often be desirable for clusters to encompass sexual networks. The ideal would be for each cluster to be self-contained in terms of sexual relations, with cluster members having sexual contacts only with other members of the same cluster.

In practice, it is very unlikely that this could be achieved except, perhaps, in very remote and isolated communities. However, the general principle may be of value in selecting clusters. For example, in a CRT of mass STD treatment for HIV prevention in Rakai, Uganda (Wawer et al. 1998), 56 trading villages situated on secondary roads were grouped into 10 clusters based on prior information regarding patterns of social relations within and between these clusters (Figure 4.2). The trial investigators report that: "In order to minimise risk of contamination due to reintroduction of STD into the intervention arm population, communities were grouped so as to be endogamous with respect to sexual contacts...The groupings...were designed to encompass patterns of maximal internal social and thus, presumably, sexual interchange (i.e., sexual networks). Communities were grouped on the basis of (i) distance to major highways and trading centres; (ii) quality of roads into the community; (iii) natural boundaries such as hills and swamps (which represent substantial barriers to mobility in Rakai); and (iv) community travel patterns for market attendance, work and social purposes (including travel to neighbouring towns to frequent discos and bars)".

Example 4.16

In the case of vector-borne diseases, such as malaria and filariasis, it is important to consider the flight patterns of insect vectors when defining clusters. To capture the true overall effects of a population-wide intervention, the clusters need to be large enough to minimise the effect of vector reinvasion from outside the cluster.

An RCT of the impact of insecticide-impregnated curtains in Burkina Faso provides a good example (Habluetzel et al. 1997). In this trial, the investigators considered randomising individual villages in order to minimise the design effect. However, they finally decided to group the villages into 16 large geographical clusters, each containing about 10 villages and covering an area of 40–80 km^2. As noted in Example 3.11, the intervention was expected to have an important *indirect effect* on malaria, acting through *mass killing* of the mosquito vectors. If villages had been chosen as clusters, it was considered that there would have been much greater scope for this effect to be diluted by reinvasion of vectors from outside the village.

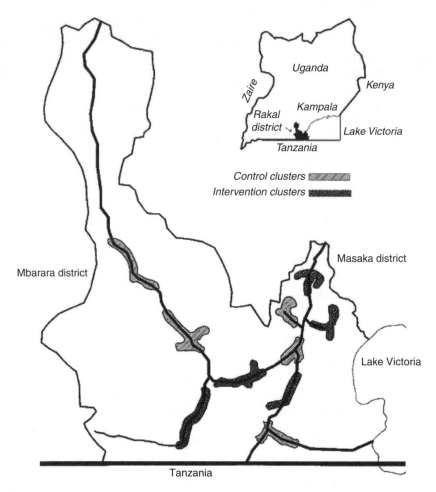

FIGURE 4.2
Map of study area of Rakai STD treatment trial showing locations of intervention and control clusters. (From Wawer, M.J., Gray, R.H., Sewankambo, N.K., et al. A randomized, community trial of sexually transmitted disease control for AIDS prevention, Rakai, Uganda. *AIDS* 1998, 12, 1211–25. With permission.)

4.4 Strategies to Reduce Contamination

4.4.1 Separation of Clusters

One of the main strategies for reducing contamination in a CRT is to select clusters for the trial that are well-separated. This is particularly useful for reducing the level of contact between intervention and control clusters (see Section 4.3.4). Additional strategies may be needed to reduce contact between trial clusters and the wider population.

The separation needed will depend on the intervention under study and, for infectious diseases, the transmission dynamics of the infection.

For example, for an educational intervention delivered in schools, it is probably sufficient to ensure that the clusters are sufficiently distant that social contact between school children in intervention and control clusters is infrequent. Much greater geographical separation may be needed for a mass media intervention. Such interventions, by their nature, tend to cover large populations.

The need for adequate separation is one of the main reasons why RCTs are often carried out in rural populations. In urban areas, adjacent neighbourhoods tend to be close together, and there is often significant mixing between their populations. For example, residents of different neighbourhoods may work together, go to school together, and use the same shops, clinics and other services, either within these neighbourhoods, on their boundaries or in the town centre. Randomisation of urban neighbourhoods within the same town may therefore result in substantial contamination. Some RCTs have randomised entire towns, although this tends to be costly and logistically difficult.

By contrast, contamination is likely to be less severe if rural villages are randomised, and costs may be considerably less. Sometimes, neighbouring villages are grouped together to form clusters, depending on the patterns of social contact between them. The Rakai trial of mass STD treatment is a good example (see Example 5.13). Study areas with well-separated communities also help to minimise contamination due to contacts between trial clusters and the wider population.

Example 4.17

Figure 4.3 shows the locations of the 12 study communities in a trial of improved STD treatment for HIV prevention in Mwanza, Tanzania, previously discussed in Example 1.1 and Example 3.14. These predominantly rural communities were specifically chosen to be well-separated to reduce the level of contamination between clusters. Three aspects of this design are worth noting in this respect:

- There were large distances between the communities in most cases (note the scale of the map). However, geographical distance is less relevant here than ease and extent of travel between communities. Where communities were relatively close, they were separated by natural barriers such as rivers or swamps, or travel between them was on poor roads with limited public transport.
- Each community in this trial was defined as the catchment area served by a health centre and its satellite dispensaries. This was done partly to facilitate the administrative delivery of the intervention through these linked health units. However, it also helped to reduce contamination by increasing the size of each cluster (see Section 4.3.4) and ensuring that neighbouring villages were grouped into the same cluster. It also accounted for the possibility that residents might visit different health units in the same cluster, depending on their personal preferences.
- While the definition of clusters in this trial was aimed at reducing contamination between intervention and control arms, the investigators were careful to collect data to monitor the degree of contamination. Records were kept of the numbers of visits to health units made by residents of other clusters. In the event, these numbers were very small, and this gave some assurance that contamination between intervention and control clusters was effectively limited.

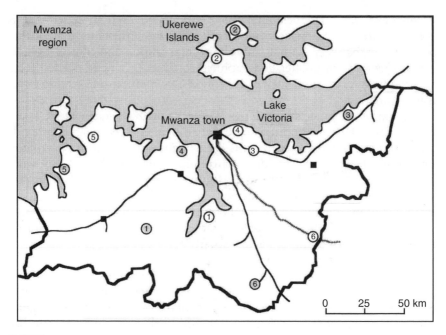

FIGURE 4.3
Map of study area of Mwanza STD treatment trial showing locations of 12 study communities. Numbered circles show six matched pairs of communities. Intervention communities are shaded. (From Hays, R., Mosha, F., Nicoll, A., et al. A community trial of the impact of improved sexually transmitted disease treatment on the HIV epidemic in rural Tanzania: 1. Design. *AIDS* 1995, 9, 919–26. With permission.)

4.4.2 Buffer Zones

In some RCTs, the clusters are defined by areas on the map which may correspond to administrative districts or arbitrary geographical zones. In many cases, these zones do not correspond to well-separated communities, particularly in rural areas where there are scattered households. In such cases, allocating neighbouring zones to different treatment arms could result in substantial levels of contamination, since there may be considerable interaction between clusters, especially along zone boundaries.

To reduce contamination, investigators have sometimes specified that the trial clusters should be separated by *buffer zones*, so that there is little or no common boundary between any two clusters.

Example 4.18

In the *MEMA kwa Vijana* trial in Tanzania, previously discussed in Example 2.4, 20 rural communities were randomly allocated to an intervention arm receiving an integrated adolescent sexual health programme or a control arm (Hayes et al. 2005). Each community in this trial corresponded roughly to an administrative area known as a "ward", mostly consisting of around five or six villages with an average population of 17,000. The study communities are shown in Figure 4.4. There were concerns that, if intervention and control communities were directly adjacent, the

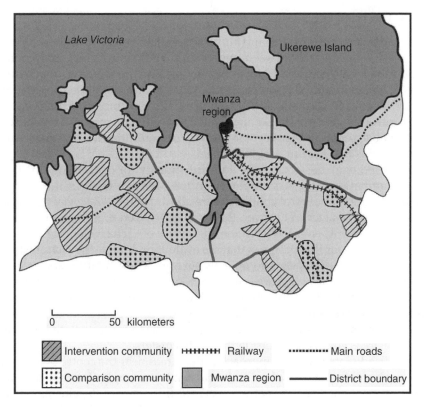

FIGURE 4.4
Map of study area of MEMA kwa Vijana adolescent sexual health intervention trial in the Mwanza Region, Tanzania showing locations of intervention and control communities. (From Ross, D.A., Changalucha, J., Obasi, A.I.N., et al. Biological and behavioral impact of an adolescent sexual health intervention in Tanzania: A community-randomized trial. *AIDS* 2007, 21, 1943–55. With permission.)

knowledge, attitudes, behaviour or HIV risk of young people in control communities might be affected through contact with their counterparts in nearby intervention communities. Therefore, in selecting the 20 study communities, an effort was made to leave gaps between them wherever possible to act as buffer zones.

Example 4.19

By contrast, consider again the CRT of vitamin A supplementation in rural Ghana discussed in Example 3.4 (Ghana VAST Study Team 1993). In this trial, no buffer zones were left between the clusters. As we have seen, vitamin A or placebo in this trial were administered by study staff to individual children depending on which cluster they lived in, and quality control studies suggested that there were few instances of children receiving the wrong product. Moreover, this trial was aimed at measuring the protection conferred by vitamin A supplementation on individual children, and population-level effects on transmission were not anticipated. Social contact between neighbouring zones was therefore not considered to be a major concern in this trial.

4.4.3 The Fried Egg Design

Well-separated communities and buffer zones serve chiefly to reduce contamination due to contacts between intervention and control clusters. Depending on the local geography, however, they may not be effective in avoiding contact between intervention or control clusters and the wider population. In the Mwanza STD treatment trial (Figure 4.3), for example, the intervention and control clusters may be far apart, but contamination may still result from contacts between intervention (or control) communities and neighbouring communities that are not part of the trial.

The "fried egg" design may be a useful strategy for controlling this type of contamination, and was employed in the Mwanza trial. In this design, the intervention or control conditions are administered *throughout* the corresponding trial clusters. However, the samples selected to measure the study endpoints are only selected from the *central area* of each cluster (Figure 4.5).

The rationale for this design is that the evaluation sample for each cluster is selected from an area that is completely surrounded by a buffer zone receiving the *same treatment condition* (intervention or control) as the evaluation sample. This helps to mimic the effect that would be seen if an intervention were to be implemented throughout a country or large region, although of course there may still be some contamination due to contacts with individuals from areas completely outside the study cluster.

One disadvantage of this approach is that areas near the centre of a cluster may not be representative of the entire cluster. For example, if the cluster is the catchment area of a health centre, areas near the centre of the cluster may be those closest to the health centre. This may mean that health-seeking behaviour in the evaluation area is different from that in the more outlying areas of

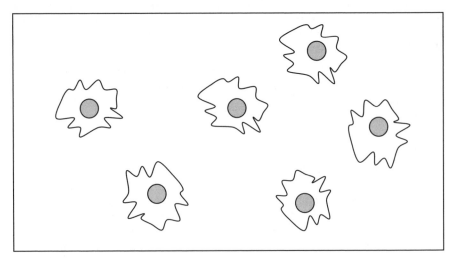

FIGURE 4.5
Schematic diagram showing "fried egg" design. White areas represent clusters allocated to intervention or control arms. Shaded areas represent areas from which evaluation samples are selected.

the cluster, so that the impact of an intervention delivered through the health centre may be over-estimated. This may be less of a problem where clusters are based on arbitrary geographical zones, where the centre of the cluster does not correspond to the central area of a well-defined community.

Example 4.20

In the Mwanza trial of STD treatment, as we have seen, the community was defined as the catchment area of a health centre and its satellite dispensaries (Grosskurth et al. 1995; Hayes et al. 1995). The impact of the intervention was measured in a cohort consisting of 1000 adults aged 15–54 years selected from each of the 10 study communities. These adults were randomly selected from the population residing within 90 minutes walking distance of the health centre. Since the communities were typically large, and the health centre was generally located fairly centrally within the community, this design corresponded roughly to the "fried egg" design described above.

TABLE 4.1

The Examples of This Chapter Classified According to the Three Levels of Design that Characterise CRTs

Example*	Randomisation Unit	Intervention Recipient	Data Collected
4.1	Village	Household	Household, individual
4.2	City	Pharmacists, sex workers	Individual (random sample of general population)
4.3	Département	General population	Patients at GP surgeries
4.4	Community	Individual (including some not randomised as lived outside study communities)	Individual
4.5	Group of households	Household	Household, individual
4.6	School	Class	Students
4.7	General practice	Patient, GP	Patient
4.8	Health centre	Personnel dealing with TB patients	Patient
4.9	Mine shaft	Individual	Individual
4.10	Household	Individual	Individual
4.11	Individual	Individual	Individual's teeth
4.15	Community (group of villages)	Individual	Individual
4.16	Community (group of villages)	Household	Individual
4.17/4.20	Community	Health unit	Individual (random sample of general population)
4.18	Community	School	Individual
4.19	Group of households	Individual	Individual

*Hypothetical examples omitted.

4.5 Levels of Randomisation, Intervention, Data Collection and Inference

We have given many examples of different choices of randomisation unit. The considerations that come into play in making these choices relate to the parameter of interest (efficacy, effectiveness, indirect effect, etc.), the logistical ease of implementing an intervention at different levels, the logistics of conducting the trial, political considerations and the possibility of contamination.

In Table 4.1, the examples of this chapter are classified according to the different levels at which design features of a CRT are exhibited. For some of the examples, there is more than one parameter of interest. Whereas, some studies may only focus on estimation of the overall effect of an intervention, which includes outcomes on all persons regardless of their exposure to the intervention, others may estimate overall, total and indirect effects. Of course, more complicated designs are possible. For example, randomisation units might be selected during a multistage sampling process, and different types of intervention might be administered at different levels of randomisation.

5

Matching and Stratification

5.1 Introduction

In a simple *unmatched* CRT design, a set of clusters is randomly allocated between two or more treatment arms. If there is substantial between-cluster variability, it may be decided to first group together clusters that are expected to be similar with respect to the outcome of interest, and to allocate the treatment within these groups. This is usually done in an attempt to prevent imbalance in important covariates between the treatment arms, and to improve the precision and power of the trial.

In this book, we shall use the term *matching* to denote trials in which the clusters are formed into groups such that only one cluster in each group is allocated to each treatment arm. For example, this would result in *matched pairs* in trials with two treatment arms, *matched triplets* in trials with three treatment arms, and so on. We shall use the term *stratification* to denote trials in which larger groups of clusters are formed, referred to as *strata*, such that in at least some strata more than one cluster is allocated to a treatment arm.

In Section 5.2 we discuss the rationale for matching in a CRT, while some of the disadvantages are explored in Section 5.3. Stratification, as an alternative to matching, is discussed in Section 5.4. In Section 5.5, we discuss practical considerations in the choice of variables to match on. Finally, in Section 5.6, we consider how to decide on the use of matching or stratification when designing a CRT.

5.2 Rationale for Matching

In this section, we show how matching can help to minimise differences between treatment arms with respect to baseline characteristics, and how matching can improve the power of study. Because there are other ways to ensure baseline comparability (see Section 6.2), the main advantage of matching or stratification lies in the potential for increased efficiency or precision of estimation.

5.2.1 Avoiding Imbalance between Treatment Arms

The key strength of the randomised controlled trial is the use of randomisation to determine the allocation of study subjects to the different treatment arms. Randomisation has three main advantages for this purpose. First and foremost, the larger the number of randomisation units, the greater the probability that the treatment groups are well-balanced with respect to both known and unknown potential confounders. Second, it is a fair and transparent procedure, which avoids conscious or unconscious bias on the part of the investigator in the selection of which subjects will receive the intervention, thus enhancing the *credibility* of the trial results. It is a convenient way to allocate treatments, and helps to maintain blinding in single- or double-blind trials. Third, it provides a formal justification for the use of some particular procedures of statistical inference.

In a conventional individually randomised trial, hundreds or thousands of subjects are typically randomised to each arm, and in these circumstances randomisation can usually be relied upon to achieve a high degree of comparability between the treatment groups. A consequence of this is that, while it is always good practice to check the data for baseline comparability, the primary analysis is often a *crude analysis* with no adjustment for covariates.

In CRTs, by contrast, it is common for only a small number of clusters to be randomised. In these circumstances, randomisation still has the advantages of fairness and transparency, but can no longer be relied upon to achieve balance between the treatment arms. This clearly calls into question one of the main benefits of the experimental approach to study design, which aims to ensure that the study groups under comparison are similar with respect to all factors apart from the intervention of interest.

Baseline comparisons showing substantial differences between the treatment arms clearly undermine the *credibility* of the trial results, since critical readers may reasonably question whether any differences in outcomes between the treatment arms might be attributable to differences in known or unknown confounders. While it is possible to carry out an *adjusted analysis* to allow for covariates which show imbalance between the treatment arms, this adds complexity to the analysis, reduces the transparency of the results and depends on additional assumptions—for example that the effects of the covariates are linear on the logistic scale (see Chapter 10 and Chapter 11).

By grouping the clusters into similar pairs (assuming two treatment arms, or larger groups if there are more than two), we can help to ensure that the treatment arms are similar at baseline, at least with respect to the characteristics we choose to match on. We return later to the question of how the matching should be performed.

Example 5.1

As we have seen in Example 4.17, the Mwanza trial of STD treatment for HIV prevention was carried out in 12 rural communities in Tanzania. These communities were widely spread over a large geographical region, and included remote rural villages, settlements along major truck routes, communities on two of the islands in Lake Victoria and villages located on the lakeshore (Grosskurth et al. 1995; Hayes et al. 1995).

Baseline data on HIV prevalence were not available at the time of randomisation in this trial. On the basis of previous epidemiological data from this and other regions, however, HIV prevalence and incidence at this early stage of the epidemic were expected to be higher in roadside settlements (HIV often spreads initially along major transport routes) and lower in the rural villages and islands. Some general geographical trends in HIV prevalence across the region were also anticipated. It was therefore decided to arrange the 12 communities into 6 matched pairs as follows:

- The two roadside settlements and two island communities formed two of the matched pairs.
- The four remote rural villages and four lakeshore villages were each matched into pairs on the basis of geographical location.

The pairing also took account of prior STD case rates reported by the health units in each community, since the intervention was to be implemented through these units. The locations of the six matched pairs are shown in Figure 4.3. On this map, Pair 2 denotes the two lake island villages, while Pair 3 denotes the two roadside settlements.

The HIV prevalences recorded during the subsequent baseline survey are shown in Table 5.1 (Grosskurth et al. 1995). Note the very wide variation in prevalence, with much higher rates in the roadside settlements and low rates on the lake islands. Had an *unmatched* design been used, both roadside settlements could easily have been allocated to the same treatment arm, and similarly for the island communities. This could have resulted in substantial baseline imbalance between the treatment arms, calling into question the results of the trial.

Following the matched design, reasonable balance was achieved with overall prevalences of 3.8 and 4.4% in the intervention and control arms, respectively. Despite this, the investigators chose to *adjust* the outcome results for the baseline prevalence in each community to allow for the residual imbalance.

TABLE 5.1

Baseline HIV Prevalence Rates (%) Observed in the Mwanza Trial of STD Treatment for HIV Prevention

Matched Pair	Intervention	Control	Type of Community
1	3.9	3.0	Rural village
2	2.0	1.6	Island
3	6.8	8.6	Roadside
4	5.4	4.3	Lakeshore
5	2.8	4.7	Lakeshore
6	1.8	4.5	Rural village
Overall	3.8	4.4	

Example 5.2

The Community Intervention Trial for Smoking Cessation (COMMIT) was carried out to assess the impact of a multi-faceted community-level intervention designed to reduce the prevalence of cigarette smoking (COMMIT Research Group 1995a, 1995b). The main focus of the intervention was on health education using a variety of approaches.

The trial was carried out in 11 matched pairs of communities, including 10 pairs in the U.S. and one in Canada. The communities in each pair were matched on geographic location, population size and socio-demographic factors. The populations of the communities varied from 49,421 to 251,208. Intervention impact was evaluated through cross-sectional telephone surveys of adults aged 25–64 years, carried out at baseline and after 5 years to measure the prevalence of smoking, and through follow-up of a randomly sampled cohort of smokers to measure smoking cessation rates.

Table 5.2 shows the prevalences of smoking at baseline and follow-up, as measured in the repeated cross-sectional surveys. The matched pairs design was successful in achieving close comparability of smoking prevalence in the intervention and control arms at baseline, with mean prevalences of 27.6 and 28.6%, respectively. Moreover, the baseline prevalences of smoking in the two communities in each matched pair tended to be quite similar. However, the overall variability in smoking prevalence between communities, from 22 to 35%, was relatively modest and so we might expect the gain from using a matched design in this trial to be somewhat less than in the Mwanza STD treatment trial.

5.2.2 Improving Study Power and Precision

The precision and power of a CRT depends on the degree of variability between clusters in the outcome of interest. In some trials, this variability

TABLE 5.2

Prevalence (%) of Cigarette Smoking in Adults Aged 25–64 Years in the 22 Study Communities of the COMMIT Smoking Cessation Trial

	Baseline Survey		Final Survey	
Matched Pair	Intervention	Control	Intervention	Control
1	28.6	27.0	21.6	22.2
2	34.8	32.6	33.8	27.8
3	25.5	28.6	24.8	26.4
4	30.0	33.6	25.0	30.0
5	30.2	32.6	24.0	30.6
6	23.5	22.3	19.3	18.3
7	27.7	27.9	25.3	22.2
8	31.4	30.6	29.3	28.3
9	24.9	28.5	20.5	27.9
10	24.0	23.0	22.0	18.8
11	23.4	28.5	19.9	27.1
Mean of prevalences	27.6	28.6	24.1	25.4

can be very substantial. In the Mwanza STD trial discussed in Example 5.1, for example, baseline HIV prevalence in the 12 study communities varied from 1.6 to 8.6% and it would be reasonable to assume at the design stage that the primary outcome (HIV incidence) might show similar variability.

Carrying out a trial in such heterogeneous communities may increase the generalisability of the findings. However, it also has the effect of increasing the value of the between-cluster coefficient of variation, k, and hence reduces the power and precision of the trial for any given sample size, as we shall see in Chapter 7.

If we group the study communities into *matched pairs*, presumed to be more similar with respect to the primary outcome, then we can carry out a *matched analysis*. There are various approaches to this analysis, as we shall see in Chapter 12, but the general principle is that comparisons are made between the intervention and control communities *within matched pairs*. It follows that the overall coefficient of variation, k, across all communities can be replaced by the coefficient of variation within matched pairs, k_m. This may be considerably smaller than k, resulting in increased power and precision.

Example 5.3

We now consider the outcome data from the Mwanza STD trial. Table 5.3 shows the cumulative incidence of HIV infection over two years of follow-up in the six matched pairs of study communities (Grosskurth et al. 1995).

Although the observed incidence rates are based on quite small numbers of HIV seroconversions, it is clear that there was substantial variability in incidence over the six communities in the intervention arm, and the six communities in the control arm. Had this trial been carried out with an unmatched design and analysis, it is very unlikely that a significant result could have been achieved with such a large degree of overlap in incidence rates. By contrast, an analysis that takes into account the matched design exploits the much smaller variation in incidence within matched pairs. Note that while baseline HIV prevalence was higher in intervention communities in half the matched pairs (Table 5.1), the HIV incidence outcome was consistently lower in the intervention community in *all six matched pairs*.

A simple approach to unmatched analysis uses the *t-test* applied to the community-level incidence rates in each treatment arm. In this case, we obtain

TABLE 5.3

Cumulative HIV Incidence Observed over 2 Years of Follow-up in the Mwanza Trial of STD Treatment for HIV Prevention

Matched Pair	Intervention	Control	Type of Community
1	5/568 (0.9%)	10/702 (1.4%)	Rural village
2	4/766 (0.5%)	7/833 (0.8%)	Island
3	17/650 (2.6%)	20/630 (3.2%)	Roadside
4	13/734 (1.8%)	23/760 (3.0%)	Lakeshore
5	4/732 (0.5%)	12/782 (1.5%)	Lakeshore
6	5/699 (0.7%)	10/693 (1.4%)	Rural village
Overall	48/4149 (1.2%)	82/4400 (1.9%)	

$t = 1.35$ on 10 df, and this is clearly very far from being statistically significant ($p = 0.21$). The corresponding matched analysis uses the *paired t-test*, which gives $t = 5.30$ on 5 df, and this is highly significant ($p = 0.003$). Clearly the matched design gave increased power in this trial.

5.3 Disadvantages of Matching

5.3.1 Loss of Degrees of Freedom

When we analyse the results of a CRT to test the effect of an intervention, we first compute a statistic representing the difference between the outcomes in the intervention and control arms. This statistic might, for example, be the difference in the proportions with the outcome of interest between the two arms, averaging over the clusters in each arm.

Consider first a simple unmatched CRT with c clusters in each arm. Let p_{ij} be the observed proportion with the outcome of interest in the jth cluster in the ith treatment arm, where $i = 1$ denotes the intervention arm, and $i = 0$ denotes the control arm. Then we compute the statistic:

$$d = \bar{p}_1 - \bar{p}_0$$

where $\bar{p}_i = \sum_{j=1}^{c} p_{ij}/c$ is the average of the observed proportions in the ith treatment arm.

As we have seen, a simple test of the null hypothesis of zero intervention effect is the *t-test* obtained as:

$$t = \frac{d}{\sqrt{\dfrac{s_1^2 + s_0^2}{c}}} \tag{5.1}$$

where s_1^2 and s_0^2 are the empirical variances of the proportions in the clusters in the two treatment arms. The denominator of Equation 5.1 is the estimated standard error of d, and is based on the variation between the c observed proportions in the intervention arm and the c observed proportions in the control arm. The total degrees of freedom for this variance estimate are:

$$df = 2 \times (c - 1) = 2c - 2$$

Now consider a matched CRT with c matched pairs of clusters. We begin by computing the difference between the proportions *within each pair*. For the jth pair, we have:

$$d_j = p_{1j} - p_{0j}$$

To test the null hypothesis based on the matched data, we can use the *paired t-test*:

$$t_m = \frac{\bar{d}}{\sqrt{\dfrac{s_m^2}{c}}} \tag{5.2}$$

where $\bar{d}$ is the average of the differences d_j and s_m^2 is the empirical variance of these differences. The denominator in Equation 5.2 is the estimated standard error of $\bar{d}$ and is based on the variation between the c pair-specific differences. The degrees of freedom for the matched test are therefore:

$$df = c - 1$$

and note that this is only half the degrees of freedom for the unmatched analysis.

Comparing Equation 5.1 and Equation 5.2, we note that in both cases the expected values of the numerators will be equal to the true intervention effect. However, the denominator of Equation 5.2 will be smaller than that of Equation 5.1 if and only if:

$$s_m^2 < s_1^2 + s_0^2$$

Assuming that s_1 and s_2 are roughly equal to a common value s, it can be shown that:

$$s_m^2 = 2s^2(1-r)$$

where r is the correlation between the observed proportions in the intervention and control clusters matched together in the same pairs. It follows that the matched test statistic t_m will generally be larger than the unmatched test statistic t_u, the difference depending on how effective the pair-matching is, as measured by the correlation coefficient r.

However, the *power* of the trial will depend not only on the expected value of the test statistic, but also on the critical value of the t distribution, which in turn depends on the degrees of freedom. Matched studies generally provide lower variance, but this is at least partly offset by the smaller degrees of freedom, $(c-1)$ instead of $2(c-1)$.

Table 5.4 shows the critical values of the t distribution for unmatched and matched CRTs with differing numbers of clusters per treatment arm.

TABLE 5.4

Critical Values of t Distribution for Unmatched, Matched and Stratified Trials for Differing Numbers of Clusters, and Break-even Correlations in Endpoints within Pairs or Strata

Clusters/ Arm	Unmatched Trial		Matched Trial			Stratified Trial*		
c	df	$t_{0.05}$	df	$t_{0.05}$	r	df	$t_{0.05}$	r
4	6	2.45	3	3.18	0.37	4	2.78	0.20
6	10	2.23	5	2.57	0.22	8	2.31	0.06
8	14	2.14	7	2.36	0.15	12	2.18	0.02
10	18	2.10	9	2.26	0.12	16	2.12	0.02
12	22	2.07	11	2.20	0.10	20	2.09	0.01

Source: Adapted from Klar, N. and Donner, A. The merits of matching in community intervention trials: A cautionary tale. *Statistics in Medicine* 1997, 16, 1753–64. Table II. They show break-even value of correlation r_{xz} between outcome (x) and matching variable (z). We show break-even value of $r = r_{xx} = r_{xz}^2$.
*Assuming two strata with equal numbers of clusters.

It also shows the break-even value of the correlation coefficient, r, assuming a two-tailed test at the 5% level and 80% power. Below this break-even value, an unmatched design would give higher power than a matched trial, because the loss in degrees of freedom would outweigh the reduction in variance. Note that as the number of clusters increases, the size of the break-even correlation decreases. This implies that in trials with few clusters, the matched design will only provide increased power if the matching is very effective. Strategies to achieve effective matching are discussed in Section 5.5.

Example 5.4

Figure 5.1 shows the observed HIV incidence rates in the intervention communities in the Mwanza trial plotted against the corresponding rates in the comparison communities in the same matched pairs. The correlation coefficient in this trial was $r = 0.94$. Clearly this greatly exceeds the break-even correlation of 0.22 for a trial with six clusters per arm, and the matched design was highly effective in this study. Matching does not often achieve such high correlations, however, and we return to this point in Section 5.5.

5.3.2 Drop-out of Clusters

It is uncommon for any trial to achieve complete follow-up of all those recruited to the study. In a conventional individually randomised trial, losses to follow-up lead to a reduction in precision and power, and raise concerns over *selection bias* since those lost to follow-up often differ systematically from those remaining in the trial.

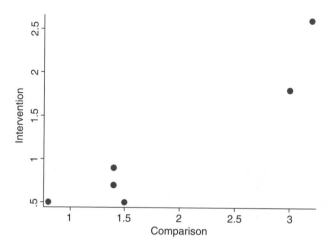

FIGURE 5.1
Cumulative incidence of HIV infection in matched pairs of communities in the Mwanza trial
of STD treatment for HIV prevention.

Losses to follow-up of individuals are also of importance in CRTs for the
same reasons. In some CRTs, however, *entire clusters* may drop out of the
trial. This may occur for several reasons:

- Communities or institutions may decide that they no longer wish to
  participate in the trial, for a range of possible reasons. For example,
  in a trial randomising GP surgeries, some GPs may decide that the
  workload involved in taking part in the trial is too disruptive, and
  may withdraw after enrolling in the trial so that no follow-up data
  are available. Or researchers may lose the trust of villagers taking
  part in a village-randomised trial, and village leaders may decide
  that the entire village should opt out of the study.

- Follow-up may become logistically impossible in some clusters. For
  example, some communities may become too dangerous to follow up
  due to war or civil strife, or access may be restricted due to weather
  or natural disasters.

- In some trials, recruitment of sufficient individuals turns out to be
  difficult in some clusters. For example, in a GP-randomised trial of
  treatment for a specific condition, no patients might present with the
  condition in some practices.

As in loss to follow-up of individuals, loss of entire clusters reduces power
and precision, as well as raising concerns over selection bias. In *matched CRTs,*
however, there is the additional problem that if a cluster is lost from the trial,
the entire matched pair is lost—since the remaining cluster no longer has

a matched cluster for comparison. Since issues of cost and logistics some-times mean that CRTs only include the minimum acceptable number of matched pairs, the loss of even one pair may mean that study power becomes inadequate.

The only exception to this is where it is decided to *break the matching* in the analysis, and this point is discussed further in Chapter 12.

5.3.3 Limitations in Statistical Inference for Matched Trials

Despite the above disadvantages, the matched pairs design has been quite widely used, especially for trials with few clusters, perhaps partly because of the intuitive attraction of a design in which pairs of similar clusters are compared. As we shall see in Chapter 12, effective methods of statistical analysis for such trials are available. However, the use of a matched design does impose a number of limitations on the statistical inference that can be carried out. We briefly review these here.

5.3.3.1 Adjustment for Covariates

Even if the matching improves the balance between the treatment arms, we may wish to carry out an adjusted analysis, both to remove the bias due to residual imbalance and to improve precision and power by reducing between-cluster variability. For *unmatched* studies, there is a range of meth-ods available to carry out such adjusted analyses, and these include regres-sion methods which allow us to analyse the effects of both individual-level and cluster-level covariates in the same model. These methods also ensure that optimal *weights* are given to the data from different clusters, in contrast with the simplest methods of analysis based on the *t-test*.

Unfortunately, these regression methods do not work well for matched studies, mainly because they involve the inclusion of additional model parameters for the matched pairs, and this violates the asymptotic assump-tions on which such methods are based, since the number of model param-eters approaches the number of clusters. There are, however, alternative methods to adjust for covariates based on cluster-level summaries and these are discussed in detail in Chapter 12.

5.3.3.2 Testing for Variation in Intervention Effect

It may be of interest to assess whether the effect of intervention varies between matched pairs. This cannot be done, however, because the differ-ence in outcomes between the clusters in each pair depends on both the size of the intervention effect *and* the intrinsic between-cluster variability within that matched pair. It is impossible to separate out these two effects with-out making additional assumptions. This difficulty results from the lack of *replication* within each matched pair, meaning that there is only one cluster per treatment arm in each matched pair.

However, it may still be possible to analyse for variations in intervention effect by grouping the matched pairs into broader *strata*, and using analysis of variance to test for interactions between intervention effect and strata.

We note that this limitation is avoided by the *stratified* CRT design, which incorporates some replication of clusters in each treatment arm within strata (see Section 5.4).

5.3.3.3 Estimation of Intracluster Correlation Coefficient and Coefficient of Variation

The *intracluster correlation coefficient*, ρ, and *coefficient of variation*, k, are important measures of the degree of clustering in a CRT, and play a central role in study design. For example, we shall see in Chapter 7 that we need estimates of ρ or k to carry out sample size calculations.

Unfortunately, it is not possible to estimate ρ or k based on data from a matched trial because, as we have already seen, the between-cluster variability is confounded with variations in the intervention effect. The only exception is if we can assume that the intervention effect is constant over all matched pairs, but this is a strong assumption that is unlikely to be realistic in most settings.

As we shall see in Chapter 12, we have methods of analysis for matched studies, including simple methods based on the *paired t-test* which do not require an estimate of either k or ρ, and so this is not a major disadvantage for the analysis of the trial in question. However, it does mean that we will have less empirical data on which to base sample size assumptions for *future* trials.

5.4 Stratification as an Alternative to Matching

The most serious disadvantage of the pair-matched design is the loss of power and precision due to the loss of degrees of freedom resulting from the lack of *replication* within each matched pair. *Stratification* is an alternative to matching which lies between the extremes of a completely unmatched design and a pair-matched design.

This design involves the grouping of available clusters into two or more *strata* that are expected to be similar with respect to the outcome of interest. The clusters within each stratum are then randomly allocated between the treatment arms. Matching is therefore an extreme form of stratification in which the number of clusters in each stratum is equal to the number of treatment arms.

Like matching, stratification aims to achieve a reduction in the variance of the estimated treatment effect. However it does have a number of advantages over the matched design:

- Fewer degrees of freedom are lost and, depending on the relative reductions in variance achieved by the two designs, this can result in the stratified design having higher power and precision than the matched design.
- Because there is replication within strata, it is possible to test for variations in intervention effect between strata.
- It may be possible to use regression methods to adjust for and analyse the effects of individual-level and cluster-level covariates, because fewer parameters are needed to model the stratum effects.
- If one cluster is lost from a stratum, this does not require the loss of data from the entire stratum (unless this stratum happens to contain only two clusters).

Table 5.4 shows the degrees of freedom and break-even values of the correlation coefficient for which the stratified design (with two strata of equal size) exceeds the power of the unmatched design. Several points are clear from this table. First, the degrees of freedom for the stratified design are intermediate between those for the unmatched and pair-matched designs. Second, the break-even correlation is much lower for the stratified design than the matched design, because fewer degrees of freedom are lost.

The pair-matched design may achieve closer matching, and therefore a higher correlation of outcomes within matched pairs, than is achieved by a broader stratification. Matching is usually imperfect, however, and in practice stratification into two or three strata may capture a large part of the reduction in between-cluster variance achieved by pair matching (Todd et al. 2003).

These considerations suggest that stratification will often be the method of choice.

Example 5.5

The benefits of the stratified design have only become clear during the past few years, and so there are relatively few CRTs with this design in the published literature compared with unmatched and pair-matched designs.

One example is provided by a further study in Mwanza Region, Tanzania. This trial, previously discussed in Example 2.4 and Example 4.18, was carried out to measure the impact of an adolescent sexual health programme on HIV incidence and other endpoints (Hayes et al. 2005). A total of 20 rural communities were selected, each comprising around five to six villages, five to six primary schools and one or two health units. A study cohort was enrolled from the final three standards (grades) at the primary schools in each community, and followed up for 3 years. There was expected to be substantial variation in HIV incidence between communities, and it was decided to use stratification to improve the power and precision of the trial.

An initial survey was carried out among young people in each community to measure the prevalence of HIV and chlamydia in young people aged 15–19 years (Obasi et al. 2001). This age-group was selected to be similar to the projected age of the main study cohort at final follow-up. HIV prevalence in this initial survey was therefore expected to be a good surrogate for (i.e., closely correlated with) the HIV incidence in the study cohort. However, HIV prevalence in this age-group was low, and prevalence estimates in each community were based on a very small number of HIV-positive individuals. Prevalence estimates were therefore too imprecise to form the basis for meaningful construction of matched pairs. It was therefore decided to form three strata:

- Stratum 1: Observed HIV prevalence in initial survey exceeds 1% (six communities).
- Stratum 2: Observed HIV prevalence in initial survey 1% or less, but with geographical factors known to be associated with higher risk (eight communities).
- Stratum 3: Observed HIV prevalence in initial survey 1% or less, and with no geographical factors known to be associated with higher risk (six communities).

Within each stratum, communities were randomly allocated to the two treatment arms using a process of *restricted randomisation* that will be described in Chapter 6.

5.5 Choice of Matching Variables

5.5.1 Estimating the Matching Correlation

Assuming that we have decided to use matching or stratification, how should the matching be carried out and what variables should we match on?

As we have seen, the effectiveness of matching is maximised if it induces a strong correlation in the endpoint of interest among clusters within pairs or strata. The strength of this correlation depends on two factors:

- The correlation between the matching variable(s) and the endpoint
- The closeness of matching on the matching variable(s)

The effect of the first of these factors can be simply presented. If r_{xz} is the correlation between the matching variable, z, and the endpoint of interest, x, and if pairs are perfectly matched on this variable, then the matching correlation is given by:

$$r = r_{xz}^2$$

While this formula helps to give a general indication of the degree of correlation that can be achieved by matching, it is in practice of quite limited value in the design of a specific trial for several reasons:

- In many cases, prior data are not available on the correlation between the matching variable and endpoint measured over the same time intervals as will apply during the trial. For example, if z is baseline HIV prevalence and x is HIV incidence during a 3-year follow-up, we would need to have prior data linking HIV prevalence to subsequent HIV incidence over a similar time period.

- Such correlations may not be stable over time. For example, the relationship between HIV prevalence and incidence is known to change over time as the epidemic is initiated, expands and finally stabilises or contracts. Even if prospective data on correlations between z and x are available, they will by definition relate to a time period prior to the trial, and may misrepresent the correlation that will be seen during the trial.

- If estimates of r_{xz} are available, they may be based on samples of different size than will apply during the proposed trial. Note that r refers to the correlation coefficient between the *observed* cluster-level endpoint measures (means, proportions or rates) in the intervention and control clusters in each matched pair. The *observed* correlation depends on the sample size for each cluster as well as the *true* correlation of the underlying measures. If based on different sample sizes, prior estimates of r_{xz} would therefore need to be adjusted to allow for this.

- Perfect matching is rarely achieved, so that r_{xz}^2 is likely to overestimate the value of r that will be achieved by matching. In addition, it is common to seek matches on several variables, with differing r_{xz} and closeness of matching for each variable, so that estimating the overall r is likely to be difficult.

Instead, we recommend that when planning a new trial, investigators should estimate the reduction in the between-cluster coefficient of variation, k, likely to be achieved by matching. In Chapter 7 we present sample size formulae based on values of k_m, the estimated coefficient of variation *within matched pairs or strata*. It is usually possible to make a plausible estimate of k_m on which to base sample size calculations. Using the unmatched k will provide a conservative estimate.

5.5.2 Matching on Baseline Values of Endpoint of Interest

Matching is most effective if the matching variable is highly correlated with the endpoint. In most cases, the closest correlation is likely to be with the baseline value of the *same endpoint*, and so this is a natural candidate for matching.

The feasibility of this will depend on the type of endpoint. If it is based on the *prevalence* of some condition at one point in time, then a cross-sectional survey at baseline would be sufficient. However, if it is based on the *incidence* of some event over an extended time period, we would need to carry out a prospective study to measure this rate *prior* to randomisation. This would greatly add to the cost and duration of the study, particularly if the follow-up period is lengthy, and this will seldom be acceptable. The only exception would be if longitudinal data are already available based on past studies or surveillance data.

Even where a cross-sectional survey is carried out to measure baseline values of the endpoint, it may not always be feasible to match on this variable. If there is a time delay between data collection and analysis, for example because of the time taken to process specimens in the laboratory, the interval between baseline survey and randomisation may be judged too lengthy.

5.5.3 Matching on Surrogate Variables

Where baseline values of the endpoint are not available, the alternative is to match on other variables that are expected to be correlated with the endpoint. These surrogate variables might be characteristics of the *cluster* (for example, size, geographic location, altitude, distance from main road), or summary measures at the cluster level of individual characteristics (for example, socio-economic status or risk factors for the disease of interest).

Where the endpoint is the *incidence* of some condition over time, we might decide to match on the *baseline prevalence* of that condition although, as we have seen, the relationship between prevalence and incidence may not be straightforward especially for epidemic (as opposed to stable endemic) diseases.

5.5.4 Matching on Multiple Variables

The strength of the correlation within matched pairs or strata may be increased by matching on more than one variable, each of which is correlated with the endpoint. Formally, if pairs are perfectly matched on all of these variables, the matching correlation r will equal R_{xz}^2 where R_{xz} is the multiple correlation coefficient between the endpoint and the set of matching variables.

When using a matched pair design, it is quite common to match on multiple variables in this way. In the case of stratification, we could form strata based on the *cross-classification* of two or more matching variables. However, this would usually result in an excessive number of strata, which should be avoided.

However, it is sometimes feasible and appropriate to define strata based on the values of two or more variables. In Example 5.5, HIV prevalence based on an initial survey together with geographical characteristics of communities was used in combination to define three strata for the trial of an adolescent sexual health programme in Mwanza.

5.5.5 Matching on Location

Formation of pairs or strata on the basis of geography or proximity is a common strategy in the design of CRTs. Many spatially related factors can account for variability in health outcomes, including socioeconomic status, organisational capacity, location of health facilities, distance to a hospital and exposure to pathogens. Stratifying on location conveniently reduces within-stratum variability with respect to such factors, and helps to ensure that they are balanced across study arms. There may also be political advantages in ensuring that the intervention is evenly spread across a study area.

Nonetheless, geographical stratification may still result in undesirable configurations. Consider a CRT with 16 randomisation units, grouped into four geographical strata (quadrants) as shown in Figure 5.2. If two units within each stratum are randomly assigned to the intervention arm, it may happen that the eight shaded units receive the intervention while the eight unshaded units are assigned to the control arm. Now suppose that there is a strong North-to-South gradient in a variable that is highly predictive of the study outcome. One might argue that there are then only three relatively independent randomisation units: The top layer of control units, the wider middle layer of intervention units and the bottom layer of control units.

Such clearly undesirable configurations can be avoided through the imposition of additional constraints, and these methods of *restricted randomisation* are discussed in Chapter 6. An extreme example of such constraints would be the designation of a "checkerboard" structure, as shown in Figure 5.3. Given this randomisation scheme, the concordance or discordance of any pair of randomisation units with respect to intervention and control status is fixed, and all that remains random is the allocation of treatment to either the shaded or unshaded units.

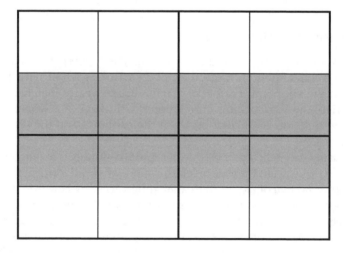

FIGURE 5.2
Example of study with 16 geographically determined randomisation units, stratified into four quadrants. Shaded areas represent intervention clusters.

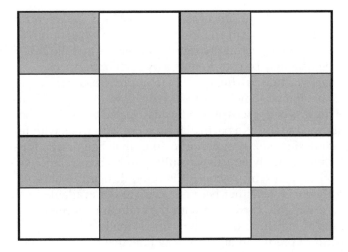

FIGURE 5.3
Checkerboard arrangement of randomisation units. Shaded and unshaded areas represent intervention and control clusters, or vice versa.

If statistical analysis is performed using the model-based perspective common to public health investigations, such an extreme constraint to the point of having only two possible randomisation outcomes does not pose any problems. If, however, we wished to adopt a strict application of randomisation-based inference, using the permutation test as discussed in Section 6.2.4 and Section 10.5.3, this scenario would not be acceptable. With only two possible randomisation outcomes, there are too few permutations to make any useful inferences.

5.6 Choosing Whether to Match or Stratify

5.6.1 Introduction

In this section, we give some general guidance on choice of design strategy for different types of CRT. As we shall see, this choice depends on the closeness of matching that can be achieved as well as the number of clusters to be randomised. We begin by considering trials with a small number of clusters, say less than 10–15 per treatment arm, and then discuss trials with larger numbers of clusters.

5.6.2 Trials with a Small Number of Clusters

The matched pairs design has been used most commonly for trials in which only a small number of clusters are randomised to each treatment arm. This is probably due mainly to concerns over imbalances between arms, which can easily occur by chance in an unmatched design when only a few clusters are randomised. Investigators are rightly concerned that the *credibility* or *face validity* of the trial may be compromised by such imbalances.

Unfortunately, while pairing is likely to improve balance, we have seen in Section 5.3 that it may sometimes reduce the power and precision of a study because of the loss of degrees of freedom associated with a matched analysis. Table 5.4 shows that this is a particular problem with trials with few clusters, and a paired design is only superior to an unmatched design for such trials if the matching is highly effective, resulting in high correlation of outcomes within matched pairs. In practice, it is often difficult to achieve matching that is highly effective, either because data are not available in advance on factors that are highly correlated with the endpoints of interest, or because the closeness of matching on those factors is inadequate. Furthermore, it is often difficult to predict in advance how effective the matching is likely to be, since we often do not have reliable data on the correlation between the matching factors and the endpoints.

By contrast, stratification loses fewer degrees of freedom, and is superior to the unmatched design even for weak matching correlations when there are more than around five clusters per arm. We therefore suggest that a stratified design is likely to be the method of choice for such trials, providing there are potential matching factors that are likely to show some correlation with the endpoint of interest. While stratification is less likely than pairing to achieve close balance between the treatment arms, we shall see in Chapter 6 that there are more effective ways of ensuring balance, based on *restricted randomisation*.

Some investigators have suggested that, for small numbers of clusters, a matched design accompanied by an unmatched analysis may be the optimal choice when the matching correlation is not strong. This method is known as *breaking the matching*, and helps to achieve balance while avoiding the loss of degrees of freedom in the analysis. However, as we have argued above, balance on a range of factors can be achieved more effectively by restricted randomisation, and study power and precision are likely to be maximised by the use of stratification. A further disadvantage of breaking the matching is that the investigator needs to specify *in advance* that an unmatched analysis will be conducted. This will result in loss of power if it turns out that the matching was highly effective. The alternative of choosing an unmatched *or* matched analysis depending on the matching correlation *observed* in the trial has been shown to increase the type 1 error above the nominal level (Diehr et al. 1995).

How many strata should be used? If there are only a few clusters, and too many strata are defined, we will again lose too many degrees of freedom with a consequent loss of study power. As a rough guideline, we suggest no more than two strata if there are six or fewer clusters per arm, and no more than three strata if there are seven to ten clusters per arm.

5.6.3 Trials with a Larger Number of Clusters

In trials with larger numbers of clusters in each treatment arm, randomisation is usually likely to achieve acceptable balance between arms even with an unmatched study design. This situation is similar to a conventional clinical trial, in which randomisation of a large number of individuals to two or more treatment arms can usually be relied upon to ensure balance on both known and unknown confounding factors.

However, matching or stratification may still be of considerable value in CRTs with a large number of clusters to increase their power and precision. They do this by reducing between-cluster variability, since clusters in the same matched pair or stratum are likely to be more similar than those in different pairs or strata. We have seen in Section 5.3 that as the number of clusters increases, the loss of degrees of freedom through use of matching or stratification has very little effect. Either of these approaches can therefore be an effective design strategy for such trials.

In most practical situations, it is likely that stratification (with, say, three of four strata) will capture most of the additional power provided by matching unless there are matching factors that are very closely related to the endpoints of interest. Given the disadvantages associated with the paired design, we suggest that stratification is likely to be the preferred design choice for these trials, as well as for trials with few clusters.

6

Randomisation Procedures

6.1 Introduction

Random allocation of experimental units to the different treatments under study is the defining feature of the randomised controlled trial. The rationale for randomisation in individually randomised trials has been widely discussed. The main reasons for adopting randomisation include the following:

- Impartiality: Random allocation provides assurance to the investigators and to the scientific community that the treatments have been allocated fairly and impartially. If non-random methods are used, it is difficult to avoid the suspicion that the investigators may have been biased, either consciously or unconsciously, in their allocation of units to treatment arms, probably in a direction that would favour the intervention under study.

- Transparency: Random allocation provides a convenient method of allocating treatments that is transparent, objective and easily described. The method could in principle be replicated by other investigators, and this is an important principle of medical experimentation.

- Balance: As noted in Chapter 5, random allocation ensures, if the sample size is large, that the treatment arms are similar with respect to all factors other than the treatment under study. In other words, they are balanced on potential confounding factors, both known and unknown. This helps to ensure the credibility or *face validity* of trial results and may also improve precision.

- Blinding: Use of a random allocation scheme that is concealed from participants or study personnel may reduce their ability to guess which participants have received which treatment condition and thus help to ensure blinding.

- Inference: The use of randomisation can provide a formal justification for the use of statistical inference to make probability statements about study hypotheses or confidence statements about parameter values. This applies particularly to the permutation test and related statistical methods. Model-based approaches to analysis do not formally rely upon randomisation, however.

All of these reasons apply also to CRTs. We have seen in Chapter 5, however, that many CRTs include a relatively small number of clusters, and this means that adequate balance may not be achieved by the use of simple *unrestricted randomisation*. This is one of the main reasons for considering the use of matched or stratified study designs. These represent special types of *restricted randomisation*, and in Section 6.2 we consider in more detail how restricted randomisation may be used in CRTs to improve balance.

In Section 6.3, we go on to discuss a number of practical issues in randomisation, including the generation and concealment of random treatment allocations, and describe approaches that have been used to involve the study communities in the randomisation process.

6.2 Restricted Randomisation

6.2.1 Basic Principles

Consider a CRT in which a total of $2c$ clusters are to be randomly allocated to two treatments A and B, with c clusters allocated to each treatment arm. The number of possible ways of choosing c of the clusters to be allocated to arm A is:

$$\text{Number of allocations} = {}^{2c}C_c = \frac{(2c)!}{c!c!}$$

Unrestricted randomisation involves randomly selecting one of these ${}^{2c}C_c$ allocations. For example, if 12 clusters are to be allocated to two treatment arms using unrestricted randomisation, there are ${}^{12}C_6 = 924$ possible allocations, and one of these is randomly selected when the trial is carried out. The same result is achieved by randomly choosing six clusters from the 12, without replacement. For example, balls numbered 1–12 could be put in a bag, and six of them drawn out without replacement to determine which clusters are to be allocated to treatment arm A.

Matched and stratified designs are examples of *restricted randomisation* since these schemes involve selecting randomly from a smaller set of allocations fulfilling certain restrictions. In the case of the matched-pairs design, we first divide the 12 clusters into six pairs which are matched on specified characteristics. Within each pair, we then randomly select one of the two clusters to be allocated to arm A. There are two possible allocations in each pair, and so the total number of possible allocations is:

$$\text{Number of allocations} = 2^c$$

In our example, there are $2^6 = 64$ possible allocations, and these are a subset of the 924 allocations possible under unrestricted randomisation.

Stratified designs impose fewer constraints, so that allocations are chosen from a larger subset of the total number possible under unrestricted randomisation. In our example, suppose that the 12 clusters are grouped into two strata, each containing six clusters. If we require an equal number of clusters in arms A and B within each stratum, the number of possible allocations is given by:

$$\text{Number of allocations} = (^6C_3)^2 = 20^2 = 400$$

While matching and stratification may help to reduce imbalances between the treatment arms, these designs can often not be relied upon to achieve adequate balance, particularly where there are several variables on which balance is required. Suppose, for example, that we have identified five important variables on which we would like our treatment arms to be balanced. These variables might be known risk factors for the disease outcome of interest. To use the matched-pairs design to achieve balance in this case, we would need to identify pairs of clusters that are well-matched on all five of these variables. In many cases, this will not be feasible. Stratified designs may also be impractical in this situation. Even if we were willing to dichotomise each of the five variables into "low" and "high" categories, we would potentially need to define $2^5 = 32$ strata, and this is an excessive number of strata unless there are a very large number of clusters.

Fortunately, there is an alternative approach to achieving overall balance between the treatment arms, which does not require us to identify subgroups of clusters that are matched on all of the balancing variables. This approach to restricted randomisation is described in the next section.

6.2.2 Using Restricted Randomisation to Achieve Overall Balance

We have previously noted the greater difficulty in achieving balance between the treatment arms in a CRT than in individually randomised trials, resulting from the relatively small number of experimental units that are randomised. Not surprisingly, therefore, the first table in most published reports of CRTs is often devoted to displaying baseline results on key variables across the various treatment arms. In this table, the investigators aim to convince readers that a reasonable degree of balance was achieved. Note that this assessment should be based on quantitative differences between the arms, and not on the results of significance tests, which are irrelevant if random allocation has been used (see Chapter 15).

Usually, most investigators and readers will feel reassured about the balance achieved in a trial if they can see that each of the variables is similarly distributed across treatment arms; for example, if the mean of each quantitative variable or the prevalence of each binary variable takes similar values in each arm. This is referred to as *overall balance*, since it does not require that there is balance within particular subgroups (e.g., the strata in a stratified design), nor that the *joint distributions* of variables show balance.

A combination of stratification and restriction for overall balance can be employed. The stratification can improve efficiency by allowing comparisons to be made within relatively homogeneous strata, while additional restriction criteria can be used to ensure overall balance. Consider the example of a pair-matched CRT in Kenya to measure the effect of an HIV preventive intervention. Beyond the pairing, further restriction of the randomisation was proposed to ensure that in exactly half the pairs, the intervention community would have a higher predicted HIV risk than its matched control community, and *vice versa* for the other pairs.

Restricted randomisation can be used to *ensure* an acceptable level of overall balance, using baseline or pre-existing data on each cluster. This is done by restricting to allocations that satisfy certain pre-determined criteria. One allocation is then selected randomly from this restricted subset. For CRTs with limited numbers of clusters, we recommend, in general, highly restricting the randomisation through constraints aimed at achieving balance on relevant cluster-level or individual-level covariates (Moulton 2004; Raab and Butcher 2001). This approach is similar to those that have been employed in a sequential manner in clinical trials, including minimisation, dynamic randomisation and adaptive assignment (Berry and Eick 1995; Pocock and Simon 1975; Signorini et al. 1993). The randomisation for most CRTs, however, occurs simultaneously for all clusters, and thus the constraints would be employed at the start of the trial to ensure balance before any intervention occurs.

The process is best illustrated by an example, which is based on an unmatched CRT.

Example 6.1

The Baltimore Drug Intervention Study planned to assess the impact of an intervention involving family and community network mobilisation on drug dependence. The primary outcome measure was to be the incidence rate of admission to treatment facilities for drug dependence. From all Baltimore City census tracts, 20 had been selected as being of particular concern. Census data were available on the following relevant covariates for each tract: total population, family income, % vacant houses, % males employed, % high school education, % receiving Public Assistance, % 15–64 years of age, and % African-American.

Using unrestricted randomisation, there are a total of $^{20}C_{10} = 184{,}756$ ways of allocating the 20 tracts to the two treatment arms, 10 to each arm. Restricted randomisation was used in this trial to ensure adequate balance on the covariates available from the census and on two additional criteria. The initial balance constraints considered were:

- Perfect balance on geographical areas that had received prior city-level special attention (10 tracts in all) or not; only allocations with five tracts of each type allocated to each arm were considered.
- Balance to within 10% on the eight census data covariates. Specifically, for each covariate, if the mean covariate value over intervention tracts divided by the mean for the control tracts was greater than 1.1 or less than 1/1.1, that allocation was excluded from consideration.
- Approximate geographical balance. The city was divided into quadrants, each containing five of the 20 study tracts. Allocations were only included if each quadrant had at least two intervention and two control tracts, corresponding to a 2:3 or 3:2 split between the arms.

A computer program was used to assess each of the 184,756 allocations against these criteria. Only 46 allocations met all the criteria. For reasons that will be discussed in Section 6.2.4, this scheme was judged to be too restrictive. The balance criteria were therefore relaxed slightly resulting in 148 allowable allocations, and one of these was randomly selected.

Note that having thus restricted the randomisation, the investigators can be completely confident that the defined balance criteria will be achieved, whichever allocation is selected. Indeed, since the criteria usually give *upper bounds* on the imbalance that will be tolerated, the actual balance on most variables will generally be *closer* than required by these bounds.

Restricted randomisation is an important method of achieving adequate balance in CRTs, particularly those with a small number of clusters. Turning back to the other reasons for use of randomisation, outlined in Section 6.1, we note that restricted randomisation still ensures *impartiality* of allocation. For most balance criteria, each allowable allocation has a mirror-image allocation in which the intervention clusters become control clusters and *vice-versa*. Since chance decides which of these is selected, impartiality is clearly achieved.

In terms of *transparency*, restricted randomisation clearly requires a more detailed explanation in the *Methods* section of reports and papers than simple unrestricted randomisation. If the procedure is not explained carefully, there is the risk that observers may suspect the investigators of manipulating the scheme to favour the results they would like to see. However, providing the balance criteria are clearly stated, it is an objective procedure that could potentially be replicated by an independent investigator, although only if provided with the covariate information required to test the criteria.

Where restricted randomisation is used as described above to achieve overall balance, this aspect of the design is generally ignored in the *analysis*. We return to this point in Section 6.2.4. This contrasts with designs employing matching and stratification, which are most often analysed using methods that take account of the matched study design in order to reduce the variance of the effect estimate.

6.2.3 Balance Criteria

Having decided to use restricted randomisation for a particular trial, we have to decide on the balance criteria that will be used. There are three general types of criteria that we may choose to include:

- Balance on covariates: Demonstrating that the treatment arms are similar with respect to important risk factors for the outcome of interest is clearly the most critical objective here, since any imbalance on such factors could lead to serious bias in estimates of intervention effects. To enhance *face validity*, however, investigators may also wish to ensure similarity on general social and demographic variables, even where these are not thought to be closely related to the outcome. Data on covariates may come from a baseline survey carried out by the investigators, from previous studies in the same clusters, or from other sources including routine or administrative data. If we rely on prior data (e.g., because baseline data from the trial will not be available in time for the randomisation) we need to recognise that, because of secular trends or random error, the baseline data are unlikely to show such close balance as required for the restricted randomisation.

- Balance on sample size: The precision and power of a study are usually maximised when sample sizes are similar in the treatment arms under comparison. In the case of CRTs, this means that both the number of *clusters* as well as the number of *individuals* should be similar across arms, since precision is influenced by variation at both levels. Note that this discussion refers to sample sizes of those surveyed to measure the impact of the intervention. The total population size of the cluster (of which the trial sample may be a subgroup) may be a further factor requiring balance, since this might be a risk factor for the outcome of interest or influence the effect of the intervention. In this sense, however, cluster size would be regarded as a covariate as discussed above.

- Balance for political or logistical reasons: Achieving a design that is acceptable to stakeholders, such as local political leaders or study participants, may be just as important for the success of a trial as the statistical considerations discussed above. This may imply additional criteria, requiring for example that each political unit in a study area receives a "fair share" of the intervention. Logistical factors may also be important. For example, each field team may cover a number of geographically neighbouring clusters. If these teams also have responsibilities for implementing or monitoring the intervention, or carrying out process evaluation, it may be important to ensure that workloads are equalised by arranging an even distribution of intervention clusters between field teams.

Having decided which variables we wish to balance, we need to construct a description of the balance criteria that need to be satisfied.

For quantitative covariates, we may specify a given upper bound on the difference in *means* across treatment arms. This upper bound may be chosen by reference to biological knowledge about the effects of covariates, in order to define limits within which an informed reader would consider that reasonable balance had been achieved. Alternatively, we could use a consistent rule for each covariate, for example requiring that the difference in means is no more than a quarter standard deviation of the variable among individuals in the population.

Similarly for dichotomous variables, we might specify upper bounds on differences in *proportions* across treatment arms. Again, we might consider applying a consistent rule across covariates, for example by requiring a difference between arms of no more than 10% in relative terms in the proportions of interest.

When there is variation in cluster size, then balancing a variable using the mean of all individuals who fall in a given study arm will not be the same thing as balancing the means of cluster-level summaries of the variables. When the analysis is one that mainly reflects population size weighting, such as Generalised Estimating Equations with adjustment for within-cluster correlation (see Chapter 11), then balance on individual-based means will be best. If, however, we plan to use the *t-test* applied to cluster-level summaries, then balancing on the means of these cluster summaries would be most appropriate. Unless there is substantial variability in cluster size and substantial between-cluster variation in the covariate of interest, the two approaches will usually give similar results.

Assuming that equal numbers of clusters are to be allocated to each treatment arm, balance on sample size is achieved by ensuring that the total sample size (overall number of individuals) allocated to each arm falls within defined limits.

Exact balance in terms of distribution across political or geographical units may not be possible. For example, if there are two treatment arms and some political units containing an odd number of clusters, an equal distribution is clearly impossible. The balance criteria will need to define an acceptable level of balance in such cases, as in Example 6.1 above. In that example, not only were there criteria that were to be balanced across all clusters in a study arm, but also one that had to be satisfied within each of four geographical strata.

Having defined a proposed list of balance criteria, a computer program can be used to test each possible allocation against these criteria, and to determine how many allocations are acceptable. If this number is too small, or renders impossible some configurations that would best be allowed, the balance criteria may need to be relaxed in order for the restricted randomisation to have greater validity of statistical inference. This point is discussed further in Section 6.2.4.

Commonly, an iterative approach is adopted:

- List the variables on which balance is required.
- Define a list of proposed balance criteria for these variables.
- Enumerate the allocations that fulfil these proposed criteria.

- If this number is too small, or important configurations are excluded, try relaxing at least some of the criteria and re-enumerate the acceptable allocations.
- If the number of acceptable allocations is very large, consideration could be given to tightening up the balance criteria.

As an example of important configurations, we would not in general want a scheme that always included a given pair of units in the same treatment arm, as this would mean that they are effectively randomised as one unit.

We give two practical examples of CRTs which have employed forms of restricted randomisation.

Example 6.2

We return to the trial of an adolescent sexual health intervention carried out in Tanzania, previously discussed in Example 5.5 and shown in Figure 4.4 (Hayes et al. 2005). In brief, 20 rural study communities were grouped into three strata based on their expected risk of HIV infection. There were six communities in the low-risk stratum, eight in the medium-risk stratum and six in the high-risk stratum.

Ten communities were to be allocated to each treatment arm. The total number of ways of allocating 20 communities to two arms, with ten communities per arm, in an unmatched design is given by:

Number of allocations using unrestricted randomisation $= {}^{20}C_{10} = 184{,}756$

This number is reduced in the stratified design to:

Number of allocations for stratified design $= {}^{6}C_3 \times {}^{8}C_4 \times {}^{6}C_3 = 20 \times 70 \times 20 = 28{,}000$

Note that these 28,000 allocations are a subset of the total of 184,756 possible allocations, satisfying the additional constraint that *exactly half* of the communities in each stratum are allocated to the intervention arm. Under unrestricted randomisation, some allocations would put *all* the communities in a stratum into the same treatment arm.

In the trial in Mwanza, further restrictions were applied to the stratified allocation as follows:

- Mean HIV prevalence in each treatment arm within 0.075% of overall mean.
- Mean prevalence of *Chlamydia trachomatis* (CT) infection in each treatment arm within 0.1% of overall mean.
- Two of the 20 communities were close to gold mines, and one of these was to be allocated to each treatment arm.
- Even distribution of intervention communities over the four administrative districts in which the trial was carried out.

HIV and CT prevalence were based on an initial survey of young people carried out in each of the study communities. Prevalences of HIV and CT (another sexually transmitted infection) were both assumed to be correlated with patterns of risk behaviour among young people in the study communities, and therefore to be predictors of the risk of acquiring HIV infection. The bounds defined above were derived through an iterative process in which different bounds were tried and the numbers of acceptable allocations examined.

The third balance criterion was chosen because gold mines are often associated with high prevalences of HIV and other sexually transmitted infections, because the large populations of well-paid migrant mine-workers attract high rates of commercial and transactional sex. Had both communities been allocated to the same treatment arm, this may therefore have undermined the credibility of the trial.

Finally, the support of district and village leaders was critical to the success of the trial. Ensuring an even distribution of the intervention communities between districts helped to convince these stakeholders that any benefits of the intervention were shared fairly.

Of the 28,000 possible allocations under the stratified design, 953 were found to satisfy the balance criteria. One of these was randomly chosen at a public randomisation ceremony.

Example 6.3

A somewhat different approach to restricted randomisation was used in a CRT of a similar school-based sexual health intervention in the U.K., known as the SHARE trial, previously discussed in Example 1.2 and Example 4.6 (Raab and Butcher 2001; Wight et al. 2002). In this trial, 25 secondary schools in South-East Scotland were to be randomly allocated to the intervention and control arms.

As in the previous example, the schools were first grouped into strata based on location and local government areas. There were five strata, containing eight, two, two, four and nine schools, and it was decided to (approximately) balance the allocation within these strata by assigning the treatments in the ratios 4:4, 1:1, 1:1, 2:2 and 4:5, respectively. Only four of the schools had more than 4% of pupils of Asian ethnicity, and the randomisation was restricted to allocations that assigned two of these schools to each treatment arm. A further constraint was that the total numbers of pupils available for the trial cohort should not differ by more than 200 between arms.

In addition, overall balance was sought on 12 other factors:

- Number of pupils estimated to be in schools and eligible for enrollment in SHARE
- Proportion of placing requests into school
- Proportion of pupils eligible for free school meals
- Proportion of Year 4 pupils staying on to Year 5
- Proportion of Year 5 pupils staying on to Year 6
- School attendance rate
- Proportion of school leavers not in employment
- Unemployment rate in school catchment area
- Deprivation score for catchment area
- Quality of sex education prior to trial
- Accessibility of family planning clinic to school pupils
- School ethos

Data were available prior to the trial for each of these factors, based on local authority or national government data, census data or information collected by the researchers from clinics or professionals. Rather than define a separate balance criterion for each factor, the researchers defined a balance score:

$$B = \sum_l w_l (\bar{z}_{l1} - \bar{z}_{l0})^2$$

where $\bar{z}_{l1}$ and $\bar{z}_{l0}$ are the means of the school-level values of variable z_l in the intervention and control arms, respectively, and the w_l are weights ($l = 1,\ldots, 12$). In the SHARE trial, the researchers used weights that were the reciprocals of the variances of the 25 school-level values. This is equivalent to standardising the variables so that they each have unit variance across the schools.

In this particular trial, the distribution of the values of balance score B over possible allocations was examined and an allocation with a low value of B was chosen. One possible approach to selection is to restrict to allocations with B less than a defined cut-off value and then to randomly choose one allocation from this restricted subset.

Note that this example illustrates a trial in which balance was sought on covariates and sample size as well as distribution among administrative areas.

6.2.4 Validity of Restricted Randomisation

When we use a restricted randomisation scheme in place of simple unrestricted randomisation, we run the risk of producing a design that is either *biased* or not *valid* (Moulton 2004). This would result in standard methods of statistical inference giving incorrect results. This risk is particularly high when strong constraints are imposed and the number of acceptable allocations is small.

A design is *biased* if there is any difference across the clusters in their probability of allocation to any given treatment. Such designs could result in *biased estimates* of intervention effect. This would occur if clusters with a higher probability of allocation to a specific treatment arm differed from other clusters in their intrinsic risk of the outcome of interest.

Biased designs do not often occur in practice, but we provide a simple example. Suppose there is a constraint to be satisfied within each stratum of a CRT with a 2:1 intervention:control allocation and strata consisting of three clusters each. In a given stratum, the cluster means of a constraining variable are 2, 8, and 8, and a balancing criterion is that within each stratum, the difference between the cluster-level means of this variable is to be no more than 4. That would require that the cluster with value 2 must be allocated to the same arm as one of the clusters with value 8; for if the cluster with value 2 were the control, then the difference would be $(8+8)/2 - 2 = 6$. In this example, the cluster with value 2 has a 100% chance of allocation to the intervention arm, while each of the other two has only a 50% chance. Clearly, if the cluster with value 2 also differs with respect to other characteristics that affect the endpoints of interest, then we are biasing the study outcome.

Note that bias cannot occur in trials in which we use *symmetric* balance criteria (see Section 6.2.2), for then a final step of the randomisation can be to assign the specific treatments to the arbitrarily labelled treatment arms. In a two-arm trial, for example, this means that every cluster has a 50% chance of receiving each treatment, and the design is therefore unbiased. For this reason, we recommend that symmetric balance criteria are used wherever possible.

More problematic is the *validity* of a design. A completely randomised design is said to be *valid* if every *pair* of clusters has the same probability of being allocated to the same treatment. Failure to satisfy this condition may result in *correlations* between the clusters in each treatment arm. Estimated variances, used to carry out significance tests and derive confidence intervals, are generally based on the assumption of *independence* between the clusters in each arm. An invalid design may therefore result in tests with incorrect Type I error, and confidence intervals with incorrect coverage (Bailey 1983, 1987).

When using restricted randomisation, researchers therefore need to assess the validity of the chosen randomisation scheme. At a minimum, this should involve checking the number of acceptable allocations. If the number of *unrestricted* allocations is large, but the number after restriction is very small (say less than 100), it is quite likely that there will be serious departures from the conditions for validity. If this is the case, we recommend relaxing the balance criteria so as to obtain a larger number of acceptable allocations, since this is likely (although not guaranteed) to result in a more uniform distribution of joint allocation probabilities.

Note that, except for very simple constraints as with randomised block designs, it will not in general be possible to achieve a perfectly valid design. Simulations have indicated, however, that it takes substantial intracluster correlation coupled with a large departure from validity to appreciably affect the Type I error (Moulton 2004).

To investigate the validity of a design more thoroughly, it is necessary to carry out a check on how many times each pair of clusters are assigned together to the same treatment arm. If a computer program is used to obtain a list of acceptable allocations, this can be adapted to also keep a count of this number for each pair of clusters. In a two-arm trial, the results can be stored in the lower triangle of a $2c \times 2c$ matrix, where c is the number of clusters allocated to each treatment arm.

Suppose n is the number of acceptable allocations under the chosen restricted randomisation scheme. Then, for a perfectly valid design, each pair of clusters should occur together in $n/2$ of these allocations. In practice, moderate deviations from this are unlikely to have serious implications for validity, but extreme deviations may have. We suggest a good starting point is to look for pairs that *never* occur together or *always* occur together. Investigation of these pairs of clusters usually identifies specific balance criteria that are responsible for this. Relaxing these criteria may solve the problem.

Note that if restricted randomisation is applied within a matched or stratified design, as in Example 6.2 and Example 6.3, the results of the validity check may identify pairs of clusters that do not satisfy the above validity check, because of constraints that are intrinsic to the matched design. For example, in a pair-matched trial, the clusters in a matched pair must *always* be allocated to different treatment arms. This will not lead to incorrect statistical inference, provided an appropriate method of analysis is used (see Chapter 12). In this case, we would be assessing validity for all pairs of clusters that are *not* in the same matched pair. Furthermore, some balance criteria *deliberately* impose constraints which mean that some pairs of clusters cannot be allocated to the same arm, as we have seen in the examples in this chapter.

The above discussion assumes that standard methods of statistical analysis will be used. These methods will be discussed in later chapters. An alternative is to use methods that specifically *take account* of the randomisation scheme. These methods of *randomisation-based inference* have the advantage that they should provide tests of correct size even though the design does not satisfy the requirements for *validity*. Disadvantages are that standard statistical software cannot generally be used for this (unless the design is very simple), and that deriving confidence intervals using this approach to inference is computationally complex. A simple application of randomisation-based inference is discussed in Section 10.5.3.

Example 6.4

We return to the example based on the Baltimore Drug Intervention Study, first discussed in Example 6.1. In that trial, 46 of the 184,756 possible allocations of the 20 study clusters satisfied the initial set of balance criteria. A 20×20 matrix (Table 6.1a) was constructed to display the number of times (out of 46) that each pair of clusters was allocated to the same treatment arm. For a perfectly valid design, this should approximate to 23 for all pairs.

The researchers examined which pairs of units *always* appeared together or *never* appeared together in the same arm. This revealed four pairs which were *never* allocated to the same arm: (1,17), (1,12), (12,14) and (14,17). Inspection of the census tract data revealed that clusters 1 and 12 had the highest percentages of vacant houses, while units 14 and 17 had the highest percentages receiving Public Assistance. It was therefore difficult for these pairs to be allocated to the same treatment arm without violating the balance criteria.

Given these data configurations, it was decided to relax the balance criteria for these two covariates, to allow $\pm 25\%$ imbalance between treatment arm means rather than the standard $\pm 10\%$ criterion adopted for the other covariates. With the adjusted criteria, there were now 148 acceptable allocations (Table 6.1b), which included 22 in which the pair (1,17) were in the same arm, 22 for (1,12), six for (12,14) and 10 for (14,17). Clearly this is not optimal, but was considered to provide sufficient opportunities for these pairs to occur together given the desire to avoid substantial imbalance on the relevant covariates.

If the outcomes in clusters that are assigned "too often" to the same treatment arm are positively correlated, there will be a slight inflation of Type I error. Conversely, if outcomes in clusters that are assigned "too often" to opposite arms are positively correlated, then the Type I error will fall slightly below its nominal value. For this reason, the former circumstance may be regarded as a more serious problem than the latter.

TABLE 6.1

Matrices Showing Number of Acceptable Allocations for Which Each Pair of Census Tracts Was Allocated to the Same Treatment Arm

(a) Matrix for 46 Allocations with all Variables Restricted to ±10% between Arms

	1	2	3	4	5	6	7	8	9	10	11	12	13	14	15	16	17	18	19	20
1	23																			
2	7	23																		
3	1	15	23																	
4	17	9	7	23																
5	7	11	15	9	23															
6	5	13	17	7	15	23														
7	17	9	7	11	5	9	23													
8	14	14	10	12	6	4	14	23												
9	9	15	15	9	11	9	13	18	23											
10	21	7	3	15	9	7	19	12	11	23										
11	14	10	8	12	16	8	8	11	6	12	23									
12	0	16	22	6	16	18	6	9	14	2	9	23								
13	14	12	10	14	4	10	16	13	14	12	5	9	23							
14	23	7	1	17	7	5	17	14	9	21	14	0	14	23						
15	11	9	11	13	13	17	9	4	5	9	12	12	14	11	23					
16	5	13	17	9	13	13	9	12	11	7	12	18	6	5	7	23				
17	0	16	22	6	16	18	6	9	14	2	9	23	9	0	12	18	23			
18	7	13	15	7	13	13	5	10	9	5	12	16	10	7	13	15	16	23		
19	20	6	4	14	8	6	14	15	12	18	13	3	13	20	10	6	3	10	23	
20	15	5	7	13	13	13	13	6	3	15	16	8	8	15	15	11	8	11	12	23

(continued)

TABLE 6.1 (*Continued*)

(b) Matrix for 148 Allocations with Restrictions for Two Variables Relaxed to ±25%, the Rest Remaining at ±10% between Arms

	1	2	3	4	5	6	7	8	9	10	11	12	13	14	15	16	17	18	19	20
1	74																			
2	29	74																		
3	21	36	74																	
4	43	34	24	74																
5	27	34	38	32	74															
6	24	41	47	27	39	74														
7	39	32	32	32	24	31	74													
8	46	43	39	35	25	12	39	74												
9	34	45	43	33	39	22	39	56	74											
10	63	28	24	40	30	29	44	39	41	74										
11	44	33	25	41	41	26	35	40	26	37	74									
12	11	46	60	20	50	55	24	31	41	16	21	74								
13	41	32	30	48	24	33	50	33	39	34	29	24	74							
14	60	29	17	51	23	22	47	44	32	59	52	3	47	74						
15	35	32	32	42	40	57	32	13	13	28	39	38	46	37	74					
16	27	42	44	30	32	41	34	43	37	30	37	52	20	23	24	74				
17	11	44	58	22	48	53	24	33	39	18	23	72	22	5	38	52	74			
18	30	37	43	27	47	36	25	34	30	23	28	49	37	24	39	37	47	74		
19	44	25	27	45	27	28	39	40	44	45	46	21	43	50	33	29	23	30	74	
20	37	24	26	40	46	43	44	21	13	38	43	32	34	41	48	32	34	43	27	74

6.2.5 Restricted Randomisation with More than Two Treatment Arms

Our examples have focused on trials with two treatment arms, but the same principles can be extended to trials with more than two arms.

Simple balance criteria, based on differences between means over the clusters in each arm, can be extended to impose bounds on the maximum difference between any two arms. In other words, constraints are placed on the difference between the treatment arms with the largest and smallest means for each covariate.

The balance score, B, could also be extended to take the form:

$$B = w_1 \sum_i (\bar{z}_{1i} - \bar{z}_{1\bullet})^2 + w_2 \sum_i (\bar{z}_{2i} - \bar{z}_{2\bullet})^2 + \cdots + w_L \sum_i (\bar{z}_{Li} - \bar{z}_{L\bullet})^2$$

where $\bar{z}_{li}$ is the mean of covariate z_l over all the study clusters in treatment arm i, and $\bar{z}_{l\bullet}$ is the mean over all the clusters ($l = 1, \ldots, L$).

6.3 Some Practical Aspects of Randomisation

6.3.1 Concealment of Allocation

In individually randomised clinical trials, it is a well-established principle that the allocation of subjects to treatment arms should in general be *concealed* until the point at which they have been enrolled to the trial. The research has shown that substantial bias is associated with inadequate concealment of allocation.

The same principle applies to CRTs. Advance knowledge of the treatment arm to which a potential cluster would be allocated may consciously or unconsciously influence the decision of the researcher or cluster representatives as to whether the cluster should be included in the trial. This may therefore result in bias.

Procedures for obtaining consent for clusters to take part in CRTs are discussed in Chapter 13. Whatever procedures are used, the aim should be to seek agreement that the cluster can be enrolled in the trial on the basis that treatments will be randomly allocated.

6.3.2 Public Randomisation

In Section 6.1, we noted that two of the advantages of randomisation are *impartiality* and *transparency*. In a conventional clinical trial, in which patients are entered into the study by medical practitioners, it can generally be assumed that these practitioners are familiar enough with the basics of trial design and randomisation that they are able to provide sufficient reassurance to their patients that fair allocation procedures will be used. Providing the protocol gives a clear description of the randomisation procedure, the research team is generally trusted to carry out this function fairly and correctly.

In some CRTs of public health interventions, by contrast, entire communities are randomised to different treatment arms. Community leaders or representatives may have little understanding of trial procedures or the principles of randomisation. Moreover, the randomisation scheme to be used is often more complex than in a conventional trial. It may involve matching or stratification and, as we have seen in this chapter, restricted randomisation may be used to improve balance between the treatment arms. These factors may give rise to suspicion among community leaders that fair procedures have not been used, or to suspicion among the scientific community that the researchers have manipulated the trial to their own ends.

For these reasons, some researchers have invested considerable effort in devising methods of carrying out the randomisation in some form of *public ceremony*. The stakeholders to be invited to such a ceremony might vary according to the context of the trial. For trials of public health interventions, in which entire communities are randomised, they might include local government representatives, community leaders, community representatives, members of the community advisory board and scientific collaborators. For trials in which medical practices, schools or other institutions are randomised, they might include doctors, head-teachers or other professionals with responsibility for the randomisation units.

Public ceremonies have taken different forms. The main aims are generally:

- To explain the background to the trial and why it is being conducted. This will probably have been done previously at the time when the study clusters are being recruited to the trial, but should be repeated at the ceremony.
- To explain the need for random allocation and the procedure to be used for this, including any form of restricted randomisation that will be applied.
- To carry out the randomisation using a transparent procedure, preferably with the involvement of key stakeholders in the randomisation process.

The exact approach used will differ according to the design and context of the trial, but we present a practical example based on one of the most "public" randomisation ceremonies that we are aware of, and which also illustrates some of the other methods discussed in this chapter.

Example 6.5

The Zambia and South Africa TB and AIDS Reduction (ZAMSTAR) trial is being carried out to measure the impact of two intensive TB control strategies on the prevalence of TB in 24 communities in Zambia (16 communities) and South Africa (eight communities) with high prevalences of HIV infection (Ayles et al. 2008; Sismanidis et al. 2008). In brief, these two strategies are:

- Intervention A: Improved case finding (ICF) for TB, including provision of TB diagnostic laboratories with public access and other community-based interventions.
- Intervention B: A package of interventions delivered to households of TB cases, who will be encouraged to provide treatment support to the case and to access other control measures against HIV and TB.

The ZAMSTAR trial will measure the effects of these interventions through a CRT with a 2×2 factorial design (see Chapter 8), with the following four treatment arms:

- Arm 1: ICF intervention only
- Arm 2: Household intervention only
- Arm 3: Both ICF and household interventions
- Arm 4: Neither intervention

The 24 communities were randomly allocated to the four treatment arms by first stratifying and then applying a system of restricted randomisation. Stratification was based on country and tuberculin skin test (TST) rate. TST rates were measured in a sample of schoolchildren in each community, and can be regarded as a measure of tuberculosis transmission rates in the community. The four strata were:

- Stratum 1: Zambian communities with high TST rates (eight communities)
- Stratum 2: Zambian communities with low TST rates (eight communities)
- Stratum 3: South African communities with high TST rates (four communities)
- Stratum 4: South African communities with low TST rates (four communities)

The total number of ways of allocating the communities to Arms 1–4 under this stratified design is given by:

Total number of allocations =

$$\frac{8!}{2! \times 2! \times 2! \times 2!} \times \frac{8!}{2! \times 2! \times 2! \times 2!} \times 4! \times 4! = 3{,}657{,}830{,}400$$

The following (symmetric) balance criteria were then applied (these are not set out in detail here):

- Similar number of communities with high estimated HIV prevalence in each arm
- Mean TST rate across communities similar in each arm
- Similar number of "open" communities (characterised by social science appraisal methods as having greater social diversity) in each arm
- Similar number of urban communities in each arm
- Political constraints to ensure an even distribution of the interventions across administrative districts

Checking all 3,657,830,400 allocations for these criteria would have been computationally very intensive. Instead, allocations were randomly selected and tested using a computer program until 1000 unique allocations were obtained meeting the balance criteria. By *unique* allocations, we mean 1000 different ways of dividing the 24 communities into four groups of six, irrespective of which treatment was to be assigned to each group. This therefore represented a total of 24,000 distinct treatment allocations (where $24 = 4!$). A computer-generated list was prepared of the 1000 unique allocations, which were numbered from 000 to 999. Each numbered line on the list showed the communities allocated to the four treatment groups which were arbitrarily labelled A–D.

The public randomisation proceeded in three steps:

Step 1

A limited number of stakeholders were invited to a preliminary meeting at which the objectives of the trial and the randomisation procedures were described in detail.

Step 2

Steps 2 and 3 were carried out in public on a football pitch during the interval of a football tournament in Zambia. A total of 24 volunteers were chosen to represent the communities, and each carried a placard with the name and number of the community (Figure 6.1).

Ten miniature footballs, numbered from 0 to 9, were placed in a sack, and three senior officials were invited to draw one football from the sack at a time, with replacement. This procedure provided a way of randomly selecting a three-digit number between 000 and 999, and identified one line on the numbered list. In the event, the number 773 was chosen.

The 24 volunteers were then asked to divide themselves into four groups labelled A–D, based on line 773 of the computer-generated list.

Step 3

In the final step, a further randomisation was carried out to determine which treatment would be allocated to each of the four groups. From two sacks with four footballs each, one representing the interventions and the other the treatment codes A–D, a single football drawn from the intervention sack was matched with a single football drawn from the code sack, without replacement. This process was carried out four times by different people. The ICF intervention was allocated to group C, the household intervention to group A, both ICF and household interventions to group D, and neither intervention to group B.

This final step was judged to be particularly important in assuring stakeholders of the fairness and transparency of the procedure. Since the stratified design and restricted randomisation constituted a relatively complex procedure, involving the use of computer programs, the observer had to take it on trust that this step had been carried out correctly. However, having divided the communities into four groups, the final step was a simple way of deciding which intervention each group

(a)

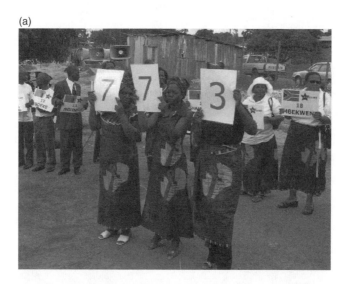

(b)

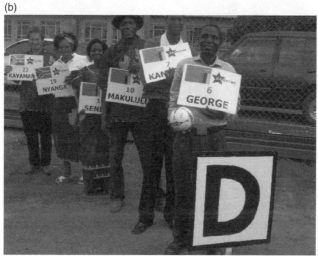

FIGURE 6.1
(a) Public randomisation ceremony in ZAMSTAR trial, showing selection of treatment allocation satisfying pre-defined balance criteria. (b) Public randomisation in the ZAMSTAR trial, showing the six communities (two in South Africa and four in Zambia) assigned to treatment arm D.

would receive. This was easy to understand, was clearly fair and was carried out by community representatives rather than the research team.

Note, however, that a slightly different approach would be needed for trials in which blindness of treatment allocation is to be preserved during the trial, for example where a placebo is used in the control arm.

7

Sample Size

7.1 Introduction

The main aim of most well-conducted randomised trials is to obtain unbiased estimates of treatment effects that are sufficiently precise to answer the research questions of interest. Eliminating or minimising bias rests on careful trial design and implementation, and relies on standard methods, such as random allocation of treatments, blinded evaluations and maximising follow-up rates. There is little point in minimising bias, however, if random errors are large due to an inadequate sample size.

The importance of adequate sample size, and the consequences of trials that are too small for their purpose, have been widely discussed. Trials that are too small have low power, meaning that there is an unacceptably high probability of obtaining a non-significant result even when an intervention actually has a medically important effect. Even if a significant result is obtained, the confidence interval on the effect estimate is likely to be wide, indicating a failure to quantify the effect accurately. Conversely, the value of a negative result is compromised, since a wide confidence interval means that we are unable to distinguish between an intervention with no effect and one with a substantial beneficial or adverse effect.

These arguments apply with equal cogency to CRTs. Indeed the expense and logistical complexity of such trials places even more responsibility on researchers to ensure that trials are designed with sufficient power to achieve their main objectives. This chapter sets out in detail the methods needed to select an appropriate sample size for a CRT. We begin in Section 7.2 with methods for unmatched studies, and provide formulae for the different types of study outcome, including event rates, proportions and means of quantitative variables. In Section 7.3, we consider extensions of these methods for matched and stratified trials. The formulae presented require estimates of the coefficient of variation, k, and in Section 7.4 we explain how such estimates may be obtained. The formulae given in Section 7.2 assume that the sample size per cluster is given, and that we need to calculate the number of clusters required per treatment arm. Sometimes, we also wish to select an appropriate sample size for each cluster, and this problem is considered in

Section 7.5. Further issues, considered in Section 7.6, include sample size for trials with more than two treatment arms, for trials with treatment arms of unequal size and for *equivalence* or *non-inferiority* trials.

A fundamental principle of CRT design is that sufficient *replication* is required to draw reliable conclusions. In an individually randomised trial of a new drug, we recognise that responses and outcomes are likely to vary between individual patients. Only by randomising a sufficient number of patients are we able to accurately measure the average outcome, and to determine whether this varies between patients in different treatment arms. In a CRT, the cluster takes the place of the individual patient. We recognise that responses and outcomes are likely to vary between clusters. Once again, only by randomising sufficient clusters to the different treatment arms can we obtain sufficiently accurate estimates of average response in each arm, and of differences between arms.

In some CRTs, there may be many thousands of *individuals* within each cluster. A common error in some CRTs in the past has been to assume that, because a large number of *individuals* are studied, the trial is adequately powered even though there may be very few clusters. This is a fallacy. An extreme case of this is a trial in which just two clusters are randomly allocated, one to each treatment arm. Such 1:1 trials have been reported quite frequently. They are equivalent to a clinical trial in which just two patients are randomly allocated to the two treatment arms. Because there is *no replication* at all within each treatment arm, we have no way of measuring and taking account of the degree of between-cluster variation, and so no statistical inference is possible with such a design. It should be clear from this discussion that we need several clusters in each treatment arm to draw any useful conclusions about the effect of an intervention.

A useful rule of thumb is to regard four clusters per arm as an absolute minimum. We shall see later that the *t-test* based on cluster-level responses is generally the preferred method of analysis for CRTs with small numbers of clusters. However, with as few as four clusters per arm, we may not wish to rely on parametric methods such as the *t-test* that require assumptions of normality of cluster-level responses. But the equivalent nonparametric method, the *Wilcoxon rank sum test*, requires a *minimum of four clusters per arm* to yield a statistically significant result. The equivalent test for matched studies, the *signed rank test*, requires a *minimum of six matched pairs*.

7.2 Sample Size for Unmatched Trials

We begin by considering the simplest CRT design with two treatment arms, equal numbers of clusters to be allocated to the two arms, and clusters of equal size. Later we consider more general designs. We present sample size formulae for the three main types of trial endpoint.

Sample size formulae for CRTs can be expressed in terms of either k, the between-cluster coefficient of variation, or ρ, the intracluster correlation coefficient. As we have seen in Section 2.3, these are two alternative measures of variability between clusters. While the approaches are essentially equivalent, we have chosen to present formulae based on the coefficient of variation k. This provides a unified set of methods covering all the main types of study endpoint (Hayes and Bennett 1999). We recall that the intracluster correlation coefficient, ρ, is not defined for person-years event rates. For completeness, however, sample size determination based on ρ is discussed briefly in Section 7.2.5.

7.2.1 Event Rates

We first consider *event rates* with a person-time denominator. These might include mortality rates, incidence rates of a severe disease or incidence rates of seroconversion to an infection. The objective of the trial is to compare the rates in the intervention and control arms.

For an individually randomised trial, a standard formula requires y person-years in each treatment arm, where:

$$y = (z_{\alpha/2} + z_\beta)^2 \frac{(\lambda_0 + \lambda_1)}{(\lambda_0 - \lambda_1)^2} \tag{7.1}$$

In this formula, $z_{\alpha/2}$ and z_β are standard normal distribution values corresponding to upper tail probabilities of $\alpha/2$ and β, respectively. This sample size gives $100(1 - \beta)\%$ power of obtaining a significant difference ($p < \alpha$ on a two-sided test) assuming that the *true* event rates in the presence and absence of the intervention are λ_1 and λ_0, respectively.

In a CRT, suppose now that there are y person-years of follow-up *in each cluster*. Then c, the required number of clusters per arm, is given by:

$$c = 1 + (z_{\alpha/2} + z_\beta)^2 \frac{(\lambda_0 + \lambda_1)/y + (k_0^2 \lambda_0^2 + k_1^2 \lambda_1^2)}{(\lambda_0 - \lambda_1)^2} \tag{7.2}$$

Here, k_0 and k_1 represent the between-cluster coefficients of variation of the *true* rates in the control and intervention arms, respectively.

We recall that the *coefficient of variation, k_0,* of the true event rates in the control clusters is defined as

$$k_0 = \sigma_{B0} / \lambda_0$$

where σ_{B0} is the standard deviation of the true rates among the control clusters. If we can assume that the intervention has a similar proportional effect across clusters (for example, reducing the true event rate by roughly 20% in each cluster), it follows that both σ_{B1} and λ_1 will be reduced by the same fraction, so that the coefficient of variation k_1 will equal the value k_0 in the control arm. In this case, Equation 7.2 simplifies to:

$$c = 1 + (z_{\alpha/2} + z_\beta)^2 \frac{(\lambda_0 + \lambda_1)/y + k^2(\lambda_0^2 + \lambda_1^2)}{(\lambda_0 - \lambda_1)^2} \tag{7.3}$$

where k is the common value of the between-cluster coefficient of variation in the two treatment arms.

As we shall see in Chapter 11, the *t-test* applied to cluster-level summaries is one of the most robust methods of analysing unmatched CRTs. When the number of clusters, and hence the *degrees of freedom* for the *t-test*, are small, the percentage points of the t distribution are appreciably larger than those of the standard normal distribution. The addition of one cluster in Equation 7.2 and Equation 7.3 is made to correct for this. The effect of this correction will be small in trials with a large number of clusters.

Note from Equation 7.2 that if there is no variation in true event rate between clusters in each arm (no "clustering"), then $k_0 = k_1 = 0$ and, ignoring the addition of one cluster, cy from Equation 7.2 reduces to the total y required by Equation 7.1. The increase in sample size needed to allow for the clustered design will depend on the relative size of the second term in the numerator, and this depends on the values of k_0 and k_1. The *design effect* can be estimated by calculating the ratio of cy obtained from Equation 7.2 or Equation 7.3 to y from Equation 7.1.

Example 7.1

We illustrate the calculation of sample size for a CRT of insecticide-treated bed-nets in Kilifi District, Kenya (Nevill et al. 1996). One of the primary objectives of this trial was to measure the impact of these nets on all-cause mortality among young children aged 1–59 months. The proposed study area was divided along administrative boundaries into zones with populations of approximately 1000 individuals of all ages, including about 200 children aged 1–59 months. The intervention was to be randomly allocated to zones, and a demographic surveillance system used to record deaths of young children in each zone occurring during a 2-year follow-up period.

Mortality data were already available for 51 of the study zones for the 2 years prior to the study, and were used to estimate k using methods described in Section 7.4. There were a total of 321 deaths over 21,646 person-years of observation, giving an overall mortality rate in these 51 study zones of:

$$r = 321 / 21,646 = 0.0148$$

or a rate of 14.8 per 1000 person-years. The estimate of k was 0.29, implying that the true cluster rates varied mostly between approximately $14.8 \times (1 \pm 2 \times 0.29)$, or from 6.2 to 23.4 per 1000 person-years.

We can now use Equation 7.3 to determine the number of zones required for the trial. Assuming that the mortality rate in the control arm remains constant at $\lambda_0 = 0.0148$, that the person-years per cluster during the trial is similar to that in the previous 2 years ($y = 21,646/51 = 424$), that the proportional effect of the intervention is roughly constant over clusters so that $k_0 \approx k_1 \approx 0.29$ and that we require 80% power ($z_\beta = 0.84$) of detecting a significant difference ($p < 0.05$, $z_{\alpha/2} = 1.96$) if the intervention reduces mortality by 30% to $\lambda_1 = 0.7 \times 0.0148 = 0.0104$, we obtain:

$$c = 1 + (1.96 + 0.84)^2 \frac{(0.0148 + 0.0104)/424 + 0.29^2(0.0148^2 + 0.0104^2)}{(0.0148 - 0.0104)^2} = 36.2$$

We would therefore select a total of 74 zones, with 37 randomised to each treatment arm, giving a total of $37 \times 424 = 15,688$ person-years per arm.

Note that in the absence of clustering, Equation 7.1 gives:

$$y = (1.96 + 0.84)^2 \frac{0.0148 + 0.0104}{(0.0148 - 0.0104)^2} = 10,205$$

person-years per arm, so that the estimated design effect is $15,688/10,205 = 1.54$.

In practice, trial size is also influenced by logistical factors and cost constraints. In the event, the bednet trial in Kilifi was carried out in a total of 56 zones, with 28 zones in each treatment arm. If the numbers of clusters and person-years are fixed, Equation 7.2 can be rearranged to derive an estimate of z_β, and hence the study power:

$$z_\beta = \sqrt{\frac{(c-1)(\lambda_0 - \lambda_1)^2}{(\lambda_0 + \lambda_1)/y + (k_0^2 \lambda_0^2 + k_1^2 \lambda_1^2)}} - z_{\alpha/2} \tag{7.4}$$

Inserting $c = 28$, $y = 424$, $\lambda_0 = 0.0148$, $\lambda_1 = 0.0104$, $k_0 = k_1 = 0.29$ and $z_{\alpha/2} = 1.96$ in Equation 7.4 we obtain $z_\beta = 0.49$ so that the power was 69%.

7.2.2 Proportions

We now consider sample size calculations for *binary* endpoints, where the objective is to compare the *proportions* of subjects with specified characteristics in the intervention and control arms. Examples would include the *prevalence* of some condition at end of follow-up (e.g., prevalence of smoking at the final survey in a smoking cessation study), or the *cumulative incidence* or *risk* of some outcome during a specified follow-up period (e.g., proportion seroconverting to HIV during a one-year period in an HIV prevention trial).

For an individually randomised trial, a standard formula requires n individuals in each treatment arm, where:

$$n = (z_{\alpha/2} + z_\beta)^2 \frac{\pi_0(1 - \pi_0) + \pi_1(1 - \pi_1)}{(\pi_0 - \pi_1)^2} \tag{7.5}$$

where π_1 and π_0 are the *true* proportions in the presence and absence of the intervention, respectively.

In a CRT, suppose now that m individuals are sampled *in each cluster*. Then c, the required number of clusters per arm, is given by:

$$c = 1 + (z_{\alpha/2} + z_\beta)^2 \frac{\pi_0(1-\pi_0)/m + \pi_1(1-\pi_1)/m + (k_0^2 \, \pi_0^2 + k_1^2 \, \pi_1^2)}{(\pi_0 - \pi_1)^2} \quad (7.6)$$

where k_0 and k_1 are the between-cluster coefficients of variation of the *true* proportions in the control and intervention arms, respectively. If the intervention has a similar proportional effect across clusters (for example, a 20% risk reduction in each cluster), then we can assume (as for event rates) that k_0 and k_1 have a common value k, and Equation 7.6 simplifies to:

$$c = 1 + (z_{\alpha/2} + z_\beta)^2 \frac{\pi_0(1-\pi_0)/m + \pi_1(1-\pi_1)/m + k^2(\pi_0^2 + \pi_1^2)}{(\pi_0 - \pi_1)^2} \quad (7.7)$$

The *design effect* can be estimated by calculating the ratio of cm obtained from Equation 7.6 or Equation 7.7 to n from Equation 7.5.

7.2.3 Means

For a *quantitative* endpoint, the objective is to compare the *mean* of the outcome variable in the intervention and control arms. Examples might include mean serum cholesterol in a trial of a dietary intervention, or mean number of sexual partners in a trial of a behavioural intervention to reduce HIV risk.

For an individually randomised trial, a standard formula requires n individuals in each treatment arm, where:

$$n = (z_{\alpha/2} + z_\beta)^2 \frac{(\sigma_0^2 + \sigma_1^2)}{(\mu_0 - \mu_1)^2} \quad (7.8)$$

where μ_1 and μ_0 are the *true* means, and σ_1 and σ_0 are the standard deviations, of the outcome variable in the presence and absence of the intervention, respectively.

In a CRT, suppose now that m individuals are sampled *in each cluster*. Then c, the required number of clusters per arm, is given by:

$$c = 1 + (z_{\alpha/2} + z_\beta)^2 \frac{(\sigma_{W0}^2 + \sigma_{W1}^2)/m + (k_0^2 \, \mu_0^2 + k_1^2 \, \mu_1^2)}{(\mu_0 - \mu_1)^2} \quad (7.9)$$

where σ_{W1} and σ_{W0} are now *within-cluster* standard deviations, and k_0 and k_1 are the between-cluster coefficients of variation of the *true* means in the control and intervention arms, respectively. If the intervention has a similar proportional effect across clusters (for example, a 10% reduction in mean blood pressure in each cluster), then we can assume that k_0 and k_1 have a common value k, and Equation 7.9 simplifies to:

$$c = 1 + (z_{\alpha/2} + z_{\beta})^2 \frac{(\sigma_{W0}^2 + \sigma_{W1}^2)/m + k^2(\mu_0^2 + \mu_1^2)}{(\mu_0 - \mu_1)^2} \tag{7.10}$$

The *design effect* can be estimated by calculating the ratio of cm obtained from Equation 7.9 or Equation 7.10 to n from Equation 7.8.

7.2.4 Variable Sample Size per Cluster

In the previous sections, we assumed an equal sample size (either number of subjects m, or person-years of observation y) in each cluster. In trials in which a random sample of subjects is selected for study within each cluster, it is usual to select samples of equal size and so the equations given above can be used without modification. This is not the case, however, in trials with clusters of different size and in which all members of each cluster are studied.

If sample sizes per cluster vary, a simple modification can be made to the equations given in Sections 7.2.1 through 7.2.3. In place of the fixed values m or y, we instead use $\bar{m}_H$ or $\bar{y}_H$ which are the *harmonic means* of the sample size in each cluster. Recall that the harmonic mean of m_j ($j = 1, \ldots, c$) is defined as:

$$\bar{m}_H = \frac{1}{\Sigma(1/m_j)/c}$$

In words, we find the (arithmetic) mean of the reciprocal of the sample size per cluster, and then take the reciprocal of this mean to obtain the harmonic mean.

7.2.5 Sample Size Calculations Based on Intracluster Correlation Coefficient

The previous sections have presented sample size formulae for unmatched CRTs based on assumed values of k, the between-cluster coefficient of variation. Alternative formulae are available based on assumed values of ρ, the intracluster correlation coefficient (Donner, Birkett, and Buck 1981; Donner and Klar 2000).

As we have noted previously, the *design effect* of a CRT is related to the intracluster correlation coefficient as follows:

$$DEff = 1 + (m - 1)\rho$$

where m is the number of individuals per cluster and ρ is the intracluster coefficient. Applying this expression to Equation 7.5 and Equation 7.8

we obtain the following formulae for the number of clusters required per treatment arm:

$$c = 1 + (z_{\alpha/2} + z_\beta)^2 \frac{[\pi_0(1-\pi_0) + \pi_1(1-\pi_1)] \times [1 + (m-1)\rho]}{m(\pi_0 - \pi_1)^2} \tag{7.11}$$

and

$$c = 1 + (z_{\alpha/2} + z_\beta)^2 \frac{(\sigma_0^2 + \sigma_1^2) \times [1 + (m-1)\rho]}{m(\mu_0 - \mu_1)^2} \tag{7.12}$$

for proportions and means, respectively. As before, the addition of one extra cluster per treatment arm is to allow for the use of the *t-test*. There is no equivalent formula for event rates because the intracluster correlation coefficient is not defined for person-years data.

Application of these formulae generally provides very similar results to those given by Equation 7.7 and Equation 7.10. In fact they are equivalent except that Equation 7.11 and Equation 7.12 assume that the value of ρ is the same in each treatment arm, whereas Equation 7.7 and Equation 7.10 assume that the value of k is the same in each treatment arm.

Recalling from Equation 2.5 that the relationship between ρ and k is given by:

$$\rho = \frac{k^2 \pi}{1 - \pi}$$

it follows that, in general, if k is constant across treatment arms then ρ will not be, and vice versa. As noted in Section 7.2.2, if the intervention is assumed to have a similar proportional effect on the outcome of interest across clusters (for example, a 20% reduction in the risk of a binary outcome in each cluster), then the value of k will be similar in both arms. There is no corresponding rationale for the assumption of constant ρ across treatment arms.

If we are unwilling to make the assumption of equal ρ across arms, we can instead use separate estimates ρ_1 and ρ_0 in the intervention and control arms, giving:

$$c = 1 + (z_{\alpha/2} + z_\beta)^2 \frac{\pi_0(1-\pi_0)[1 + (m-1)\rho_0] + \pi_1(1-\pi_1)[1 + (m-1)\rho_1]}{m(\pi_0 - \pi_1)^2}$$

and

$$c = 1 + (z_{\alpha/2} + z_\beta)^2 \frac{\sigma_0^2[1 + (m-1)\rho_0] + \sigma_1^2[1 + (m-1)\rho_1]}{m(\mu_0 - \mu_1)^2}$$

It can be shown that these formulae are now exactly equivalent to Equation 7.6 and Equation 7.9 based on separate values of k in the two treatment arms.

One advantage of the above formulae based on ρ is that researchers have published estimated values of the intracluster correlation coefficient for different endpoints and study populations, and these may be useful in guiding investigators when planning new CRTs. For example, Littenberg and MacLean (2006) present ICC estimates for 112 variables based on data from adult diabetes patients in 73 primary care practices in Vermont and surrounding areas in the USA; while Adams et al. (2004) analyse ICCs for 1039 variables based on data from 31 cluster-based studies in primary care settings, predominantly in the UK. Importantly, Adams and colleagues note that ICC estimates for the same endpoints varied considerably between studies.

While published estimates of ρ may be useful in planning a study of the same endpoint in the same study population, we caution against assuming that similar values would apply for different endpoints, or for the same endpoint in different settings. The ICC is a measure of between-cluster variation, and the extent of such variation may differ substantially across different study populations. Turner, Thompson, and Spiegelhalter (2005) show how ICCs from disparate studies may be combined in a Bayesian framework: an informative prior distribution for the ICC in the planned study is derived using subjective weights that give less weight to endpoints and populations deemed to be less relevant.

For binary data, estimated values of ρ may of course be readily converted to estimates of k using Equation 2.5. Regardless of how a value of ρ, k or the design effect is chosen when planning a study, this choice represents an important assumption that should be verified, when feasible, during the conduct of the study as we discuss in Chapter 14.

7.3 Sample Size for Matched and Stratified Trials

7.3.1 Matched Trials

In Chapter 5, we discussed the potential role of a matched design in improving *balance* between the treatment arms and increasing the *power* and *precision* of the study. To briefly summarise our main conclusions, we noted that for CRTs with a small number of clusters, pair-matching should generally be undertaken only if the clusters can be matched on factors that are *closely correlated* with the primary outcome of interest. We also provided a table showing *break-even* values of the *matching correlation* (the correlation in the cluster-level outcome of interest between the clusters in each matched pair) above which pair-matching will provide greater power and precision than an unmatched trial.

While these considerations are useful for a general discussion of design options, they are of limited value in the calculation of sample size for a specific matched trial. This is because prior estimation of the matching correlation is quite difficult in practice, for several reasons:

- We do not match clusters directly on the outcomes of interest, but on *proxy* variables for those outcomes, the so-called *matching factors*. It is difficult to know, at the start of the study, how closely correlated the matching factors and outcomes will be.

- Even if we match directly on baseline values of the primary endpoint variable in each cluster, correlations at follow-up may be different from those at baseline, both because of random sampling error (each cluster value is based on a finite sample) and because of underlying secular changes which may differ between clusters in ways that are difficult to predict.

- The matching correlation coefficient *r*, as presented in Chapter 5, is based on *observed* (rather than *true*) values of the endpoint in each cluster. These observed values will be subject to random error that will depend on the sample size *within* each cluster (i.e., *m* or *y* in Section 7.2). As we shall see in Section 7.5, the process of sample size selection may involve consideration of both the number of *clusters* and the number of individuals or person-years *within* each cluster. Use of the matching correlation in sample size determination therefore introduces an element of circularity, since the correlation will itself depend on the sample size chosen.

Instead, we recommend use of the following sample size formulae, which are simple extensions of Equation 7.3, Equation 7.7 and Equation 7.10:

7.3.1.1 Event Rates

$$c = 2 + (z_{\alpha/2} + z_\beta)^2 \frac{(\lambda_0 + \lambda_1)/y + k_m^2 \, (\lambda_0^2 + \lambda_1^2)}{(\lambda_0 - \lambda_1)^2} \qquad (7.13)$$

7.3.1.2 Proportions

$$c = 2 + (z_{\alpha/2} + z_\beta)^2 \frac{\pi_0(1 - \pi_0)/m + \pi_1(1 - \pi_1)/m + k_m^2 \, (\pi_0^2 + \pi_1^2)}{(\pi_0 - \pi_1)^2} \qquad (7.14)$$

7.3.1.3 Means

$$c = 2 + (z_{\alpha/2} + z_\beta)^2 \frac{(\sigma_{W0}^2 + \sigma_{W1}^2)/m + k_m^2 \, (\mu_0^2 + \mu_1^2)}{(\mu_0 - \mu_1)^2} \qquad (7.15)$$

In each case, there are just two changes to the formulae for unmatched trials. First, instead of adding one extra cluster per treatment arm, we add two extra clusters to allow for the loss of degrees of freedom when using the *paired t-test*. Second, the coefficient of variation k is replaced by k_m, the coefficient of variation in true rates (or means or proportions) between clusters *within matched pairs*, in the absence of intervention.

Estimates of k_m might be based on baseline data on the chosen matched pairs, as discussed in Section 7.4.2. Alternatively, the researcher might explore sample size requirements for a range of plausible assumptions about k_m. This is illustrated in the following example.

Example 7.2

We return to the trial of STD treatment for HIV prevention in Mwanza, Tanzania, previously discussed in Example 1.1, Example 4.17 and Example 5.1. In this trial, 12 rural communities were formed into six matched pairs on the basis of geographical location, type of community (roadside, rural, islands) and prior STD case rates at local clinics (Hayes et al. 1995). One community in each pair was randomly chosen to receive the intervention which consisted of improved STD treatment services delivered through government health units, and a randomly sampled cohort of 1000 adults (aged 15–54 years) was followed up in each community to record the incidence of HIV infection over a 2-year period.

Since there was a single follow-up survey after 2 years, the endpoint in the Mwanza trial was *binary* (infected or not infected among those initially HIV-negative). The outcome was therefore a *proportion* rather than an *event rate* as in the Kilifi trial, where there was continuous surveillance to record the times at which child deaths took place.

No prior data were available on HIV incidence in the Mwanza trial communities, although rural HIV prevalence among adults was known to be 3–4% from a previous region-wide sample survey, and a study in neighbouring Kagera Region had documented an annual HIV incidence in adults of around 1%. Since there were no direct data on the outcome of interest, sample size estimates had to be based on *plausible* estimates of π_0, π_1 and k_m.

The trial protocol required 80% power of detecting a 50% reduction of annual HIV incidence from an assumed 1% in the control arm ($\pi_0 = 0.02$ over 2 years) to 0.5% in the intervention arm ($\pi_1 = 0.01$). Thus, with $m = 1000$ adults followed up in each cluster, the number of clusters required per treatment arm in a matched design was given by:

$$c = 2 + (1.96 + 0.84)^2 \frac{0.02 \times 0.98 / 1000 + 0.01 \times 0.99 / 1000 + k_m^2 (0.02^2 + 0.01^2)}{(0.02 - 0.01)^2}$$

Table 7.1 shows the numbers of clusters required for a range of values of k_m. A value of $k_m = 0.25$ was chosen as a plausible estimate. This would imply that, within matched pairs, cluster-level HIV incidence in the absence of intervention would vary from 50 to 150% of an average stratum-specific value ($1 \pm 2 \times 0.25$). With this value of k_m, we obtain $c = 6.8$, and would therefore select seven matched pairs.

TABLE 7.1

Number of Clusters Required per Treatment Arm to Detect a 50% Reduction in HIV Incidence over 2 Years from 2 to 1%, Based on a Random Cohort of 1000 Adults in Each Cluster and Various Values of k_m

Coefficient of Variation, k_m	80% Power	90% Power
0	4.3*	5.1*
0.10	4.7	5.6
0.15	5.2	6.3
0.20	5.9	7.2
0.25	6.8	8.4
0.35	9.1	11.5
0.50	14.1	18.2

Note: The next integer value above the number shown would usually be chosen.

* Including two extra clusters added to allow for use of paired *t*-test.

Note that, ignoring clustering and applying Equation 7.5, we would require:

$$n = (1.96 + 0.84)^2 \frac{0.02 \times 0.98 + 0.01 \times 0.99}{(0.02 - 0.01)^2} = 2313$$

giving a design effect of $7000/2313 = 3.0$.

In the event, six matched pairs were chosen in this trial. In addition, allowance is needed in the sample size calculation for *losses to follow-up* in the trial cohort and for the fact that some individuals were already HIV-positive baseline. The final analysis was based on 8549 initially HIV-negative cohort members who were successfully followed up for HIV seroconversion, or an average of $m = 8549/12 = 712$ per cluster.

The actual power of the trial could be computed retrospectively by reversing Equation 7.14 to obtain:

$$z_\beta = \sqrt{\frac{(c-2)(\pi_0 - \pi_1)^2}{\pi_0(1-\pi_0)/m + \pi_1(1-\pi_1)/m + k_m^2 (\pi_0^2 + \pi_1^2)}} - z_{\alpha/2} \qquad (7.16)$$

Inserting $c = 6$ and $m = 712$ in Equation 7.16, and assuming $k_m = 0.25$, we obtain $z_\beta = 0.39$, giving a power of 65%.

Methods of choosing m, the sample size in each cluster, are discussed in Section 7.5.

7.3.2 Stratified Trials

As we noted in Chapter 5, stratified trials with more than two clusters per stratum may often be the best compromise between a completely unmatched trial, in which power may be lost as a result of substantial between-cluster variation (large k), and a pair-matched trial in which the loss in degrees of freedom can sometimes outweigh the reduction in k.

To a reasonable approximation, Equations 7.13 through 7.15 can be used for stratified trials, but with k_m now taken as the coefficient of variation between clusters *within strata*. Estimation of k_m for stratified trials is discussed in Section 7.4. The value of k_m for a stratified design will generally lie between the k_m for a pair-matched design and the k for an unmatched design.

Since fewer degrees of freedom are lost in the stratified design, the addition of *two* clusters per treatment arm will be conservative. The appropriate correction will fall somewhere between one and two, depending on the number and size of the strata.

7.4 Estimating the Between-cluster Coefficient of Variation

As we have seen, the *design effect* associated with cluster randomisation depends critically on the variation between clusters in the outcome of interest. Use of the sample size formulae presented in Section 7.2 and Section 7.3 requires an estimate of this variation as measured by k, the between-cluster coefficient of variation. In this section, we discuss how to obtain estimates of k.

7.4.1 Unmatched Trials

We recall that the coefficient of variation in the ith treatment arm, k_i, is defined as σ_{Bi}/λ_i, σ_{Bi}/π_i or σ_{Bi}/μ_i for outcomes measured as event rates, proportions and means, respectively. The values of λ_i, π_i or μ_i need to be specified in any case, as these are intrinsic to any sample size calculation. For CRTs, we additionally need to estimate σ_{Bi} in order to obtain a value for k_i.

In many cases, empirical data on between-cluster variation of the outcome of interest are not available at the time when a CRT is being designed. If it is not feasible to carry out preliminary research to obtain such data, the best that can be done is to examine the required sample size for various plausible values of k based on expert judgement. An example is given to illustrate this.

Example 7.3

It is proposed to carry out a CRT to measure the impact of vitamin A supplementation on all-cause child mortality. On the basis of prior mortality rates in the study area, child mortality (in children aged 1–4 years) is expected to average 40/1000 person-years in the control arm, so that $\lambda_0 = 0.040$.

Discussion with researchers who have previously worked in the study area reveals that there are substantial variations in socioeconomic status in different parts of the study area, and it is assumed that there are corresponding geographical variations in mortality rates. Informed judgement suggests that mortality could easily vary between 20/1000 person-years and 60/1000 person-years in different clusters.

On this basis, the investigators obtain an initial estimate of k by taking $\sigma_{B0} = 0.010$, since if the cluster-level mortality rates are approximately normally distributed, 95% of them will be expected to fall within two standard deviations $(2 \times 0.010 = 0.020)$ of the mean. This implies that $k_0 = \sigma_{B0}/\lambda_0 = 0.010/0.040 = 0.25$. For comparison, k values of 0.1 or 0.5 would imply cluster-level mortality rates in the control arm ranging approximately from 32 to 48, or from 0 to 80 per 1000 person-years, respectively.

As a rough guideline in the absence of data, experience from field trials suggests that k is often ≤ 0.25, and seldom exceeds 0.5 for most health outcomes. For a non-negative response variable that is approximately normally distributed, it is uncommon for the standard deviation to exceed half the mean, otherwise negative values would occur. Values of k in excess of 0.5 can sometimes occur, however, especially if the distribution of cluster values is skewed.

Sometimes investigators are in a more fortunate position, and have some prior data on between-cluster variation, either from the proposed study clusters or from comparable units in a different but similar population. In the vitamin A trial, for example, there might be mortality data from areas of similar size in a different part of the same country. Note that some caution is needed in the latter case, as geographical variations may themselves vary between different parts of a country.

Data may not be available on the actual outcome of interest, but on a proxy for that outcome. In an HIV prevention trial, for example, data may available from previous surveys in the study area, or from the baseline survey of the trial, on cluster-level HIV prevalence rates. We might be willing to assume that the variation in HIV prevalence as measured by the coefficient of variation k is similar to that for HIV incidence. However this may not be valid since the relationship between the prevalence and incidence of an infectious disease is complex, and varies at different stages of an epidemic.

When estimating k from empirical data on cluster-level rates, proportions or means, the first step is to compute the empirical variance of the cluster-specific results, s^2. It is important to remember that k and σ_B are based on *true* cluster-level values, whereas the empirical variance s^2 is based on *observed* values for each cluster, and incorporates the random sampling error in these values. To estimate σ_B and hence k, we therefore need to subtract an estimate of this random error component. We give formulae for rates, proportions and means.

7.4.1.1 Event Rates

Suppose that we have data from c clusters, and that the observed rate in the jth cluster is r_j $(j = 1, \ldots, c)$. Then the empirical variance of the observed rates is obtained as:

$$s^2 = \sum (r_j - \bar{r})^2 / (c - 1)$$

where $\bar{r} = \Sigma r_j / c$ is the mean of the cluster-specific rates.
It can be shown that the expected value of s^2 is given by:

$$E(s^2) = \lambda \sum (1 / y_j) / c + \sigma_B^2 = \lambda / \bar{y}_H + \sigma_B^2 \tag{7.17}$$

where λ is the true mean rate, y_j is the person-years of follow-up in the jth cluster, and $\bar{y}_H$ is the harmonic mean of the y_j. In this expression, the first term represents the *Poisson* variation in the *observed* cluster rates. Hence we can estimate 2B σ_B^2 as:

$$\hat{\sigma}_B^2 = s^2 - \frac{r}{\bar{y}_H}$$

and hence $\hat{k} = \hat{\sigma}_B / r$, where r is the overall rate computed from all clusters combined.

Example 7.4

In the planning of the trial of impregnated bednets in Kilifi, first discussed in Example 7.1, data were available on child mortality from 51 of the proposed study zones. Over all these zones, there were a total of 321 deaths over 21,646 person-years of observation, giving an overall child mortality rate of $r = 321/21,646 = 0.0148$. The empirical standard deviation of the observed mortality rates across zones was $s = 0.00758$, and the harmonic mean of the person-years per zone was $\bar{y}_H = 379$.

Hence k was estimated as follows:

$$\hat{\sigma}_B^2 = 0.00758^2 - 0.0148 / 379 = 1.84 \times 10^{-5}$$

Therefore

$$\hat{k} = \frac{\sqrt{1.84 \times 10^{-5}}}{0.0148} = 0.29$$

and this was the estimate used in calculating the number of clusters required for the trial.

7.4.1.2 Proportions

The expected value of s^2, the empirical variance of cluster proportions, is now:

$$E(s^2) = \pi(1 - \pi) / \bar{m}_H + \sigma_B^2$$

where π is the true mean proportion and $\bar{m}_H$ is the harmonic mean of the sample size in each cluster. In this expression, the first term represents the *binomial* variation in the *observed* cluster proportions. Hence we can estimate σ_B^2 as:

$$\hat{\sigma}_B^2 = s^2 - \frac{p(1-p)}{\bar{m}_H}$$

and $\hat{k} = \hat{\sigma}_B / p$, where p is the overall proportion computed from all clusters combined.

7.4.1.3 *Means*

The expected value of s^2, the empirical variance of cluster means, is now:

$$E(s^2) = \sigma_W^2 / \bar{m}_H + \sigma_B^2$$

where σ_W^2 is the *within-cluster* variance of the (quantitative) response variable. Hence:

$$\hat{\sigma}_B^2 = s^2 - \hat{\sigma}_W^2 / \bar{m}_H$$

where $\hat{\sigma}_W^2$ is the usual estimate of within-cluster variance, and $\hat{k} = \hat{\sigma}_B / \bar{x}$ where $\bar{x}$ is the overall mean computed from all clusters combined.

An alternative approach for quantitative endpoints is to use *mixed effects analysis of variance*, with the cluster means analysed as random effects. This will give a more precise estimate of σ_B, particularly if sample sizes vary substantially between clusters.

7.4.2 Matched and Stratified Trials

If a matched or stratified design is used, the sample size calculation requires an estimate of k_m, the within-pair or within-stratum coefficient of variation between clusters in the absence of intervention. Often, empirical data to estimate k_m will not be available, and we will have to rely on assessment of sample size for a range of plausible values of k_m as illustrated in Example 7.2.

If we are fortunate, we may be able to use prior data on the endpoint of interest from clusters grouped according to the pre-defined strata or pairs. These might be baseline prevalences or means, or event rates measured over a previous time period. If we are willing to assume that the between-cluster variation in the endpoint at follow-up will be roughly similar, we can use estimates of k_m based on these prior data to guide our choice of sample size.

7.4.2.1 *Event Rates*

Suppose that in the sth stratum, we have data from c_s clusters, and that the observed rate in the jth cluster in the sth stratum is r_{sj} $(j=1,\ldots,c_s)$. Then the empirical variance of the observed rates in this stratum is obtained as:

$$s_s^2 = \sum (r_{sj} - \bar{r}_s)^2 / (c_s - 1)$$

where $\bar{r}_s = \sum r_{sj} / c_s$ is the mean of the cluster-specific rates.

Then, modifying Equation 7.17 appropriately, we obtain:

$$E(s_s^2) = \lambda_s / \bar{y}_{Hs} + \sigma_{Bs}^2$$

where λ_s is the true mean rate in the sth stratum, $\bar{y}_{Hs}$ is the harmonic mean of the person-years of observation in the clusters in this stratum and σ_{Bs}^2 is the between-cluster variation in true rates within this stratum. Hence we can estimate σ^2_{Bs} as:

$$\hat{\sigma}^2_{Bs} = s^2_s - \frac{r_s}{\bar{y}_{Hs}} \qquad (7.18)$$

and hence $\hat{k}_s = \hat{\sigma}_{Bs} / r_s$, where r_s is the overall observed rate in the sth stratum.

Assuming that the within-stratum coefficient of variation, k_s is roughly constant across strata, a simple pooled estimate of the value of k_m, the within-stratum coefficient of variation, can be obtained as:

$$\hat{k}_m = \sum \hat{k}_s / S$$

where S is the number of strata.

7.4.2.2 Proportions and Means

Similar methods can be used, but with Equation 7.18 replaced by:

$$\hat{\sigma}^2_{Bs} = s^2_s - \frac{p_s(1-p_s)}{\bar{m}_{Hs}}$$

and

$$\hat{\sigma}^2_{Bs} = s^2_s - \frac{\hat{\sigma}^2_{Ws}}{\bar{m}_{Hs}}$$

for proportions and means, respectively, with the obvious notation.

Sometimes matched pairs are formed on the basis of baseline values of the endpoint of interest. For example the observed baseline rates could be placed in ascending order, and clusters with adjacent values chosen to form matched pairs. While it would be possible to obtain an estimate of k_m based on the observed baseline values in these matched pairs, it is important to recognise that this will be an *underestimate* of the *true* value of k_m. This is because when we match clusters based on observed values, the *true* difference between the matched clusters will on average be greater than the observed difference (this is a form of *regression to the mean*). Methods are available to adjust for this effect (Hughes 2005).

7.5 Choice of Sample Size in Each Cluster

For the sample size equations presented in Section 7.2, we assumed that the sample size per cluster was fixed and showed how to estimate the required number of clusters, c. This is the most useful formulation in trials where the sizes of clusters are defined in advance and in which *all* subjects in each cluster are selected for study.

In other trials, however, we may be able to manipulate the sample size in each cluster (*y* or *m*) as well as the number of clusters (*c*). This would be the case if cluster boundaries are arbitrary, and if we wish to explore the consequences of different choices of cluster size. It would also be the case if we are considering selecting a *sample* of subjects for study within each cluster, rather than carrying out measurements on the entire cluster.

For a given number of clusters and overall sample size, maximum statistical efficiency in a CRT is obtained if we select an equal sized sample from each cluster. Recalling that there is likely to be between-cluster variation in the endpoints of interest and, possibly, in the effects of the intervention, each cluster gives us an independent estimate of the mean outcome over all clusters. Spreading the sampling effort uniformly over clusters minimises the standard error of our estimates, and maximises the power of detecting a significant difference between the sets of clusters in each treatment arm. This differs from standard *cluster sampling* methodology, where we often select samples proportional to the size of each cluster in order to obtain an efficient estimate of the overall population mean. The inferential task is different in a CRT.

As noted in Chapter 2, a simple expression for the *design effect* of a CRT is given by:

$$DEff = 1 + (m-1)\rho$$

where *m* is the sample size per cluster and ρ is the intracluster correlation coefficient. This means that, if all else remains equal, the statistical efficiency of a trial is always increased by reducing the sample size per cluster and selecting a *larger number of clusters*. However, we also noted that the situation may be more complex than this, since ρ (and *k*) as well as the intervention effect may vary with cluster size, and there may also be cogent logistical, financial and other reasons for choosing larger clusters.

Setting aside these issues for the time being, we can explore different design options by inserting different possible values of *m* or *y* in Equation 7.3, Equation 7.7 or Equation 7.10, and calculating the corresponding values of *c*.

Example 7.5

In our discussion of the Mwanza trial of STD treatment, we used the equation:

$$c = 2 + (z_{\alpha/2} + z_\beta)^2 \frac{\pi_0(1-\pi_0)/m + \pi_1(1-\pi_1)/m + k_m^2(\pi_0^2 + \pi_1^2)}{(\pi_0 - \pi_1)^2} \tag{7.19}$$

to estimate the number of matched pairs required for 80% power assuming that $\pi_0 = 0.02$, $\pi_1 = 0.01$, $m = 1000$ and $k_m = 0.25$. The computed value of *c* was 6.8 suggesting that around seven matched pairs were required.

The total population of each community in the Mwanza trial averaged around 25,000 and so there was considerable scope for sub-sampling within each cluster. To guide the choice of m, the sample size per cluster, curves were plotted showing the numbers of clusters required for a range of values of m and k_m, and these are shown in Figure 7.1.

A number of points are clear from this diagram. First, the required number of clusters increases quite substantially as the between-cluster variability k_m increases. Second, the required number of clusters can be decreased (for given k_m) if the sample size per cluster is increased. Third, the effect of increasing the sample size per cluster is subject to *diminishing returns*, particularly for large values of k_m. The reason for this can be seen by examining Equation 7.19. As m increases, the first two terms in the numerator (representing the binomial sampling error within each cluster) decrease, but the last term (representing between-cluster variation) remains constant. As the first two terms approach zero, increasing m has no further effect on c.

In our example, assuming that $k_m = 0.25$, it is clear that as the sample size per cluster increases from 100 to 500, there is a substantial reduction in the number of clusters required. However, little is gained by increasing the sample size per cluster beyond about $m = 750$. In the Mwanza trial, it was decided to select a random study cohort of 1000 from each study community. This would allow for losses to follow-up and exclusion of subjects who were already HIV-positive at baseline.

An alternative approach is to compute the study power for various combinations of c, m (or y) and k, using Equation 7.4 and Equation 7.16 or their equivalents, and displaying the results as *power curves*.

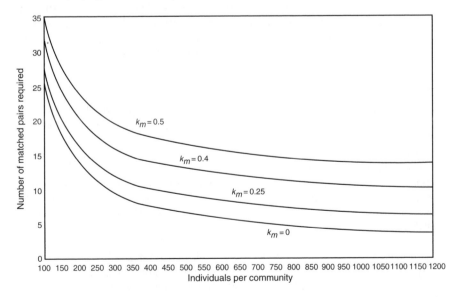

FIGURE 7.1
Sample size requirements for Mwanza STD treatment trial. Graph shows number of matched pairs of communities and number of individuals per community required to detect reduction in HIV incidence over 2 years from 2 to 1% for various values of k_m. (From Hays, R.J., and Benenett, S. Simple sample size calculation for cluster-randomized trials. *International Journal of Epidemiology* 1999, 28, 319–26. With permission.)

7.6 Further Issues in Sample Size Calculation

We briefly discuss some miscellaneous issues in sample size calculation, most of which also apply to conventional individually randomised trials.

7.6.1 Trials with More than Two Treatment Arms

Given the expense and logistical complexity associated with CRTs, and the challenge in gathering enough clusters to achieve sufficient power for comparison of two treatment arms, CRTs with more than two arms are relatively uncommon, and CRTs with more than three arms *very* uncommon.

If the decision is taken to adopt this design, it is important to specify in advance which comparisons the study is to be powered for. Sample size calculations will generally proceed by considering pair-wise comparisons between specific treatment arms.

In a three-arm trial, there are commonly two alternative interventions (A and B), which are compared with a single control arm (C). The trial may be powered for pair-wise comparisons of arms A and C, and arms B and C. It is important to recognise that this may not provide adequate power for a direct comparison of arms A and B. If both interventions are effective in reducing the rates of a disease endpoint, then the expected difference between arms A and B may be smaller than the expected difference between either of these arms and the control arm. Furthermore, the overall event rate will be smaller in these two arms, thus requiring a larger sample size. For these reasons, if the direct comparison of two intervention arms is of interest, it is important to carry out a separate sample size calculation for this comparison.

Example 7.6

In the HIV prevention trial in Masaka District, Uganda, previously discussed in Example 3.14, 18 rural parishes were arranged in six *matched triplets* and randomly allocated to three treatment arms. Arm A received a community-based Information, Education and Communication (IEC) intervention designed to promote safer sexual behaviour (Kamali et al. 2003). Arm B received the IEC programme *plus* improved syndromic treatment services for STDs. Arm C was the control arm and received general community development activities (unrelated to HIV). A cohort of adults was followed up in each parish to measure effects of the interventions on HIV incidence.

The trial was powered to detect a 50% reduction in HIV incidence between either of the intervention arms and the control arm. While direct comparison of arms A and B would also be of interest, in order to examine the effect of *adding* improved STD treatment to the IEC intervention, the study was not powered for this comparison.

7.6.2 Trials with Treatment Arms of Unequal Size

The sample size equations given in Section 7.2 assume that equal numbers of clusters are to be allocated to each treatment arm. Sometimes, investigators prefer an unequal allocation ratio, usually allocating more clusters to the arm expected to be more acceptable or to provide greater benefit to participants or their communities. The arguments for and against this design choice have been widely discussed in the context of conventional clinical trials. It is a less common choice in CRTs, perhaps because a larger total number of clusters is needed with an unequal allocation ratio. Given the challenges in including a sufficient number of clusters in most CRTs, it is probably best to opt for the statistically most efficient design, with equal numbers of clusters in each arm, unless there are particularly compelling arguments for unequal allocation.

Suppose that in an unmatched two-arm CRT we have decided on an allocation ratio of n, with c_0 clusters allocated to the control arm and $c_1 = nc_0$ clusters allocated to the intervention arm. For event rates, Equation 7.2 now becomes:

$$c_0 = 1 + (z_{\alpha/2} + z_\beta)^2 \frac{(\lambda_0 / y + k_0^2 \lambda_0^2) + (\lambda_1 / y + k_1^2 \lambda_1^2) / n}{(\lambda_0 - \lambda_1)^2} \tag{7.20}$$

The equations for other types of endpoint and for matched and stratified studies can be modified similarly.

As a rough approximation, the total number of clusters has to be multiplied by the factor:

$$F = (n+1)^2 / 4n$$

Note that this reduces to $F = 1$ for $n = 1$, while for $n = 2$ we obtain:

$$F = (2+1)^2 / 8 = 1.125$$

For example, if we require a total of 16 clusters with an equal allocation of eight clusters to each arm, we would instead require 18 clusters with 6 in one arm and 12 in the other.

7.6.3 Equivalence Trials

Previous sections have focused on *superiority trials*, in which the objective is to demonstrate a difference in outcome between treatment arms. In some trials, usually referred to as *equivalence trials* or *non-inferiority trials*, the objective is instead to demonstrate that a new intervention is *no worse than* an existing intervention. For example, we may wish to compare a new treatment with an existing treatment which is known to be highly effective but which has unpleasant side effects or is very expensive. To support a change of policy to use the new treatment, it may be sufficient to show that the new treatment is *as effective or almost as effective as* the existing treatment.

There are various alternative formulations of test hypotheses and sample size calculations for equivalence trials. We illustrate a common approach based on a simple example with a proportion as endpoint.

Example 7.7

Suppose the existing cure rate associated with a treatment is 80% and we wish to demonstrate that this falls no lower than 70% with a new treatment which is considerably less toxic. We plan to carry out an unmatched CRT in which medical practices are randomised to the new or existing treatments, with $m = 100$ patients followed up in each practice and an assumed k of 0.10.

Writing $\Delta = \pi_1 - \pi_0$, where Δ is the true difference in cure rates between the new (π_1) and old (π_0) treatments, the null hypothesis for such an equivalence trial would usually be specified as H_0: $\Delta \leq -0.1$, and the alternative hypothesis as H_1: $\Delta > -0.1$. The null hypothesis represents *inferiority* of the new treatment, and we therefore require high power (say 80%) of rejecting this hypothesis (and concluding that the two treatments are equivalent) if the true cure rates are similar (say $\pi_1 = \pi_0 = 0.8$).

Thus, with an appropriate modification of Equation 7.7, we require c clusters per arm, where c is given as:

$$c = 1 + (z_\alpha + z_\beta)^2 \frac{2\pi_0(1-\pi_0)/m + 2k^2\pi_0^2}{\Delta^2}$$

$$= 1 + (1.64 + 0.84)^2 \frac{2 \times 0.8 \times 0.2/100 + 2 \times 0.1^2 \times 0.8^2}{0.1^2} \qquad (7.21)$$

$$= 10.8$$

Note that while formally the null hypothesis, as specified, implies a *one-sided* significance test, some investigators would prefer to ensure high power of excluding a 10% lower cure rate on the new treatment using a *two-sided* test. This would ensure that a standard 95% confidence interval on Δ would exclude -0.1 with 80% probability, and would require use of $z_{\alpha/2} = 1.96$ in Equation 7.21, giving $c = 13.5$.

7.6.4 Power and Precision

We have provided formulae based on achieving adequate power of rejecting a specified null hypothesis. While this is the most common approach to sample size determination, the primary objective in some trials may be to *measure the size of the treatment effect* rather than to *test the null hypothesis*.

A simple approach in this case is to choose c so that the estimated variance of the treatment effect is reduced below a cut-off value chosen by the investigator. As we shall see in a later chapter, there are different ways of measuring the treatment effect. If it is represented by the absolute *difference* in outcomes between treatment arms (for example, $\Delta = \lambda_1 - \lambda_0$ for event rates), the estimated variance can be obtained as:

$$Var(\hat{\Delta}) = \frac{(\lambda_0 + \lambda_1)/y + k^2(\lambda_0^2 + \lambda_1^2)}{c} \qquad (7.22)$$

with equivalent formulae for other types of endpoint.

We can give a rough indication of the precision of the estimated treatment effect if the standard approach based on power calculations is used. Ignoring the addition of one extra cluster to allow for use of the *t-test*, the number of clusters is chosen by setting:

$$(z_{\alpha/2} + z_{\beta})^2 \times Var(\hat{\Delta}) = \Delta^2$$

Rearranging this equation, we obtain:

$$SE(\hat{\Delta}) = \frac{\Delta}{z_{\alpha/2} + z_{\beta}}$$

For example, if we choose c so as to obtain 80% power of a significant difference ($p < \alpha$ on a two-sided test), we have $z_{\alpha/2} = 1.96$ and $z_{\beta} = 0.84$, so that:

$$SE(\hat{\Delta}) = \Delta / 2.8 = 0.36\Delta$$

and this would often be regarded as adequate precision for an estimate of treatment effect.

7.6.5 Assumptions about Intervention Effects

In Section 7.2, we have shown that estimates of between-cluster variation of the endpoint of interest in the treatment arms under comparison are needed to derive sample size requirements. In the most general forms of these equations (Equation 7.2, Equation 7.6 and Equation 7.9), we specify separate estimates of the coefficient of variation, k_1 and k_0, in the intervention and control arms respectively. In Equation 7.3, Equation 7.7 and Equation 7.10, we provide simplified versions of the formulae based on the assumption that k_1 and k_0 are roughly equal to a common value k.

While we may have some empirical data from which to estimate k_0, for example from prior or baseline data from the same clusters, it is extremely unlikely that we will have data on the between-cluster variation in the intervention arm. We therefore need to make some plausible assumption about the value of k in this arm. Constancy of k across arms will occur if the intervention has a *fixed proportional effect* on the endpoint of interest in each cluster.

As an example, suppose the true cluster-specific mortality rates in the absence of intervention vary between 20 and 40 per 1000 person-years, and suppose that the effect of intervention is to halve each of these mortality rates. The true rates after intervention will range from 10 to 20 per 1000 person-years. Both the mean rate and the standard deviation of the rates will be reduced by 50% and hence the coefficient of variation k will remain unchanged.

An alternative assumption is that the *absolute effect* of intervention is constant across clusters, rather than the *proportional effect*. In this case, $\sigma_{B1}^2 = \sigma_{B0}^2$, and hence for rates we can assume $k_1^2\lambda_1^2 = k_0^2\lambda_0^2$, with equivalent results for other types of endpoint.

Often the intervention effect will show some *variation* between clusters. In this case, the result will generally be a higher k in the intervention arm than implied by the above assumptions. Unless the variation in treatment effect is substantial, the effect on sample size is likely to be fairly modest. However, the cautious investigator may prefer to use the more general forms of Equation 7.2, Equation 7.6 and Equation 7.9, trying different plausible values of k_1 and exploring the consequence for the number of clusters required.

8

Alternative Study Designs

8.1 Introduction

So far, we have focused mainly on CRTs with the simplest types of study design, in which clusters are randomised to just *two* treatment arms. The great majority of CRTs fall into this category, and this is perhaps not surprising given the limitations in numbers of clusters imposed by cost and logistical constraints in many such studies.

In this chapter, we briefly consider alternative study designs that may be used in CRTs. We first discuss basic design choices concerning the treatment arms to which clusters are randomised. We consider trials with more than two treatment arms, *factorial trials, crossover trials* and the *stepped wedge* design in which the intervention is introduced incrementally in one cluster after another. We go on to consider the choice of sampling design used to evaluate the impact of an intervention, comparing designs based on cross-sectional samples and those relying on follow-up of a study cohort.

The analysis and interpretation of data from studies with these alternative designs is not always straightforward. Investigators would generally be advised to use simpler designs unless there are cogent reasons for adopting these more complex designs.

8.2 Design Choices for Treatment Arms

8.2.1 Trials with Several Treatment Arms

Trials with more than two treatment arms were previously discussed in Section 7.6.1. As noted there, CRTs with more than three arms are uncommon, because it is usually not feasible to enrol a sufficiently large number of clusters to provide an adequate sample size in each treatment arm.

CRTs with three arms are more common, and these follow two main approaches:

- Trials in which two different interventions (in arms A and B) are each compared with a single control arm (C). Such a trial, through sharing of the control arm, is clearly more cost-effective than carrying out two independent trials, since there is a sizeable reduction in the total number of clusters randomised. A further advantage is that this design also allows a direct comparison of the two interventions. However, if this is a stated objective of the trial, it is important for a separate sample size calculation to be carried out for this comparison. Where a binary outcome is of interest, and where each intervention is partially effective in reducing the proportion with this outcome as compared with the control arm, direct comparison of arms A and B may require a much larger sample size than comparison of either arm with arm C.

- Trials in which a more *intensive* intervention is provided in arm A than arm B, and where a *dose response* analysis may be of interest. Arm A may receive the same type of intervention but at a higher level of *intensity*, or may receive an *additional* intervention over and above that provided in arm B. As before, direct comparison of arms A and B with arm C may be of interest, but it is likely that direct comparison of arms A and B will also be important, to determine whether the more intensive intervention has a greater effect. As before, this will require a specific sample size calculation for this comparison.

The reader is referred to Example 7.6 for illustration of a CRT with three treatment arms.

8.2.2 Factorial Trials

Increases in efficiency and financial savings can sometimes be achieved by combining the study of multiple interventions in the same trial using a *factorial* design. Suppose there are two interventions of interest, I_1 and I_2. Then the basic layout of the 2×2 factorial trial is shown in Figure 8.1.

In this design, there are four treatment arms. Arm A serves as the control arm and receives neither of the experimental interventions; arm B receives the first intervention, I_1; arm C receives the second intervention, I_2; and arm D receives both interventions, I_1 and I_2. In a CRT with this design, similar numbers of clusters would usually be randomised to each of these four arms.

Such designs are used in two slightly different contexts, and we consider these in turn.

8.2.2.1 Independent Effects

First, suppose we can assume that the effects of interventions I_1 and I_2 are *independent*, by which we mean that the effect of I_1 on the outcome of interest

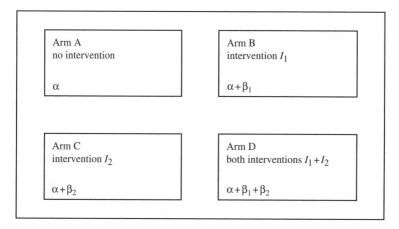

FIGURE 8.1
Basic layout of a 2 × 2 factorial trial and true means in each treatment arm under assumption of independent intervention effects.

is the same irrespective of whether or not I_2 is present, while the effect of I_2 is the same irrespective of whether or not I_1 is present. For example, for a quantitative endpoint our model for the true mean μ in any given treatment arm would be:

$$\mu = \alpha + \beta_1 z_1 + \beta_2 z_2 \qquad (8.1)$$

In this equation, z_1 and z_2 are indicator variables denoting the presence or absence of interventions I_1 and I_2, α is the mean in the control arm which receives neither intervention, and β_1 and β_2 represent the independent effects of the two interventions.

Figure 8.1 shows the true means in the four treatment arms under this model. It is clear from this that we can estimate β_1, the effect of I_1, by comparing either arms A and B, or arms C and D. Our best estimate of β_1 would be obtained by pooling these two comparisons, and treating the study as a trial of intervention I_1 *stratified* on the presence or absence of I_2. Conversely, the effect of I_2 can be estimated by comparing arms A and C, and arms B and D, and treating the study as a trial of I_2 stratified on the presence or absence of I_1.

By way of illustration, suppose we randomise 10 clusters to each of the four treatment arms. Then estimation of each intervention effect is based on comparison of the 20 clusters with that intervention and the 20 clusters without that intervention. This means that we have essentially achieved two trials for the price of one. We can proceed by calculating the required sample size for each of these two component trials, and selecting the larger of the two.

There are some additional considerations for trials where the endpoints are rates or proportions. First, the assumption of independent effects in Equation 8.1 will depend on which measure of effect is used. Table 8.1 shows

TABLE 8.1

Illustrative Example Showing True Rates in Four Arms of a 2×2 Factorial
Trial Assuming Independent Effects on the (a) Ratio or (b) Absolute Scales.

		I_1				I_2	
(a)		Absent	Present	(b)		Absent	Present
I_2	Absent	100	70	I_2	Absent	100	70
	Present	50	35		Present	50	20

an example in which intervention I_1 alone reduces the rate of an endpoint by
30%, while I_2 alone reduces it by 50%. In Table 8.1a, the effects are independent on the *ratio* scale, since the effect of I_1 is still to reduce the rate by 30%
(from 50 to 35) in the presence of I_2. In Table 8.1b, the effects are independent
on the *absolute* scale, since the effect of I_1 is to reduce the rate by 30 irrespective of the presence of I_2. The factorial design could reasonably be used in
either of these cases, but the method of analysis should take into account the
assumed effect of the combined interventions.

Secondly, if both interventions have some effect on the endpoint, the
sample size calculation needs to take this into account. Taking Table 8.1a as
an example, the sample size calculation for a simple trial with two treatment
arms to measure the effect of I_1 (in the absence of I_2) would take $\lambda_0 = 100$
and $\lambda_1 = 70$. In a 2×2 factorial trial, however, we have to take account of the
reduced rates in arms C and D due to the effect of I_2. As a result, the overall
values of λ_0 and λ_1 would be reduced to 75 and 52.5, respectively. If these
values are inserted in Equation 7.3, it can be shown that this results in a
somewhat larger sample size than for the simple two-arm trial.

It remains the case, however, that for a relatively modest increase in overall
sample size, the effects of two interventions can be measured rather than one.
Similar considerations apply to CRTs where the endpoint is a proportion.

8.2.2.2 Non-independent Effects

In some cases, we may expect the effect of one intervention to depend on
whether another intervention is also provided. We might expect the effects
of the two interventions to be *antagonistic*. For example, either I_1 or I_2 might be
effective in reducing the risk of some disease outcome, but once one of these
interventions is in place, the other might have little or no additional effect.
Alternatively, we might expect the effects to be *synergistic*, so that I_2 has a
greater effect if I_1 is already in place.

In the case of such *non-independent effects*, the factorial design may be
adopted—not to improve efficiency by answering two questions in one
study—but in order that the *joint effects* of the two interventions can be measured explicitly. In this case it is the various *pairwise* comparisons between
arms that are of interest. Thus, referring to Figure 8.1, comparison of arms A
and B, and of arms C and D, tells us about the effect of I_1 in the absence and

presence of I_2, respectively. Comparison of arms A and C, and of arms B and D, tells us about the effect of I_2 in the absence and presence of I_1, respectively. We may also wish to compare arms B and C, to examine which single intervention provides the better outcome, or arms A and D to look at the overall effect of providing both interventions.

Not all of these comparisons may be of interest in any specific trial. The investigator needs to define which are of interest, and the sample size can then be calculated based on these pairwise comparisons, using the methods presented in Chapter 7.

If it is specifically desired to determine whether the effects are non-independent, this will impose more stringent sample size requirements. With obvious notation, this would require examination of the contrast $(D - C) - (B - A)$. There are four terms in this contrast, each subject to random sampling error. Sample sizes to formally test departures from a null hypothesis of independence of effect (i.e., of no *interaction* between the two interventions) may be very substantial.

We have made a clear distinction between settings where intervention effects are expected to be *independent* or *non-independent* relative to a specified scale (ratio or absolute). In practice, researchers often have limited prior knowledge of how effects are likely to combine, or of whether independence can reasonably be assumed. If the effects of one intervention are likely to be in the same direction regardless of the presence of the other intervention, even if not of equal magnitude, researchers may be prepared to take the risk of adopting a factorial design based on the assumption of independence, recognising that the measured effect can then be construed as the *average* of the effects of one intervention in the absence and presence of the other. It is important to recognise, however, that the power of the test of interaction needed to assess the assumption of independence may be very low in these circumstances.

Example 8.1

We return to the Zambia and South Africa TB and AIDS Reduction (ZAMSTAR) trial, first described in Example 6.5 (Ayles et al. 2008). This trial is being carried out to measure the impact of two intensive TB control strategies on the prevalence of TB in Zambia (16 communities) and South Africa (eight communities):

- Intervention A: Improved case finding (ICF) for TB, including provision of TB diagnostic laboratories with public access and other community-based interventions.
- Intervention B: A package of interventions delivered to households of TB cases, who will be encouraged to provide treatment support to the case and to access other control measures against HIV and TB.

TB transmission is driven mainly by untreated smear-positive cases passing on the infection to other community members. TB prevalence, the primary endpoint in this trial, is driven by the incidence of new cases (which depends in turn on the infection rate) and on the rate at which these cases are removed through diagnosis and treatment.

The two interventions in this trial were intended to work through different but complementary mechanisms. The ICF intervention aimed to increase the proportion of TB cases diagnosed, and to diagnose them at an earlier stage in order to reduce the infectious period. The household intervention aimed to enhance the cure rate of diagnosed cases. It also involved provision of isoniazid prophylaxis against TB in at-risk members of the household, including children as well as those found to be HIV-positive. Thus it was argued that the effects of the two interventions might be independent, or possibly synergistic—for example, larger numbers of cases diagnosed as a result of the ICF intervention would then be eligible for the household intervention, increasing its community-level impact.

Despite the possibility of synergy between the two interventions, the researchers powered the 2×2 factorial trial based on the assumption of independent effects. The prevalence of the primary endpoint (culture-positive TB after 3 years of follow-up) in adults was expected to be approximately 1%, and the trial was powered to detect 30% reductions in this endpoint due to each intervention. The effects were assumed to be multiplicative, that is to be independent on the ratio scale, as shown in Table 8.2.

The sample size calculation is illustrated for the ICF intervention. The overall true prevalences in the control (ICF$-$) and intervention (ICF$+$) clusters were estimated to be $\pi_0 = 0.85\%$ and $\pi_1 = 0.595\%$, respectively. Impact was to be measured in a random sample of $m = 5000$ adults in each cluster and the between-cluster coefficient of variation was assumed to be $k = 0.20$. Then rearranging Equation 7.7, we obtain:

$$z_\beta = \sqrt{\frac{(c-1)(\pi_0 - \pi_1)^2}{\pi_0(1-\pi_0)/m + \pi_1(1-\pi_1)/m + k^2(\pi_0^2 + \pi_1^2)}} - z_{\alpha/2} \qquad (8.2)$$

With $c = 12$ and $z_{\alpha/2} = 1.96$ (for $p < 0.05$ on a two-sided test) we obtain $z_\beta = 1.20$, implying a power of 88% for this comparison.

In addition to the primary analysis based on stratified comparison of each intervention using all 24 clusters, the researchers planned to carry out a secondary analysis in which the six control clusters (receiving neither intervention) would be compared with the six clusters receiving both interventions. This would allow assessment of the combined effects of the ICF and HH interventions. Inserting $c = 6$, $\pi_0 = 1.0\%$, $\pi_1 = 0.49\%$ and $k = 0.20$ in Equation 8.2, we obtain $z_\beta = 2.09$ and a power of 98%. Despite the high power for this latter comparison, the researchers note that the trial was not powered to detect interaction (non-independence) between the effects of the two interventions.

TABLE 8.2

Prevalence of TB in Adults in the Four Arms of the ZAMSTAR Trial Based on Assumption of Independent Intervention Effects

	HH$-$	HH$+$
ICF$-$	1.0%	0.7%
ICF$+$	0.7%	0.49%

8.2.3 Crossover Design

The most common study design, for both individually randomised and cluster randomised trials, is the *parallel group* design, in which each cluster is randomly allocated to one of the treatment arms and remains in that arm throughout the trial.

As an alternative to this simple design, individually randomised trials sometimes adopt the *crossover* design, in which each individual patient receives two treatments, one after the other, usually in random order so that the effects of any time-trends are controlled for. An analogous design can also be used for CRTs, as shown in Figure 8.2. In Figure 8.2a, we see the standard parallel group design, in which 12 clusters are randomly allocated to two arms, six to each arm, and followed up for a specified time period. In Figure 8.2b, we see the equivalent crossover design, in which each cluster receives both treatments during successive time periods, usually with a *washout period* in between to try and avoid *carry-over effects*. In the illustration, the total person-years of observation are 12 for each design.

An important advantage of the crossover design is that comparisons can be made *within clusters* rather than *between clusters*, and this may reduce random error and thus increase the precision and power of a trial for a given number of person-years of observation. Also, as shown in Figure 8.2, only half the total number of clusters need to be recruited to achieve the same number of person-years.

There are also some important disadvantages. First, the overall duration of the study is likely to be greater. Interventions often take time to have their full effect, and this means that each cluster would need to remain in each arm for a sufficient time for the full effect to be observed. Because there would

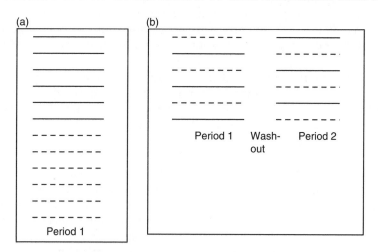

FIGURE 8.2
Illustration of (a) parallel group and (b) crossover designs for a CRT with 12 clusters and 12 person-years of observation. Solid lines denote intervention arm and dashed lines control arm. The periods are of 1 year duration.

usually be equal periods of follow-up in the two treatment arms, the overall duration of the study may be double that of a parallel group design. Second, there are often concerns about *carry-over* effects, even if a washout period is incorporated. In interventions where individuals are trained to adopt new practices or behaviours, carry-over effects seem particularly likely in clusters where the intervention period precedes the control period, and the crossover design is unlikely to be the approach of choice for this type of trial.

8.2.4 Stepped Wedge Design

The *stepped wedge design* is a modification of the crossover design. In this design, all the clusters commence the trial in the control arm. The intervention is then introduced gradually at regular intervals during the trial, either one cluster at a time or in small groups of clusters, until by the end of the trial it is in place in *all* the clusters.

Thus, the stepped wedge design is a one-way crossover, since there are no clusters that start in the intervention arm and then move to the control arm. This means that such designs are particularly susceptible to bias introduced through secular trends in the outcome of interest. CRTs often take place over a period of years, increasing the opportunity for a gradual overall improvement or deterioration in outcomes. Care must be taken in the analysis which is best done, not by comparing before-and-after observations within each cluster, but by comparing during each time period clusters in the intervention phase with those that have not yet entered the intervention phase.

An important feature of this design is that the order in which the intervention is introduced should be chosen at random. Otherwise, confounding can be introduced through variables related to the order of introduction. For example, if a respiratory disease vaccine is introduced in the northern areas of a country, and then progressively deployed in a southerly direction, this could coincide with a north–south seasonal wave of disease that might distort the measured effect of the vaccine.

The basic design is shown in Figure 8.3, for a trial with 10 clusters. At the start of the trial, all 10 clusters are in the control arm. In the first month, the intervention is introduced into one cluster and an additional cluster receives the intervention every month so that by month 10, all the clusters are receiving the intervention.

Note that, in both stepped wedge trials and crossover trials, the individual patients under study in a cluster during the control and intervention phases may be the same or different, depending on the context of the study. For example, in trials involving long-term follow-up of patients with chronic diseases, many of the individuals are likely to be the same. By contrast, in trials of treatments for acute conditions, where patients may be recruited and outcomes observed after a short interval of time, separate patients may be observed during the control and intervention phases.

The main reason for adopting this design is usually to help address ethical concerns (see Chapter 13). Where there is already considerable evidence that

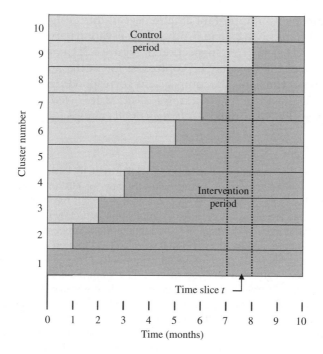

FIGURE 8.3
Schematic diagram of stepped wedge trial with 10 clusters. Statistical comparisons are made between intervention and control clusters within vertical time-slices as shown.

the intervention may have a beneficial effect, perhaps based on short-term endpoints or using an intervention approach that would not be feasible for community-wide adoption, assigning some communities to a control arm for the full duration of the trial may sometimes be judged ethically or politically unacceptable. It is often the case, however, that an intervention cannot readily be delivered simultaneously throughout a large area. In practice, interventions are often phased in gradually using a stepwise approach, to avoid overstretching human or financial resources and to ensure adequate levels of supervision and monitoring. Through random selection of the sequence of implementation, the stepped wedge design provides a fair and acceptable way of deciding which communities will benefit first from the intervention, while at the same time providing the opportunity to obtain an unbiased measure of the treatment effect.

A further advantage of the stepped wedge design, in trials where there is an intervention and control arm, is that carry-over effects are likely to be minimal since the intervention period is *after* the control period in each cluster. This is not the case, of course, in trials comparing two "active" treatment conditions. In any case, investigators still need to consider whether it would be desirable to incorporate a *wash-out period*, depending on the nature of the treatment arms.

As noted above, an important *disadvantage* of this design is that there is a systematic difference in calendar time of observation between the two treatment arms, as is clear from inspection of Figure 8.3. General time-trends in the outcomes of interest may be controlled for in the analysis, and this is done by making time-specific comparisons corresponding to vertical "slices" of Figure 8.3. However, where a *closed cohort* is followed up over time, the results may still be distorted by *cohort attrition* effects.

Example 8.2

Suppose we are carrying out a stepped wedge trial to look at the effects of community-wide provision of antiretroviral therapy for HIV-infected individuals who are eligible for treatment. A stepped wedge design has been adopted for ethical reasons, because it is planned to implement antiretroviral therapy nationally in a phased manner during a specified time period. Suppose that the primary endpoint is progression to AIDS and that we plan to follow up a closed cohort of HIV-positive subjects sampled from each community.

As shown in Figure 8.3, analysis of the primary endpoint would be based on comparing rates of progression to AIDS in those in the intervention and control arms in each time interval, represented by the vertical slices in the diagram. But to be in the at-risk population in the control arm at time *t*, subjects would have had to survive in the AIDS-free state in the absence of antiretroviral therapy for the entire time period, whereas in the intervention arm they would have had access to treatment for some of this period and fewer are likely to have progressed to AIDS. The consequence is that cohort attrition is likely to be greater in the control arm, potentially leading to a lack of comparability between the two at-risk populations in any particular time-slice.

In terms of statistical efficiency, if the analysis is based on *between-cluster* comparison within each time-slice, then the stepped wedge design has a larger variance than the simple parallel group design. This is easy to see, because the variance of an observed difference between two treatment arms is minimised when there is an equal number of observations (or person-time) in each arm. In a stepped wedge trial, this will only be the case in the "middle time-slice" where there are equal numbers of clusters in the intervention and control arms. In all other time-slices, the variance of the difference will be greater than for a parallel group design. It can be shown that the *design effect* of a stepped wedge trial relative to a parallel groups design increases with the number of "steps" (Table 8.3). For values of between 10 and 20, the design effect is around 1.4 meaning that the effective sample size for this design is about 70% of that of a parallel group design (since $1/1.4 = 0.71$). As the number of steps increases still further, the design effect approaches a limit of 1.5.

It may be possible to recover some of this loss of efficiency by carrying out an analysis that takes account of *within-cluster* comparisons before and after intervention. Using a design effect of 1.5 would therefore be a *conservative* approach to setting sample size requirements for a stepped wedge trial. Methods for the analysis of stepped wedge trials are discussed in Chapter 12.

Two modifications of the stepped wedge design can aid in the interpretation or analysis of the results. One is to include some clusters that are always in the control phase (never receive the intervention until, perhaps, the very end of the study) or always in the intervention phase. These clusters allow secular trends to be

TABLE 8.3

Design Effect of Stepped Wedge Design Relative to Parallel Groups Design

Number of Steps	Design Effect
3	1.12
5	1.25
10	1.39
15	1.40
20	1.42
40	1.46

Note: Assumes equal-sized steps distributed uniformly in time.

evaluated. The other approach is to incorporate a lengthy period of observation for all clusters before the beginning of any intervention. Such a *burn-in period* can be useful to help identify long-term secular trends and makes the analysis more convincing if a clear *change-point effect* is seen. It also helps to ensure that there is uniform ascertainment of the outcome variable across the clusters. This may be of some importance as, in some studies, it may take many months for a disease surveillance system to be fully operational.

Example 8.3

The THRio trial is being carried out in Rio de Janeiro, Brazil, to measure the effect of providing isionazid prophylactic treatment (IPT) to prevent active TB in HIV-positive patients attending public clinics for treatment (Moulton et al. 2007). Data from individually randomised trials have demonstrated that IPT given to HIV-positive subjects who are tuberculin skin test positive is effective in reducing the incidence of active TB. However, these studies were carried out prior to the widespread availability of antiretroviral therapy in developing countries, and no such trials have been carried out in HIV-positive patients receiving antiretroviral treatment. Such treatment is now freely available to all patients who need it in Rio de Janeiro, and the THRio trial is designed to measure the effect of IPT in this patient population.

While IPT is already recommended for such patients in Brazil, preliminary studies have shown that it is rarely used in practice. Because it is government policy, however, it was judged unacceptable to carry out a standard parallel group trial with a control group that would not be offered this intervention until the end of the trial. Instead, a stepped wedge design was used so that the intervention would be introduced to clinics in a stepwise manner during the 2.5 years of the trial.

A total of 29 public clinics providing care for HIV-infected patients, including free access to antiretroviral therapy when eligible, were selected for the trial. These clinics were located in different parts of the municipality of Rio de Janeiro, each providing care to an average of around 200 HIV-infected patients.

In this trial, the first two clinics started to receive the intervention immediately, and two more clinics will receive it every 2 months, until all clinics are receiving it after 29 months (Figure 8.4). The intervention involves carrying out tuberculin skin testing of all HIV-infected patients and offering isoniazid prophylaxis to skin-test

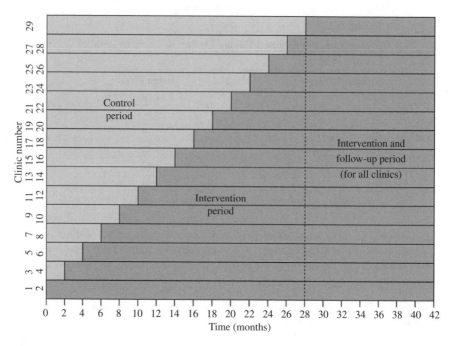

FIGURE 8.4

Schematic diagram of the THRio stepped wedge trial of a TB preventive therapy intervention in Rio de Janeiro. Clinics 1 and 2 entered the intervention period in first month of the trial (September 2005). Clinics 3 and 4 entered the intervention period in month 3. Two clinics will continue to be phased-in to the intervention period every 2 months through January 2008. Prior to starting the intervention, all events and person time accumulating within a clinic will be attributed to the control arm of the study (light shading). Once a clinic begins the intervention, all events and person time will be attributed to the intervention arm of the study (dark shading). After 29 months (January 2008), all clinics will have begun the intervention. Follow-up will continue through month 42.

positive patients after prior screening to exclude active TB. The primary endpoint will be the incidence of new confirmed cases of TB, using strict case definitions, and this endpoint will be measured at clinic level using routine patient records. Recording of endpoints will be carried out throughout the trial, both before and after the intervention is introduced in each clinic, using identical procedures to ensure a valid comparison. Follow-up will continue in all clinics until month 42, although the main analysis will be restricted to the first 28 months and will involve comparison of incidence in control and intervention clinics in each time-slice.

The sample size calculations took into account the estimated between-cluster variance, based on prior clinic data on TB incidence, and the design effect associated with the stepped wedge design (Moulton et al. 2007).

Example 8.4

The Gambia Hepatitis Intervention Study (GHIS), which commenced in 1986, was the first CRT to adopt the stepped wedge design (Gambia Hepatitis Study Group 1987). At the time this study was planned, there was strong evidence that infection with hepatitis B virus (HBV) was causally implicated in the development of chronic liver disease and liver cancer. A new HBV vaccine had recently become available and clinical trials had already established its immunogenicity and demonstrated a strong preventive effect against acute hepatitis B and chronic carriage of HBV. However, these trials were too short to establish the long-term immunogenicity of the vaccine or its efficacy in preventing liver cancer. The GHIS trial was designed to determine the effects of infant HBV vaccination on these outcomes in The Gambia, West Africa.

At the time the trial was designed, the new vaccine was still very expensive and in short supply, and there was little prospect that it would be provided on a large scale in developing countries for some years. This provided the ethical justification for a controlled trial. Several considerations led to the choice of a stepped wedge design for this trial. Individual randomisation was ruled out because of the logistical complexity of randomising 120,000 infants each requiring four vaccine doses over a 9-month period. The investigators therefore chose a CRT design based on randomising the 17 mobile vaccination teams that provided immunisations to infants throughout The Gambia. A parallel group design was considered initially, but there were concerns about denying vaccination to the control group, covering half the country, for the entire 4 years of accrual to the trial when vaccination was known to be of benefit at least in the short-term. This led to adoption of the stepped wedge design, whereby vaccination was introduced by one new vaccination team every 3 months, with the order of introduction decided at random. It was hoped that by the end of accrual to the trial, after 4 years, price and availability of the vaccine would have improved sufficiently for national vaccination to be maintained indefinitely at that time, and this turned out to be the case.

The GHIS trial is unusual in that the primary endpoint will be the incidence of liver cancer when the vaccinated and control infants reach middle age. Detailed records were kept of all 120,000 infants registered during the 4 years of accrual to the trial, half of whom were given the HBV vaccine. A strengthened cancer surveillance system has been established and will be used to identify cases of liver cancer occurring in the future, and linkage with study records will be carried out to determine which study group and treatment arm each case belonged to. Surveys will also be carried out periodically to estimate appropriate denominators for the calculation of rates. The analysis will be based on vertical time-slices and will involve comparison of cancer incidence in vaccinated and control children born during the same time interval.

Since the endpoints will be measured 30 years or more after accrual to the trial, and since HBV vaccination is unlikely to influence short-term survival of infants, differential cohort attrition does not appear to be a concern in this trial.

8.3 Design Choices for Impact Evaluation

8.3.1 Introduction

As we have seen, the impact of the intervention in a CRT is often measured in a *sample* of individuals selected from each cluster, rather than in the entire cluster. There are two main approaches to the sampling of these individuals.

First, we might take repeated cross-sectional samples from each cluster at different time-points. Second, we might choose to use a cohort design whereby a randomly selected cohort of individuals are followed up over time to record the main outcomes of interest. Even if the *entire* cluster is to be studied, rather than a random sample, we still need to decide whether impact will only be measured in the cohort of subjects seen at baseline and who are still present at follow-up, or whether new entrants to the cluster will also be surveyed. We briefly discuss the advantages and disadvantages of these alternative approaches.

8.3.2 Repeated Cross-sectional Samples

Cross-sectional samples may be used to assess intervention effect on quantitative endpoints; for example, to test whether there is a difference between mean cholesterol in clusters receiving a dietary intervention and control clusters. They may also be used to assess effects on the *prevalence* of a binary outcome at follow-up; for example, the proportion of students who are smokers following an educational programme to discourage cigarette smoking.

Cross-sectional samples cannot generally be used to measure impact on the risk or rate of events occurring during follow-up, which require a *cohort* design. An exception to this for infectious diseases is where a biological marker exists for recent infection. For example, *detuned assays* for HIV infection exploit the fact that it takes several months for a full antibody response to the virus to be mounted (Hargrove et al. 2008; McDougal et al. 2005). The assay involves carrying out two separate antibody tests on each serum sample. The first is a sensitive test which detects all subjects who are HIV-infected, apart from a short *window period*. The second "detuned" test is less sensitive, and only detects infections after a delay of some months. By combining the results from the two tests, subjects who are positive on the first and negative on the second are assumed to represent *recent* HIV infections. Using information on the *average* period between seroconversion on the sensitive and detuned assays, such data can thus be used to obtain an indirect measure of HIV incidence.

If a cross-sectional design is used, at least two cross-sectional samples are usually selected, one at baseline and one at follow-up. Even where the primary endpoint can be measured using follow-up data alone, a baseline sample is usually advisable. The limited number of clusters in most CRTs means that randomisation cannot be relied upon to ensure baseline balance between treatment arms. A baseline survey allows us to examine the balance achieved, information that is likely to be of key importance in reporting the results of a CRT. If imbalance is substantial, adjustment for baseline values can then be incorporated in the analysis.

An important advantage of the cross-sectional design is that it does not suffer from the *attrition* due to losses of follow-up from a longitudinal cohort. It is also possible, if desired, to include in the sample subjects who have entered the cluster during the study, for example in-migrants to the study population. When interpreting the results for such individuals, however, it may be necessary to take into account their degree of exposure to the intervention, particularly for interventions of long duration.

In some CRTs, several cross-sectional samples are selected at different time points during the follow-up period. This might be done to evaluate how the intervention effect varies over time, which may be the case for several reasons:

- Cumulative exposure to the intervention may increase over time. For example, in a community-wide health education programme which continues over 3 years, a greater effect may be seen after 2 or 3 years than after 1 year, because the population will have been more heavily exposed to the intervention messages. Similarly in a vaccine trial, effects may increase with repeated doses of the vaccine.
- The delivery and quality of the intervention may improve over time as staff become more familiar with it.
- In the case of infectious disease interventions, population-level effects may increase over time. For example the long-term effect of a vaccine with limited efficacy may be to eliminate the infection of interest, due to *herd immunity*, but this will take time to occur.
- We may also wish to examine how long the effect persists after an intervention ceases.

Investigators need to give careful consideration to the most appropriate choice of time points to illuminate these types of time-specific effects. It is also important to recognise that the effect measure at each time point is subject to random error, and the power to detect statistically significant differences between these may be low unless sample sizes are large. For example, suppose we wish to compare the effect of intervention on the prevalence of some attribute at two different time points. Then using the absolute difference in the mean prevalence across clusters as our effect measure, the measure of interest is:

$$d = (\bar{p}_{12} - \bar{p}_{02}) - (\bar{p}_{11} - \bar{p}_{01}) \tag{8.3}$$

where $\bar{p}_{it}$ is the prevalence at time point t in treatment arm i. This *interaction* effect contains four random quantities and its variance is thus roughly twice that of each individual comparison. If measurement of changes in intervention effect is an important objective of the trial, sample sizes need to be chosen specifically to address this objective.

8.3.3 Cohort Follow-up

The alternative to repeated cross-sectional samples is to recruit a *cohort* of individuals that are followed up over time to measure the impact of intervention. The cohort might consist of the *total population* of each cluster at baseline, or may be selected randomly from that population.

A cohort design allows us to measure intervention effects on an *event rate* of interest during a specified follow-up period. It also allows direct measurement of the *change* in a specified variable in individual subjects. It is well known in clinical trial design that cohort follow-up provides a more efficient estimate of mean change than repeated cross-sectional samples. Using similar notation to Equation 8.3, the estimated intervention effect on the mean change in a quantitative variable x from baseline to follow-up is given by:

$$d = (\bar{x}_{11} - \bar{x}_{10}) - (\bar{x}_{01} - \bar{x}_{00})$$

In an individually randomised trial, the variance of this effect is given by:

$$Var(d) = [(\sigma_{11}^2 + \sigma_{10}^2 - 2\sigma_{11}\sigma_{10}\rho) + (\sigma_{01}^2 + \sigma_{00}^2 - 2\sigma_{01}\sigma_{00}\rho)] / n = 4\sigma^2(1-\rho) / n$$

if we can assume that the variance of x is roughly similar at each time point and in each treatment arm. In this equation, n is the sample size in each treatment arm at each time-point and ρ is the correlation coefficient between baseline and follow-up values of x for the same individual. The correlation ρ is generally positive, and so the variance is reduced relative to an estimate based on repeated cross-sectional samples with $Var(d) = 4\sigma^2/n$. In a CRT, the situation is more complex, since the reduction in variance will depend on how the between-cluster variance of *change in x* compares with the between-cluster variance of individual values of x.

Similarly, for a binary endpoint, a cohort design can be used to measure the incidence of that endpoint *in those initially negative*; for example, the cumulative incidence of HIV infection among those HIV-negative at baseline. It can be shown again that the cohort estimate of incidence is more precise than indirect estimates of incidence obtained by comparing baseline and follow-up *prevalence* in repeated cross-sectional samples.

Follow-up of a cohort also enables analyses that take into account the degree to which individuals are actually exposed to the intervention. Thus, per-protocol and as-treated analyses can be carried out to estimate the maximum potential intervention effect, and dose-response analyses within the treatment arm can also be performed. This can be especially useful when there is much variability in the uptake or distribution of an intervention, or when multiple treatments or media exposures are possible.

The cohort design also has a number of important *limitations* that investigators need to bear in mind. First, the field work involved in tracing and identifying the same individuals over a prolonged time period is logistically more complex than carrying out simple cross-sectional surveys. Second, *cohort attrition* may lead to selection bias in outcome measures since those lost to follow-up are often systematically different from those successfully followed up. Effect measures may also be biased, especially if cohort attrition is *differential* between treatment arms. Of course, coverage may also be incomplete in cross-sectional surveys, but losses are usually greater in a cohort design and increase over time. Third, the *generalisability* of findings from a cohort design may be questionable, since the results will relate to a subgroup of the population who remain in the population throughout the study period and who are successfully followed up on repeated occasions. In discussing the interpretation of trial findings, investigators will need to consider whether the characteristics of this subgroup are likely to influence the effect of the intervention. Fourth, the incidence of disease endpoints is sometimes found to decrease systematically over time, particularly in a *closed cohort*. This is because the most susceptible members of the cohort are likely to acquire the endpoint early during follow-up, so that the "survivors" who remain under follow-up are at progressively lower risk. This effect needs to be taken into account when making assumptions about expected disease rates in sample size calculations. Finally, data on some outcomes may be distorted in a cohort of individuals that are surveyed repeatedly. For example, responses to questions about health-related behaviours may be influenced by responses given at previous surveys, and the quality of information given may fall if individuals become fatigued with the research.

Part C

Analytical Methods

9

Basic Principles of Analysis

9.1 Introduction

This part of the book focuses on the analysis of CRTs. A wide range of analytical methods have been proposed for this purpose, and it is not necessary for the practitioner to have a detailed understanding of all such methods. Rather than providing an encyclopaedic review of available methods, our aim is to provide the reader with a limited number of analytical tools that have proven to be robust and efficient and that cover the main types of CRT study design.

Chapter 9 is a preliminary chapter that outlines some of the basic principles underlying the analysis of CRTs. After discussing the different types of *experimental and observational units* in CRTs, we focus on the importance of arriving at a clear definition of the *parameters of interest*, which are usually alternative measures of intervention effect. As we shall see, a clear formulation of the *statistical model* is the key to this step. We go on to discuss the two main approaches to analysis, based on *cluster-level summaries* or *individual-level data*. Finally, we outline the role of analyses carried out on *baseline* data.

Chapter 10 and Chapter 11 provide more detailed accounts of cluster-level analysis and individual-level analysis of unmatched studies, while Chapter 12 discusses analytical methods for other CRT designs including matched and stratified studies.

9.2 Experimental and Observational Units

As we have seen, the key difference between a CRT and an individually randomised trial is that the intervention is randomly allocated to clusters of individuals rather than to individual subjects. The cluster therefore constitutes the *experimental unit* in a CRT. Random allocation of clusters to treatment arms aims to ensure that the *clusters* in each treatment arm are as far as possible similar, although we have seen that this aim may be only partly achieved if the number of clusters is small, as in some CRTs.

Even more importantly, random allocation ensures that any difference that does exist between the treatment arms, apart from the effect of intervention, is due to chance. The extent of this random error can be quantified by using statistical inference based on a model which states that the cluster-level results for each treatment arm come from the same distribution, in the absence of an intervention effect. By quantifying this random error at the cluster-level, we are then able to make inferences about the intervention effect. Thus, while there are different approaches to analysis, the underlying principle is that intervention effects are measured by analysing the variation between cluster-level outcomes.

While the cluster is always the *experimental unit* in a CRT, observations may be made at different levels and there may therefore be several different types of *observational unit*. In the simplest case, observations may be made only on the individual subjects in each cluster. More often, however, data will also be collected on cluster-level variables and, in some CRTs, there may also be intermediate levels of observation.

Example 9.1

Consider a CRT of impregnated bednets for the reduction of child mortality from malaria in which the cluster is a group of neighbouring villages served by a primary health care facility. Observations may be made at several levels:

- Individual: The primary endpoint will be recorded by following up children aged 0–4 years to record the rate of child mortality. In addition, individual-level data may be collected on possible confounding factors such as age, sex, weight, height and immunisation status.
- Household: Relevant variables at household level might include indicators of socioeconomic status (type of housing, occupation or educational level of household head), ethnic group and measures of treatment-seeking behaviour for common illnesses.
- Village: Distance from health facility might be recorded as a proxy for ease of accessing treatment for malaria. Size of village and adjacency to vector breeding sites might also be important indicators of malaria risk.
- Cluster: Type of health care facility (e.g., hospital, health centre or dispensary) may be relevant.

Example 9.2

In a CRT of a school-based health education programme, in which the intervention is randomly allocated to schools, units of observation might include:

- Individual pupil: e.g., age, sex, ethnicity, socioeconomic status of family.
- Class: e.g., grade, stream, size, number of students, number of sessions delivered.
- School: e.g., urban/rural, type of school, size of school.

Data from all these levels may be used when making inferences about the main parameters of interest.

9.3 Parameters of Interest

An important step in the conduct of any trial is to make a clear statement of the main objectives of the study. In the protocol, these objectives are likely to be presented verbally. Two examples of primary objectives might be

- To measure the effect of a new strategy for treatment of back pain in primary care on the mean pain score reported by patients with lower back pain
- To determine whether regular mass treatment to eliminate intestinal worm infections in young children has any effect on the incidence of other infectious diseases

To ensure that the parameter of interest is clearly specified, it is usually helpful to write down the proposed statistical model. In the case of a CRT, this model needs to take account of between-cluster variability. The terms of this model can then be used to specify the parameters of interest.

To illustrate this process, we will consider the simplest case of an unmatched CRT with two treatment arms, in which the parameter of interest is based on follow-up data at one time-point (or during one follow-up interval) on an endpoint compared between the intervention and control arms. The appropriate statistical model depends on the type of endpoint, and we consider *event rates*, *proportions* and *means* in turn.

9.3.1 Event Rates

Let λ_{ij} be the true rate of the endpoint of interest among individuals in the jth cluster in the ith treatment arm ($i=1$: intervention; $i=0$: control), and suppose there are y_{ij} person-years of observation in this cluster. Then the simplest statistical model states that d_{ij}, the number of *events* in this cluster, follows the *Poisson* distribution with mean:

$$E\left(d_{ij}\right) = \lambda_{ij} y_{ij}$$

where

$$\lambda_{ij} = \alpha + \beta_i + u_{ij} \tag{9.1}$$

In each treatment arm, the u_{ij} are assumed to be identically and independently distributed with mean 0 and variance σ_{Bi}^2, while β_0 is assumed to be 0. In this model, α and β_i are *fixed effects* while the u_{ij} are *random effects* that represent the between-cluster variability in each treatment arm.

From Equation 9.1 we can see that, since $E(u_{ij}) = 0$, the mean rate across clusters is given by:

$$\lambda_0 = E(\lambda_{0j}) = \alpha$$

in the control arm, and:

$$\lambda_1 = E(\lambda_{1j}) = \alpha + \beta_1$$

in the intervention arm.

In this model, the clusters in each treatment arm are assumed to represent a random sample from a notional wider population of clusters that are similar to those selected for the trial. In the control arm, the parameter α represents the expected rate in a randomly selected individual (or more strictly a randomly selected unit of person-time) from a randomly selected cluster. It follows that α is also the expected rate for a randomly chosen individual from the study population. To see this, suppose we have a randomly selected individual with person-time y_{ijk} and suppose d_{ijk} is the number of events observed in this individual. (This will generally be 0 or 1, and we consider the special problem of analysing trials where individuals can experience repeated events in a later chapter.) Then

$$E(d_{ijk} \mid \lambda_{ij}) = \lambda_{ij} \times y_{ijk}$$

and the unconditional expectation is given by:

$$E(d_{ijk}) = E(\lambda_{ij}) \times y_{ijk} = \lambda \times y_{ijk}$$

Given this statistical model, different parameters representing the intervention effect may be of interest. With the model written as in Equation 9.1, the most natural parameter is the *rate difference*: $\beta_1 = \lambda_1 - \lambda_0$

However, it is perhaps more common when dealing with event rates to work in terms of the *rate ratio*, and this can be obtained by rewriting the model as:

$$\log(\lambda_{ij}) = \alpha + \beta_i + u_{ij} \tag{9.2}$$

Note that this model implies a different distribution for the u_{ij} since these random effects now represent the between-cluster variation in the log-rate rather than the rate as in Equation 9.1. With this formulation, we have:

$$E(\log \lambda_{0j}) = \alpha \text{ and } E(\log \lambda_{1j}) = \alpha + \beta_1$$

so that α represents the mean of the log-rates in the absence of intervention in the notional universe of clusters of which the study clusters are regarded as a random sample, while $\alpha + \beta_1$ represents the mean of the log-rates in the presence of the intervention. In this model, $\exp(\beta_1)$ therefore represents the *rate ratio* for the effect of intervention, but based on *geometric means* of the rates over the clusters in each treatment arm.

As an approximation, this parameter may also be regarded as the *rate ratio* for randomly selected individuals in the population with and without the intervention, or λ_1/λ_0. In fact, if we make the additional assumption that the effect of the intervention is to multiply the rate by a constant factor in every cluster, it can be shown that this relationship holds exactly.

The models of Equation 9.1 and Equation 9.2 can be extended in various ways. If there are more than two treatment arms, additional β_i terms can be used to represent the effects of each treatment. We can also allow for the effects of confounding factors and other variables of interest, by introducing further regression terms. For example, Equation 9.2 could be extended to:

$$\log(\lambda_{ijk}) = \alpha + \beta_i + \sum \gamma_l z_{ijkl} + u_{ij} \tag{9.3}$$

In this equation, we assume that there are a number of additional variables z_1 $(l=1, ..., L)$, and that z_{ijkl} is the observed value of z_l in the kth individual (or kth element of person-time) in the jth cluster in the ith treatment arm. Note that some of the z variables may be measured at the cluster level, others may be measured at the individual level, and others may take time-varying values for each individual.

9.3.2 Proportions

Let π_{ij} be the true *proportion* of subjects with an endpoint of interest among individuals in the jth cluster in the ith treatment arm ($i=1$: intervention; $i=0$: control), and suppose there are m_{ij} individual subjects in this cluster. Then the simplest statistical model states that d_{ij}, the number of subjects with the endpoint of interest in this cluster, follows the *binomial* distribution with mean:

$$E(d_{ij}) = m_{ij}\pi_{ij}$$

where

$$\pi_{ij} = \alpha + \beta_i + u_{ij} \tag{9.4}$$

By analogy with the previous section, $\pi_0 = \alpha$ represents the probability that the endpoint is observed in a randomly selected individual in the absence of intervention, while $\pi_1 = \alpha + \beta_1$ represents this probability in the presence of the intervention. The parameter β_1 is the *risk difference*, $\beta_1 = \pi_1 - \pi_0$. As before, the model can alternatively be written in terms of log-proportions as:

$$\log(\pi_{ij}) = \alpha + \beta_i + u_{ij} \tag{9.5}$$

In this model, exp (β_1) represents the *risk ratio* for the effect of intervention, based on the *geometric means* of the risks in the clusters in each treatment arm. As before, exp (β_1) is approximately equal to the risk ratio for randomly selected individuals in the population with and without the intervention, and this holds exactly if the intervention has the same proportional effect in every cluster.

The effects of additional variables can be modelled by incorporating additional regression terms as in Equation 9.3.

Fitting the models denoted by Equation 9.4 and Equation 9.5 may be problematic because of *boundary effects* since π is constrained to lie between 0 and 1, whereas fitted values might fall outside this range, particularly when the effects of additional variables are modelled. For this reason, when ratio effects are of interest, it is more common to use the *random effects logistic regression model*:

$$\text{logit}(\pi_{ij}) = \log\left(\frac{\pi_{ij}}{1 - \pi_{ij}}\right) = \alpha + \beta_i + u_{ij} \tag{9.6}$$

or, more generally:

$$\text{logit}(\pi_{ijk}) = \log\left(\frac{\pi_{ijk}}{1 - \pi_{ijk}}\right) = \alpha + \beta_i + \sum \gamma_l z_{ijkl} + u_{ij} \tag{9.7}$$

Because logit(π) can take any negative or positive value, there are no boundary constraints and statistical inference based on this model therefore tends to be more stable. If we plan to use this model, however, we need to be aware that interpretation of the parameters, and in particular the parameter β_1 representing the effect of intervention, is more complex than in the case of individually randomised trials or conventional epidemiological studies. In such studies, β_1 would represent the *log-odds ratio*, exp(β_1) representing the *odds ratio* of the endpoint of interest in the exposed compared with the unexposed.

In a CRT, the situation is complicated by the random effect terms u_{ij} in the model. We can define two alternative odds ratios, with distinct meanings, only one of which is related simply to the parameter β_1 in the model.

9.3.2.1 Cluster-specific Odds Ratio

Suppose we restrict attention to subjects in the *same* cluster, who therefore share the same value of u_{ij}. Although, in any given trial, this cluster will only appear in one of the two treatment arms, the models of Equation 9.6 and Equation 9.7 will provide predicted values of the log-odds of the endpoint in that cluster in both the presence and absence of the intervention. For example, using Equation 9.6 we obtain:

$$\text{logit } (\pi_{ij}) = \alpha + u_{ij} \tag{9.8}$$

in the absence of the intervention, and

$$\text{logit } (\pi_{ij}) = \alpha + \beta_1 + u_{ij} \tag{9.9}$$

in the presence of the intervention, respectively. Subtracting Equation 9.8 from Equation 9.9, we see that the α and u_{ij} terms cancel out, and we obtain:

$$\log OR = \beta_1$$

as the *log-odds ratio* of the endpoint among subjects *within any given cluster*. The corresponding odds ratio is known as the *cluster-specific odds ratio*, denoted by OR_{CS}. This may be estimated directly from the random effects logistic regression model described above.

9.3.2.2 Population-average Odds Ratio

Consider a randomly selected individual from a randomly selected control cluster in the defined study population. The probability of the endpoint in that individual is given by:

$$E\ (\pi_{0j}) = \pi_0$$

The corresponding probability for individuals in intervention clusters is given by:

$$E\ (\pi_{1j}) = \pi_1$$

Then the *population-average odds ratio* is defined as:

$$OR_{PA} = \frac{\pi_1(1 - \pi_0)}{\pi_0(1 - \pi_1)}$$

This *OR* cannot be directly estimated from the random effects logistic regression model. To see why this is, note that from Equation 9.8:

$$E\ (\text{logit } \pi_{0j}) = \alpha$$

But, in general, we cannot derive an exact expression for $E\ (\pi_{0j}) = \pi_0$ in terms of $E\ (\text{logit } \pi_{0j})$. Similarly, we cannot derive an exact expression for $E\ (\pi_{1j}) = \pi_1$ in terms of $E\ (\text{logit } \pi_{1j})$.

We shall see in Chapter 11 that some analytical methods, in particular *generalised estimating equations (GEE)*, are not based on the random effects logistic regression model, and provide a direct estimate of OR_{PA}.

The difference between OR_{CS} and OR_{PA} is usually quite small, and OR_{CS} always takes a slightly more extreme value than OR_{PA}, meaning that OR_{CS} is further from 1. The distinction between these two parameters and their interpretation is perhaps best understood through a simple numerical example.

Example 9.3

Suppose we have three equal-sized clusters, and that the probabilities of the endpoint of interest in the absence of intervention are 0.6, 0.4 and 0.2, respectively. Suppose that the effect of intervention is to halve the *odds* of the endpoint in each cluster. Then the resulting probabilities would be as shown in Table 9.1.

If an individual is randomly selected from the combined population of the three clusters, the probability of the endpoint for that individual will be the average of the three cluster-specific probabilities, namely 0.400 in the absence of intervention and 0.263 in the presence of intervention. The *cluster-specific odds ratio* in this example is clearly 0.50, while the *population-average odds ratio* is $(0.400/0.600)/(0.263/0.737) = 0.54$, as shown.

Note that the difference between the two odds ratios is quite small, and that the cluster-specific *OR* is slightly more extreme (further from 1) than the population-average *OR*.

The interpretation of the two parameters should be clear from this illustration. The cluster-specific *OR* denotes the effect on the odds of the endpoint if the intervention is applied in any given cluster. The population-average *OR* denotes the effect on the odds in the combined population of all the clusters.

9.3.3 Means

Suppose the endpoint of interest is a quantitative variable x and let μ_{ij} be the true *mean* of that variable among individuals in the jth cluster in the ith treatment arm ($i=1$: intervention; $i=0$: control). A simple statistical model states that x_{ijk}, the value of x in the kth individual in that cluster, follows the normal distribution with mean:

$$\mu_{ij} = \alpha + \beta_i + u_{ij} \tag{9.10}$$

TABLE 9.1

Illustrative Data for Three Clusters Showing the Difference between Cluster-specific and Population-average Odds Ratios

Cluster	Without Intervention		With Intervention		
	Probability	Odds	Probability	Odds	OR
1	0.600	1.500	0.429	0.750	0.50
2	0.400	0.667	0.250	0.333	0.50
3	0.200	0.250	0.111	0.125	0.50
Average	0.400		0.263		0.54

and variance σ_W^2, where the suffix denotes the *within-cluster* variance. In each treatment arm the u_{ij} are assumed to be identically and independently distributed with mean 0 and variance σ_{Bi}^2, while β_0 is assumed to be 0. As before, α and β_i are *fixed effects* while the u_{ij} are *random effects* representing the between-cluster variability.

By analogy with previous sections, $\mu_0 = \alpha$ represents the expected value of x in a randomly selected individual in the absence of intervention, while $\mu_1 = \alpha + \beta_1$ represents this value in the presence of the intervention. The parameter β_1 is the *mean difference*, $\beta_1 = \mu_1 - \mu_0$. As before, the effects of other variables can be taken account of by introducing additional regression terms as follows:

$$\mu_{ijk} = \alpha + \beta_i + \sum \gamma_l z_{ijkl} + u_{ij}$$

Ratio measures of effect are uncommon when dealing with quantitative endpoints, except for variables that are analysed naturally on a logarithmic scale. For example, plasma viral loads (PVL) in HIV-infected patients vary over several orders of magnitude, and are usually measured on a log-scale. Variables of this kind would usually be handled by defining x as the logarithm of the underlying variable, e.g., $x = \log_{10}$ (PVL). The model remains as in Equation 9.10, but now μ_1 and μ_0 represent the log of the *geometric mean* of the endpoint variable in the presence and absence of intervention, and $\exp(\beta_1)$ represents the ratio of the geometric means.

9.3.4 More Complex Parameters

In the above sections, we have considered the simplest effect measures based on comparisons between the treatment arms at a *single time-point* or (in the case of measures based on risks or rates of disease endpoints) within a *single time-interval*.

Some CRTs use more complex study designs in which measurements of the endpoint of interest are taken over multiple time-points or time-intervals, either in the same individuals or in independent samples. The latter design includes studies where *repeated cross-sectional surveys* are carried out at different follow-up times.

As in the case of simpler designs, investigators need to specify in advance the main parameters of interest. As before, writing down the statistical model may help in formulating a clear and explicit definition of these parameters. We give an example to illustrate this.

Example 9.4

An in-school health education programme is devised to discourage secondary school students from taking up cigarette smoking. A total of 30 schools are randomised to receive the new programme (15 schools) or to act as controls (15 schools). In each school, 50 students are randomly sampled at the end of Year

11 when they are mostly aged 16 years, and asked about their current smoking behaviour. These surveys are carried out at baseline (prior to the onset of the intervention) and then at yearly intervals for three further years, with a fresh sample of Year 11 students sampled at each survey.

The observed effect of the programme is expected to increase over time, for two reasons: (i) the programme is designed to be delivered during dedicated sessions in Years 9–11 of secondary school, so that students surveyed in the first follow-up survey will only have received 1 year of the intervention, whereas in subsequent surveys they will have received two or three years of intervention; (ii) effects may also increase as teachers become more familiar with the intervention materials, and possibly through peer pressure as behavioural norms start to change as a higher proportion of school students will have received the intervention.

It may be decided to carry out a separate analysis of each follow-up survey, so that the parameter of interest would be a simple risk-based effect measure (risk difference, risk ratio or odds ratio) based on a single survey as discussed in Section 9.3.2. Alternatively, the investigators may wish to exploit the availability of repeated data from each school which should provide greater power to detect an effect of intervention. Let π_{ijt} be the true proportion of students who are cigarette smokers at the end of Year 11 in the jth school in the ith treatment arm at time t, where $t=0$ denotes the baseline survey, and $t=1$, 2 or 3 denotes the three follow-up surveys. One of several possible statistical models is as follows:

$$\pi_{ijt} = \alpha_t + \beta_i t + u_{ij}$$

where u_{ij} is a random effect corresponding to the jth school in the ith treatment arm, and has mean 0 and variance σ_{Bi}^2, and $\beta_0 = 0$. Then the parameter β_1 represents the _slope_ of the intervention effect where the latter is assumed to be zero at baseline and to increase linearly over time. The incorporation of separate α terms for each time-point allows us to distinguish intervention effects from any secular trends in smoking practices, which will be estimated based on data from the control schools. This model can be made more general by adding a random effect to β_i, yielding

$$\pi_{ijt} = \alpha_t + (\beta_i + v_{ij})t + u_{ij}$$

where $v_{0j} = 0$, which allows the slope of the intervention effect to vary across schools.

Statistical approaches to allow for _baseline differences_ between treatment arms are discussed in detail in later chapters. Baseline data on variables other than the outcome of interest are usually accounted for by adding the variables as covariates in the model. Baseline data on the outcome of interest can be handled by: (i) including them as a model covariate; (ii) analysing the _change_ in the outcome from baseline to follow-up; (iii) including the baseline data as a response variable in a longitudinal regression model, and measuring the intervention effect by fitting an interaction term between treatment arm and measurement time.

9.4. Approaches to Analysis

There are two main approaches to the analysis of data from CRTs, and these are introduced here and presented in more detail in the next two chapters.

9.4.1 Cluster-level Analysis

This approach is conceptually very simple, and is believed to perform well under a wide range of conditions. It is essentially a *two-stage process*.

In the first stage, a summary measure is obtained for each cluster, and this is usually based on data collected on the endpoint of interest among individuals in that cluster. For example, in a trial of a smoking cessation programme, this could be the proportion of smokers in each cluster that quit smoking. Thus, the total experience of the individuals in the trial is reduced to $2c$ numbers, if there are c clusters in each of two study arms.

At the second stage, we compare these two sets of cluster-specific measures using an appropriate statistical method. The most common approach is to use a simple *two-sample t-test*. Sometimes we start by making a logarithmic transformation, especially if the cluster-specific observations have a skewed distribution. The t distribution can be used both to carry out a *significance test* of the null hypothesis of no intervention effect, and to obtain a *confidence interval* for the parameter of interest.

The methods based on the t-test have been shown to be highly robust to departures from the underlying assumptions. However, a more conservative option is to use alternative *nonparametric* methods such as *Wilcoxon's rank sum test* or a *permutation test*. All these alternatives are discussed in more detail in Chapter 10.

Allowance can be made for covariates by carrying out an individual-level regression at the first stage of analysis, ignoring the clustering of the data. All variables of interest are entered into the regression model *except* for the intervention effect. Then the summary measure for each cluster is the *residual* based on comparison of the observed outcome in that cluster and the predicted outcome in the absence of an intervention effect. If there is truly an intervention effect, then the residuals will tend to differ systematically between the two treatment arms, and comparison of the residuals at the second stage, using the t-test or other methods, provides measures of intervention effect that are adjusted for the covariates considered in the first stage.

9.4.2 Individual-level Analysis

While the cluster-level approach to analysis is *robust*, it may not be statistically the most *efficient* approach, especially where the clusters are of widely varying size. The unpaired *t*-test is based on the assumption that the cluster summary measures are identically distributed and have equal variance. If cluster sizes vary, this latter assumption is clearly invalid, and greater power and precision would potentially be achieved if the analysis were weighted to take into account the different variances.

Such weighting is incorporated automatically when we carry out regression analyses based on individual-level data in a *one-stage process*. It is *essential* that the regression method chosen takes proper account of between-cluster variation. The most common choices of regression model are those based on the *random effects models* presented in Sections 9.3.1 through 9.3.3. These include *random effects Poisson regression* for event rates, *random effects logistic regression* for proportions, and *linear mixed models* for quantitative outcomes. *Generalised estimating equations* (GEE) provide a useful alternative for all three types of outcome (Zeger and Liang 1986) and also provide *population-average* rather than *cluster-specific* odds ratios.

An important advantage of individual-level regression methods over the simpler two-stage methods is that the effects of modelled covariates (which may be measured at cluster or individual level) are estimated and presented simultaneously with the intervention effects. This is not the case in a two-stage analysis, since the second stage involves comparison of cluster-level summary estimates from which the effects of other covariates have already been removed.

An important disadvantage of individual-level regression methods is that they do not appear to perform robustly when there are a relatively small number of clusters. Formally, both the one-stage and the two-stage methods are valid asymptotically, that is when there are a very large number of clusters per treatment arm. However, the two-stage methods seem to perform much more robustly for small numbers of clusters.

We therefore recommend use of the two-stage methods for CRTs with fewer than 15–20 clusters per treatment arm. For larger numbers of clusters, either approach can be used, but individual-level regression is likely to be more efficient, especially if cluster sizes vary substantially.

9.5 Baseline Analysis

Chapters 10–12 focus on methods for the final analysis of a CRT aimed at making inferences about the effects of the intervention on the endpoints of interest. Here we briefly consider the role of analyses carried out on *baseline data* before the intervention is applied.

There are three main reasons for carrying out baseline analysis of a CRT. The first is to characterise the study population in which the trial is being conducted. Issues surrounding the generalisability of trial findings depend to a considerable extent on the characteristics of the study population and so it is important that these are described adequately when a trial is reported. Baseline findings may also help in planning the later stages of the trial. For example, if baseline data are collected on the endpoints of interest, these may be used to refine sample size estimates and to make decisions about sampling procedures at final follow-up.

Secondly, we have emphasised repeatedly that CRTs are susceptible to imbalances between the treatment arms unless a large number of clusters are randomised. Baseline comparisons between arms are the main tool for identifying such imbalances. We have discussed a number of design options that can be used to reduce imbalances but, whether or not these are used, it is important to report a comparative analysis of baseline data so that the reader can judge the degree of comparability achieved.

There are some important general principles that apply in reporting such analyses in any randomised trial. First, the variables to be reported should preferably be defined in an analytical plan *before* the analysis is carried out. It is common for a large number of variables to be recorded and analysed, and it will only be feasible for some of these to be presented. Predefining these variables protects the investigator from allegations that they have been selective in reporting variables for which good comparability was achieved. Second, it is not appropriate to carry out or report the results of *significance tests* comparing the treatment arms, whether or not these make allowance for between-cluster variation. Since the allocation of clusters between arms is carried out randomly, it is known that any differences that do occur *must* have occurred by chance. This means that the null hypothesis is known to be true, so there is no logic in testing it. One could argue that what is being tested is whether the randomisation procedure was carried out correctly, but this is better addressed by documenting and evaluating the procedure. The point of displaying between-arm comparisons is not to carry out a significance test, but to describe in quantitative terms *how large* any differences were, so that the investigator and reader can consider how much effect this may have had on the trial findings.

Finally, some investigators use the findings of the baseline analysis to decide which variables need to be adjusted for in the final analysis. Random allocation guarantees an unbiased comparison of the treatment arms in the limited sense that the average treatment effect would converge to the true value if the trial were repeated a very large number of times. *Conditional* on the particular allocation chosen, however, the treatment effect will be biased if there is imbalance in a covariate which is a risk factor for the outcome of interest. Such covariates play the role that *confounders* play in observational studies, and so it is important to adjust for their effects.

Note that a covariate will confound the treatment effect *only* if it is a risk factor for the outcome of interest, and this cannot be assessed from the baseline analysis. However, it is usually possible for the investigator to reach a judgement based on prior evidence as to whether a covariate that shows imbalance between treatment arms is also likely to influence the outcome. In some trials, baseline data are used in this way to finalise the analytical plan by clearly identifying those covariates that will be adjusted for in the final analysis. Providing the analytical plan is finalised before the final results are analysed, this protects the investigator against allegations that they have carried out a large number of analyses adjusting for different covariates, and selectively presented those showing the most favourable results.

10

Analysis Based on Cluster-level Summaries

10.1 Introduction

As we have seen in previous chapters, a key feature of a CRT is that observations on individuals in the same cluster are likely to be correlated. When data from a CRT are analysed, it is therefore essential to use statistical methods that take such correlations into account. If data on individuals are analysed using standard methods that assume independence of observations, the consequence will be that standard errors of estimates are underestimated and the significance of any effects exaggerated.

In Section 9.4, we noted that there are two main approaches to the analysis of CRTs that make allowance for intracluster correlation. The first is based on analysis of *cluster-level summary measures* of the endpoints of interest, and is discussed in this chapter. The second is based on regression analysis of individual-level observations using regression methods that allow for clustering, and is discussed in Chapter 11.

We begin with cluster-level analysis for two main reasons. First, this is conceptually a simple approach. Since the clusters are the *experimental units* in a CRT, it seems logical to obtain a measure of the endpoint of interest for each of these units and then to compare these between treatment arms. Second, the approach has been shown to be *robust*, providing valid results in a wide range of circumstances. By contrast, the more sophisticated methods based on individual-level regression may be more efficient when there is a large number of clusters and when the underlying assumptions are fulfilled, but are not always reliable when the number of clusters is small as in many CRTs.

A common objection to cluster-level analysis is that information is wasted when the data are reduced to a set of summary measures. Investigators note that, in a trial with 10 clusters per arm but following many thousands of individuals, the final analysis is based on two columns of 10 numbers. This objection, however, is not valid. The power of the study and the precision of the effect estimates will depend on the observed variability in the outcome between clusters. The observed between-cluster variance will be reduced if a large number of individuals are studied in each cluster.

To see this algebraically, note from Section 7.4.1 that for a quantitative outcome, the expected value of s^2, the empirical variance of cluster means, is given by:

$$E(s^2) = \sigma_W^2/\bar{m}_H + \sigma_B^2 \qquad (10.1)$$

where $\bar{m}_H$ is the (harmonic) mean of the sample size in each cluster. Thus, the variance of the cluster summaries is expected to reduce as the sample size in each cluster increases. We can see from Equation 10.1 that the variance of the cluster means incorporates *both* the within-cluster *and* between-cluster variance in the outcome. Similar results apply to other types of endpoint.

In this chapter, we first consider in Section 10.2 how to compute *point estimates* of the intervention effect. In Section 10.3, we then describe how to obtain significance tests and confidence intervals for the intervention effect using statistical inference based on the *t* distribution, while Section 10.4 presents an alternative method based on a *quasi-likelihood* approach. In Section 10.5, we discuss methods of adjusting for covariates based on cluster-level summaries. Section 10.6 presents nonparametric alternatives to the methods based on the *t*-test. Finally, in Section 10.7, we discuss how to analyse whether the effect of an intervention varies between different subgroups of clusters or individuals.

10.2 Point Estimates of Intervention Effects

10.2.1 Point Estimates Based on Cluster Summaries

We first consider estimates based on unweighted averages of cluster-level summaries. Suppose r_{ij} is the observed *rate* of an event of interest in the *j*th cluster in the *i*th treatment arm ($i=1$: intervention; $i=0$: control). Then we can estimate the mean rate in each treatment arm as:

$$\bar{r}_i = \frac{1}{c_i}\sum r_{ij}$$

where c_i is the number of clusters in the *i*th treatment arm.

Depending on the parameter of interest (see Chapter 9), we can then use these mean rates to obtain *difference* or *ratio* estimates of the intervention effect, as follows:

$$\text{Estimated rate difference} = \bar{r}_1 - \bar{r}_0$$

$$\text{Estimated rate ratio} = \frac{\bar{r}_1}{\bar{r}_0}$$

Similar estimates can be derived based on observed *proportions* and *means*. Writing p_{ij} as the observed proportion and $\bar{x}_{ij}$ as the observed mean in the jth cluster in the ith treatment arm, we have:

$$\text{Estimated risk difference} = \bar{p}_1 - \bar{p}_0$$

$$\text{Estimated risk ratio} = \frac{\bar{p}_1}{\bar{p}_0}$$

$$\text{Estimated mean difference} = \bar{x}_1 - \bar{x}_0$$

The estimated ratio of means is rarely of interest. An exception is when the dependent variable is best analysed on a logarithmic scale, as with antibody response to a vaccine. Then inference is carried out using the difference of the means on the log scale, as discussed in Section 9.3.3, and this corresponds to the ratio of geometric means on the original scale.

10.2.2 Point Estimates Based on Individual Values

Alternative estimates of intervention effects may be obtained by replacing the means of the cluster summaries in Section 10.2.1 by the overall rates, proportions or means computed from all the individual values.

Consider estimates based on *proportions* as an example. The overall observed proportion in each arm, p_i, is obtained by dividing the number of individuals with the condition of interest (summed across all clusters) by the total number of individuals in these clusters. This proportion is a *weighted average* of the cluster proportions, with the weights provided by the sample size for each cluster:

$$\text{Overall proportion} = p_i = \frac{\sum_j m_{ij} p_{ij}}{\sum_j m_{ij}}$$

Note that if the cluster size (or the sample size selected in each cluster if subsampling is carried out) is constant, the two estimates p_i and $\bar{p}_i$ will be equal, and the two approaches will provide identical point estimates of intervention effects.

It is more common for the cluster sizes to vary and, in this case, the two approaches will yield different estimates of intervention effects. Often, the difference between the two is relatively small, and either can be presented. Sometimes, however, there is a more substantial discrepancy between the two estimates. This will occur if there are substantial differences between cluster sample sizes (the m_{ij}) *and* if there is an association between the cluster size and the outcome of interest.

For example, suppose we are carrying out a village-randomised trial of an intervention against child mortality. Suppose there is considerable variation in the sizes of the villages and that *all* children in each village are followed up for mortality, so that the cluster sample sizes vary substantially. Suppose also that mortality rates are higher in the smaller villages, perhaps because of poorer socioeconomic status or access to services in such villages. In these circumstances, the overall mortality rate (which gives more weight to larger villages) will clearly be lower than the unweighted mean of the cluster mortality rates.

Both of these measures may be appropriate depending on our objectives. The overall rate, based on individual values, is a consistent estimator of the mortality rate in the entire study population or, equivalently, the expected rate in a single individual randomly selected from the study population. By contrast, the mean of the cluster rates is a consistent estimator of the cluster-level mortality rate or, equivalently, the expected rate in a single individual randomly selected from a randomly selected village.

Overall rates, proportions and means are equivalent to the standard *ratio estimates* obtained from *cluster sampling theory*. Use of this approach is most appropriate if our chosen clusters are randomly selected from a well-defined study population of interest. This is sometimes, but not always, the case as illustrated by these examples.

Example 10.1

In the trial of vitamin A supplementation in children in Ghana, discussed previously in Example 3.4 and Example 4.19, we noted that the study clusters were obtained by dividing the entire study area into arbitrary geographical zones (Ghana VAST Study Team 1993). This is a clear example where the study clusters represent a cluster sample from the entire study population, and where it is appropriate to give weights proportional to size of cluster when estimating the overall mortality. The *overall rate* (weighted by cluster size) would thus be preferred in this context.

Example 10.2

In the trial of improved STD treatment for HIV prevention in Tanzania, previously discussed in Example 1.1 and Example 4.17, the 12 study communities were chosen to represent different types of community (roadside, lakeshore, island or rural villages) (Grosskurth et al. 1995; Hayes et al. 1995). However, these were widely-separated communities that were arbitrarily selected for logistical and other reasons, and could in no sense be regarded as a representative sample of all communities in Mwanza Region. For example, roadside communities would form a relatively small proportion of the regional population, but accounted for two out of 12 trial communities. In addition, a sample of equal size was then chosen in each community, so that the sample did not reflect the varying population of the communities. In this case, the unweighted mean of cluster summaries may be a more appropriate measure.

The above discussion refers to the difference between point estimates of the rate, proportion or mean in each treatment arm. In practice, we are usually more interested in estimates of intervention effect. For ratio measures of effect, such as the *rate ratio* or *risk ratio*, these may be less affected by the weighting used for estimation than the estimate for each treatment arm, unless the intervention effect *also* varies by cluster size.

10.2.3 Using the Logarithmic Transformation

When using means of cluster summaries to obtain effect estimates, it is advisable first to inspect the *distribution* of the observed summary measures within each treatment arm. These distributions are sometimes markedly *skewed*, and this is especially common for rates (which are bounded below by zero) and proportions (which are bounded below by zero and above by one). Skewness of the data has two consequences for the analysis. First, the means of the cluster summaries may be unduly influenced by one or more *outlying* values in the tail of the distribution, leading to instability of the estimates. Second, the inferential procedures to be presented in the next section assume that the observed cluster summaries are normally distributed, and while the *t*-test is remarkably robust to departures from this assumption, it would be preferable to avoid situations where the distribution is markedly asymmetric.

If the cluster summaries are positively skewed (displaying a long right tail), we may consider applying a logarithmic transformation to the rates or proportions prior to analysis. For rates, for example, this would entail computing:

$$l_{ij} = \log(r_{ij})$$

for each cluster, and then working with the l_{ij} which are likely to be more symmetrically distributed than the r_{ij}. It is common in statistical practice to use the natural logarithm (ln), although the choice of logarithmic base has no effect on the effect estimates.

Note that by taking the mean of the log-rates over clusters, we obtain the log of the *geometric mean*, $\bar{r}_{Gi}$, of the rates in each treatment arm:

$$\bar{l}_i = \frac{1}{c_i}\sum l_{ij} = \log\left(\prod r_{ij}^{1/c_i}\right) = \log(\bar{r}_{Gi})$$

It follows that the difference between $\bar{l}_1$ and $\bar{l}_0$ gives the log of the ratio of these geometric means:

$$\bar{l}_1 - \bar{l}_0 = \log(\bar{r}_{G1}) - \log(\bar{r}_{G0}) = \log\left(\frac{\bar{r}_{G1}}{\bar{r}_{G0}}\right)$$

This provides a convenient basis for statistical inference on the effect estimate. This point is explored in more detail in Section 10.3.4.

10.2.4 Case Studies

In this chapter, we shall use two case studies to illustrate the statistical procedures presented here.

Example 10.3

We return to the trial of impregnated bednets in northern Ghana, previously discussed in Example 4.5 (Binka et al. 1996). The study area was divided into 96 clusters of geographically contiguous households, with an average of about 1400 persons per cluster. In a public randomisation ceremony, 48 of the clusters were randomly selected to receive impregnated bednets and a demographic surveillance system was set up to record births, deaths and migrations. Follow-up continued for 2 years, at the end of which impregnated bednets were provided to all compounds in the control clusters.

The observed mortality rate in children aged 6–59 months in each cluster was calculated using a person-years denominator obtained from the demographic surveillance data. Table 10.1 shows the recorded deaths, person-years and mortality rates observed in each cluster. Note the substantial variation in person-years of follow-up, which ranged from 187.0 to 564.0 between clusters. Note also the marked variation in mortality rates, which ranged from 5.0 to 54.5 per 1000 person-years

TABLE 10.1

Mortality Rates Observed among Children Aged 6–59 Months in the 96 Clusters of the Ghana Bednet Trial

Intervention Clusters ($c_1 = 48$)			Control Clusters ($c_0 = 48$)		
Death	Person-years	Rate/1000 Person-years	Deaths	Person-years	Rate/1000 Person-years
5	261.3	19.1	13	564.0	23.0
10	440.3	22.7	10	378.0	26.5
8	358.8	22.3	12	244.3	49.1
8	258.3	31.0	14	537.6	26.0
2	402.0	5.0	9	213.9	42.1
11	394.2	27.9	16	440.7	36.3
9	470.4	19.1	10	230.9	43.3
4	454.2	8.8	9	276.6	32.5
12	220.3	54.5	4	305.6	13.1
7	340.9	20.5	5	224.8	22.2
4	426.1	9.4	7	273.2	25.6
7	287.1	24.4	3	371.1	8.1
15	461.5	32.5	6	455.0	13.2
10	331.8	30.1	10	259.4	38.6
11	416.3	26.4	12	528.0	22.7
4	262.2	15.3	5	238.0	21.0
8	382.3	20.9	11	358.3	30.7

(continued)

TABLE 10.1 *(Continued)*

Intervention Clusters ($c_1 = 48$)			Control Clusters ($c_0 = 48$)		
Death	Person-years	Rate/1000 Person-years	Deaths	Person-years	Rate/1000 Person-years
9	379.6	23.7	10	394.3	25.4
3	211.9	14.2	5	270.2	18.5
12	278.5	43.1	8	346.6	23.1
3	226.9	13.2	5	345.8	14.5
7	385.0	18.2	14	335.9	41.7
12	420.3	28.6	8	283.0	28.3
6	273.8	21.9	22	539.1	40.8
7	352.2	19.9	6	243.2	24.7
7	388.4	18.0	0	286.5	0
4	290.1	13.8	11	266.9	41.2
10	414.8	24.1	11	265.1	41.5
9	268.7	33.5	4	305.8	13.1
9	387.0	23.3	9	376.2	23.9
8	362.2	22.1	8	459.1	17.4
5	340.8	14.7	12	394.9	30.4
9	355.1	25.3	8	311.8	25.7
18	474.5	37.9	4	187.0	21.4
9	308.8	29.1	10	328.5	30.4
7	367.5	19.0	10	332.2	30.1
9	220.8	40.8	14	381.0	36.7
9	318.0	28.3	6	346.5	17.3
9	400.2	22.5	10	403.0	24.8
9	468.6	19.2	1	233.4	4.3
10	356.0	28.1	21	462.2	45.4
3	247.6	12.1	12	378.5	31.7
6	236.7	25.4	29	408.8	70.9
15	394.4	38.0	12	259.6	46.2
10	390.0	25.6	9	398.6	22.6
13	302.4	43.0	10	347.4	28.8
7	507.8	13.8	9	394.1	22.8
7	344.7	20.3	7	310.5	22.5
396	16841.1	23.5	461	16494.8	27.9

in the intervention arm, and from 0 to 70.9 per 1000 person-years in the control arm. Some of these latter variations may simply reflect random variation in rates but, as we shall see later, the extent of variation was more than could be explained solely by chance, indicating true between-cluster variability in mortality rates.

Table 10.2 shows summary measures for the two treatment arms. The overall rates in the two treatment arms, obtained by summing deaths and person-years across clusters, were 23.51 per 1000 person-years in the intervention arm and 27.95 per 1000 person-years in the control arm. In comparison, the means of the cluster summaries were 23.97 per 1000 person-years and 27.92 per 1000 person-years, and are very similar to the overall rates in this case.

Estimated intervention effects are also shown in Table 10.2. Rate differences and rate ratios are again very similar in this study, irrespective of whether overall

TABLE 10.2

Estimated Child Mortality Rates by Treatment Arm and Estimated
Intervention Effects in the Ghana Bednet Trial

	Intervention Arm	Control Arm	Effect Estimates
Number of clusters	48	48	
Total deaths	396	461	
Total person-years	16841.1	16494.8	
Analyses based on individual-level data			
Overall rate (/1000 person-years)	23.51	27.95	
Rate difference (/1000 person-years)			−4.44
Rate ratio			0.841
Analyses based on cluster summaries			
Mean of cluster rates	23.97	27.92	
SD of cluster rates	9.73	12.75	
Rate difference (/1000 person-years)			−3.95
Rate ratio			0.859

rates or means of cluster summaries are used. The rate ratio of 0.859 based on cluster summaries corresponds to a 14% reduction in all-cause child mortality. Adjustment for covariates including age is considered in the next section.

Figure 10.1 shows histograms of observed cluster rates in the two treatment arms. There is only slight positive skewness in this study, and it is unlikely that logarithmic transformation would provide more symmetric distributions. An additional problem in this case is the existence of one cluster with zero events in the control arm, since the logarithm of zero does not have a finite value. There are various heuristic ways of dealing with this problem if it is desired to apply a log transformation. One possibility is to add 0.5 to the number of events in each cluster before dividing by the person-years to obtain the observed rate.

Example 10.4

Project SHARE was previously discussed in Example 1.2 and Example 4.6 (Wight et al. 2002). In this CRT in Scotland, 25 secondary schools were randomly allocated to an intervention arm, receiving a specially designed sexual health education programme, or to a control arm. A total of 8430 students were enrolled in the study cohort and 5854 (67%) were successfully followed up after 2 years. A wide range of outcomes were examined, but we shall focus on effects on sexual health knowledge, onset of sexual activity and regret of sexual experience.

For each student, a score was calculated at follow-up based on responses to eight questions on practical knowledge about sexual health. The score could range from − 8 (poor) to + 8 (good). Table 10.3 shows that in both sexes the mean knowledge score was higher in the intervention arm, although the difference in scores was greater among male students. Although the numbers of students per school at follow-up ranged from 71 to 410, effect estimates were fairly similar whether overall mean scores or means of cluster summaries were analysed.

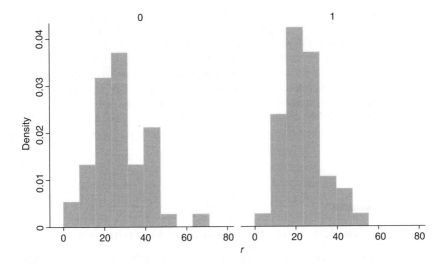

FIGURE 10.1

Histograms showing distribution of mortality rates in clusters in the intervention (1) and control (0) arms in the Ghana bednet trial.

TABLE 10.3

Selected Outcomes of Trial of a School-based Sexual Health Programme in Scotland

	Intervention Arm	Control Arm	Effect Estimates[c]
Number of clusters	13	12	
Enrolled in cohort	4197	4233	
Followed up after 2 years	2689	2812	
Sexual health knowledge score			
Males	*1200*	*1343*	
Overall mean score (SD)	4.35 (2.26)	3.66 (2.31)	0.69
Mean of cluster summaries (SD)	4.24 (0.35)	3.62 (0.43)	0.62
Females	*1489*	*1469*	
Overall mean score (SD)	5.11 (2.26)	4.61 (2.38)	0.50
Mean of cluster summaries (SD)	4.95 (0.58)	4.58 (0.55)	0.37
Onset of sexual activity[a]			
Males	*1117*	*1246*	
Overall proportion	23.5%	23.9%	0.98
Mean of cluster proportions (SD)	24.2% (5.0)	25.6% (10.9)	0.95
Regret of first sex with most recent partner[b]			
Males	*157*	*170*	
Overall proportion	9.6%	19.4%	0.49
Mean of cluster proportions (SD)	9.2% (8.6)	17.6% (12.5)	0.52

[a]Among those not sexually active at enrolment.
[b]Among those reporting more than one partner.
[c]Mean difference for knowledge score and risk ratio for other two variables.

Also shown in Table 10.3 are results for two binary outcomes for male students only. There was no effect on the proportion of students commencing sexual activity during follow-up, with overall proportions of 23.5% in the intervention arm and 23.9% in the control arm, and a risk ratio of 0.98. There was, however, some effect on regret of sexual intercourse. When students reporting more than one partner were asked if they had regretted their first sexual intercourse with their most recent partner, overall proportions were 9.6% in the intervention arm and 19.4% in the control arm, with a risk ratio of 0.49. For both these variables, results were broadly similar when means of cluster summaries were analysed.

10.3 Statistical Inference Based on the *t* Distribution

In the previous section, we discussed how to obtain point estimates of intervention effect based on cluster-level summaries. These estimates are clearly subject to random sampling error, and methods of statistical inference are needed to provide *confidence intervals* for the effect measures and to carry out *significance tests*. In this section, we describe the simplest approach to inference which is to apply the *t-test* to the cluster-level summaries.

10.3.1 Unpaired *t*-test

In most CRTs, we wish to carry out a significance test of the *null hypothesis* which states that there is no difference between treatment arms. If the clusters are randomly allocated to treatment arms, and if there is no effect of intervention, it follows that the observed cluster-level rates (or proportions or means) can be regarded as two independent random samples drawn from the same distribution with the same true mean. Consequently the *unpaired t-test* can be used to test this null hypothesis.

For rates, the test statistic is obtained as:

$$t = \frac{\bar{r}_1 - \bar{r}_0}{s\sqrt{\dfrac{1}{c_1} + \dfrac{1}{c_0}}} \tag{10.2}$$

where s^2 is the pooled estimate of the variance of observed cluster-specific rates within treatment arms, computed as

$$s^2 = \frac{\sum_{i,j}(r_{ij} - \bar{r}_i)^2}{c_1 + c_0 - 2} \tag{10.3}$$

The resulting test statistic is compared with the t distribution with $(c_1 + c_0 - 2)$ df. The extension to proportions and means is accomplished by substituting the cluster-level p_{ij} or $\bar{x}_{ij}$ for the rates r_{ij} in Equation 10.2 and Equation 10.3.

The validity of the t-test depends on two key assumptions, first that the observed cluster rates are normally distributed and second that the variance of this distribution is constant across treatment arms. Under the null hypothesis, the second of these assumptions is guaranteed by the random allocation of clusters between treatment arms. The assumption of normality is more problematic, but simulations have shown that the t-test is remarkably robust to deviations from normality, even for quite small numbers of clusters, particularly when the numbers of clusters in the two treatment arms are equal.

10.3.2 Confidence Intervals Based on Cluster Summaries

In addition to testing the evidence against the null hypothesis, it is important to compute a confidence interval which represents the precision in the effect estimate. We consider confidence intervals for *difference* and *ratio* effect measures, in turn.

10.3.2.1 Rate Difference

As a simple extension of Equation 10.2, we can obtain a 95% confidence interval for the true rate difference as:

$$(\bar{r}_1 - \bar{r}_0) \pm t_{v,0.025} \times s \sqrt{\frac{1}{c_1} + \frac{1}{c_0}} \tag{10.4}$$

where $t_{v,0.025}$ is the upper 2.5% point of the t distribution with $v = c_1 + c_0 - 2$ df, with equivalent formulae for the risk difference or mean difference.

Note that this formula assumes equal variances for the rates in the intervention and control arms. While this assumption is reasonable under the null hypothesis of no intervention effect, it may not be when there is a non-null effect that we are trying to quantify. For example, if the effect of intervention is to reduce the rate of an outcome, the variance will often be smaller in the intervention arm than in the control arm. A robust alternative to Equation 10.4 is to compute the variance of the rate difference based on separate estimates of the variances in the two treatment arms as follows:

$$(\bar{r}_1 - \bar{r}_0) \pm t_{v,0.025} \times \sqrt{\frac{s_1^2}{c_1} + \frac{s_0^2}{c_0}}$$

An adjustment can be made to the degrees of freedom to allow for the use of separate variance estimates, as discussed in Example 10.5.

10.3.2.2 Rate Ratio

We saw in Section 10.2.1 how to compute the rate ratio based on cluster summaries as:

$$RR = \frac{\bar{r}_1}{\bar{r}_0}$$

Ratio estimates of this kind tend to have *skewed* distributions, and it is usual to work instead in terms of the logarithm of RR, which is likely to have a more symmetric distribution. Using a Taylor series approximation, it may be shown that the variance of $\log(RR)$ is given by:

$$Var(\log RR) = Var(\log \bar{r}_1) + Var(\log \bar{r}_0) \approx \frac{Var(\bar{r}_1)}{\bar{r}_1^2} + \frac{Var(\bar{r}_0)}{\bar{r}_0^2}$$

and this can be estimated by

$$V = \frac{s_1^2}{c_1 \bar{r}_1^2} + \frac{s_0^2}{c_0 \bar{r}_0^2} \qquad (10.5)$$

Then a 95% confidence interval for the logarithm of the rate ratio can be obtained as

$$\log(RR) \pm t_{v,0.025} \times \sqrt{V}$$

or, equivalently, a confidence interval for the rate ratio can be obtained by dividing and multiplying the estimated RR by the error factor

$$EF = \exp\left(t_{v,0.025} \times \sqrt{V}\right)$$

Although, strictly, the statistic $\log(RR)/\sqrt{V}$ derived from Equation 10.5 does not follow the t distribution, simulations have shown that this approximation is robust under a wide range of conditions, and is more robust than using percentage points from the standard normal distribution in place of $t_{v,0.025}$.

Once again, equivalent formulae can be used to obtain confidence intervals for *risk ratios* (ratios of proportions).

10.3.3 Case Studies

Example 10.5

We return to the trial of bednets for the reduction of child mortality in Ghana, discussed in Example 10.3. The key statistics based on cluster-level rates are presented in the bottom half of Table 10.2. The mean rates in the intervention and control arms of this trial were 23.97 and 27.92 per 1000 person-years, respectively, giving an estimated rate difference of –3.95 and rate ratio of 0.859.

To test the null hypothesis of no intervention effect, we carry out an unpaired *t*-test. First we compute the pooled standard deviation, either directly from Equation 10.3 or by taking the weighted average of the standard deviations in each treatment arm from Table 10.2:

$$s^2 = \frac{(c_1-1)s_1^2 + (c_0-1)s_0^2}{c_1+c_0-2} = \frac{47\times 9.73^2 + 47\times 12.75^2}{48+48-2} = 128.6$$

giving an estimated pooled SD of $s=11.34$. Then from Equation 10.2 we compute

$$t = \frac{23.97-27.92}{11.34\times\sqrt{1/48+1/48}} = \frac{-3.95}{2.315} = -1.707$$

and referring this value to tables of the *t* distribution with $\nu=94$ df, we obtain a two-sided *p*-value of 0.091. Thus, while there is a trend towards lower child mortality in the bednet arm in this unadjusted analysis, this difference may have occurred by chance.

Box 10.1 shows how this analysis may be carried out in Stata. The *collapse* command is used to obtain cluster-level mortality rates from data on individual children, and the *t-test* command is used to compare means of cluster rates across treatment arms.

From Equation 10.4, a 95% confidence interval for the rate difference is obtained as $-3.95\pm 1.986\times 2.315$, or $(-8.55, 0.65)$, where 1.986 is the upper 2.5% point of the *t* distribution with 94 df. The same confidence interval can be obtained from the Stata output in Box 10.1. The data are therefore consistent with excess mortality in the control arm of up to around 9/1000 person-years or, at the other extreme, a small excess in the intervention arm.

BOX 10.1

```
· use ghana.bednet.dta
· collapse (mean) bednet (sum) outcome follyr, by(cluster)
· gen r=outcome/follyr
· ttest r, by(bednet)
```
Two-sample *t* test with equal variances

Group	Obs	Mean	Std. Err.	Std. Dev.	[95% Conf. Interval]	
0	48	.0279224	.0018401	.0127486	.0242206	.0316242
1	48	.0239716	.0014044	.0097297	.0211463	.0267968
combined	96	.025947	.001169	.0114537	.0236263	.0282677
diff		.0039509	.0023148		-.0006452	.0085469

```
      diff = mean(0) - mean(1)                          t =  1.7068
Ho: diff = 0                         degrees of freedom =      94

   Ha: diff < 0           Ha: diff != 0              Ha: diff > 0
Pr(T < t) = 0.9544   Pr(|T| > |t|) = 0.0912     Pr(T > t) = 0.0456
```

Note that there is some difference in variance between the two treatment arms. If we wish to use separate variance estimates in the two arms, we may use the *unequal* option in Stata. In this example, the effect on the results is negligible.

The point estimate of the rate ratio is $RR = 0.859$. From Equation 10.5, a confidence interval for the RR can be obtained by computing

$$V = \frac{9.73^2}{48 \times 23.97^2} + \frac{12.75^2}{48 \times 27.92^2} = 0.00778$$

giving an error factor of

$$EF = \exp(1.986 \times \sqrt{0.00778}) = 1.191$$

Multiplying and dividing the point estimate by 1.191, this yields an approximate 95% confidence interval for the rate ratio of (0.721, 1.023), and note that this interval includes the null hypothesis value of 1.0.

Note that if the cluster-randomised design is ignored, and we carry out a standard χ^2 test for the comparison of two rates, using the data in the top half of Table 10.2, we obtain:

$$\chi^2 = 6.20 \text{ on 1 df}$$

giving a *p*-value of 0.013. The corresponding 95% confidence interval around the point estimate of $RR = 0.841$ is (0.734, 0.964). Note that the *p*-value is much smaller than the value 0.091 based on the *t*-test, and the confidence interval is narrower. This demonstrates how analyses that fail to take account of the clustered design give results that exaggerate the significance of treatment effects and the precision of estimated effect measures.

Example 10.6

We return to the results of Project SHARE presented in Example 10.4. We saw from Table 10.3 that there was increased knowledge of sexual health in the intervention arm in both girls and boys. To test whether this difference was statistically significant in boys, we perform the *t*-test as follows:

$$t = \frac{4.24 - 3.62}{0.39 \times \sqrt{1/13 + 1/12}} = \frac{0.62}{0.156} = 3.97$$

with 23 df, giving a two-sided $p < 0.001$. In this equation, 0.39 is the pooled estimate *s* of the standard deviation, obtained from:

$$s^2 = \frac{12 \times 0.35^2 + 11 \times 0.43^2}{12 + 11} = 0.152$$

A 95% confidence interval for the mean difference in knowledge score can be obtained as $0.62 \pm 2.07 \times 0.156$, or (0.30, 0.94). From the corresponding data for girls, we obtain $t = 1.62$ and $p = 0.12$, with a 95% confidence interval for the mean difference of $(-0.10, 0.83)$. We conclude that there was strong evidence of an effect on knowledge in boys but weaker evidence in girls.

Note that if no allowance is made for clustering, and the unpaired t-test is applied directly to the individual scores for girls in Table 10.3, we obtain $t = 5.85$ on 2956 df and $p < 0.001$. This illustrates again the misleading conclusions that may be drawn if a CRT is analysed without taking account of the clustered design.

Applying the t-test to the cluster proportions for onset of sexual activity and regret of sexual intercourse among boys, we obtain $t = 0.42$ (23 df, $p = 0.68$) and $t = 1.99$ (23 df, $p = 0.058$), so that there was some indication that regret of sexual intercourse was decreased in the intervention arm. Effect measures for these binary outcomes could include the risk difference, risk ratio or odds ratio. In Table 10.3, we have shown risk ratio estimates. Confidence intervals can be obtained as in Example 10.5. For onset of sexual activity, for example, we obtain:

$$V = \frac{5.0^2}{13 \times 24.2^2} + \frac{10.9^2}{12 \times 25.6^2} = 0.0184$$

giving an error factor of

$$EF = \exp(2.07 \times \sqrt{0.0184}) = 1.324$$

Multiplying and dividing the point estimate of 0.95 by 1.324 we obtain a 95% confidence interval of $(0.72, 1.26)$. Similarly for regret of sexual intercourse we obtain a 95% confidence interval of $(0.36, 0.76)$.

10.3.4 Using the Logarithmic Transformation

In Section 10.2.3, we noted that if the distribution of cluster summaries is positively skewed, it may be appropriate to apply a logarithmic transformation to the summaries before proceeding with the analysis. For example, working with $l_{ij} = \log(r_{ij})$, we noted that

$$\bar{l}_1 - \bar{l}_0 = \log\left(\frac{\bar{r}_{G1}}{\bar{r}_{G0}}\right)$$

gives us the log of the rate ratio based on the *geometric means* of cluster rates.

If a log transformation is appropriate, a significance test can be carried out by applying the t-test to the log-transformed values. This may help to ensure that the variances of the cluster summaries in the two treatment arms are similar as well as providing a more symmetric distribution of cluster summaries, thus improving the validity of the t-test.

When a log transformation is used for statistical inference, this provides a simple confidence interval for the $\log(RR)$, and hence the RR. A 95% confidence interval for the $\log(RR)$ is given by

$$(\bar{l}_1 - \bar{l}_0) \pm t_{v,0.025} \times s_l \sqrt{\frac{1}{c_1} + \frac{1}{c_0}} \tag{10.6}$$

where s_l is the pooled standard deviation of the log-transformed cluster summaries:

$$s_l^2 = \frac{\sum_{i,j}(l_{ij} - \bar{l}_i)^2}{c_1 + c_0 - 2}$$

The corresponding 95% confidence interval for the *RR* is obtained by exponentiating Equation 10.6:

$$\exp\left[(\bar{l}_1 - \bar{l}_0) \pm t_{v,0.025} \times s_l \sqrt{\frac{1}{c_1} + \frac{1}{c_0}}\right]$$

10.3.5 The Weighted *t*-test

Application of the *t*-test to cluster-level summaries is a robust method for the analysis of CRTs, in the sense that it provides reliable *p*-values and confidence intervals with approximately correct coverage. However, it may not be fully efficient in terms of providing optimal power and precision. The *t*-test described in previous sections gives equal weight to each cluster, even though some clusters may be much larger than others and thus provide more information on the outcomes and effects of interest.

It is theoretically possible to use a *weighted* alternative to the unweighted *t*-test which weights clusters according to the information they provide. For proportions, the weighted *t*-test is obtained as:

$$t_W = \frac{\bar{p}_{W1} - \bar{p}_{W0}}{s_W \sqrt{\dfrac{1}{\sum w_{1j}} + \dfrac{1}{\sum w_{0j}}}} \tag{10.7}$$

where $\bar{p}_{W1}$ and $\bar{p}_{W0}$ are weighted averages of the proportions in each arm computed as:

$$\bar{p}_{Wi} = \frac{\sum_j w_{ij} p_{ij}}{\sum_j w_{ij}} \tag{10.8}$$

and the empirical variance estimate is now obtained as:

$$s_W^2 = \frac{\sum_{i,j} w_{ij}(p_{ij} - \bar{p}_{Wi})^2}{c_1 + c_0 - 2} \tag{10.9}$$

The extension to means and rates is obvious. Optimal weights are chosen as the reciprocal of the variance of each cluster summary. It can be shown that these are given for proportions and means by:

$$w_{ij} = \frac{m_{ij}}{1 + \rho_i(m_{ij} - 1)}$$

where ρ_i is the ICC, which may or may not differ between treatment arms. The ICC is undefined for person-years rates, but the corresponding weights for rates are as follows:

$$w_{ij} = \frac{y_{ij}}{1 + \dfrac{\sigma_{Bi}^2}{\lambda_i} y_{ij}}$$

If there is little clustering, and ρ or σ_B^2 are close to zero, each cluster is weighted by its sample size, m_{ij} or y_{ij}. The denominators of the weights represent the *design effect*, which is influenced by both the between-cluster variability and the cluster size. As the cluster size and the between-cluster variability increase, the weights tend to a constant so that equal weights are used across all clusters. Under these circumstances, Equation 10.7 through Equation 10.9 reduce to Equation 10.2 and Equation 10.3 for the unweighted *t*-test.

While the weighted *t*-test in principle offers improved precision, this depends on having an accurate estimate of ρ or σ_B^2. Unfortunately, this is generally not possible with a small number of clusters and, if the weights are not estimated accurately, the precision of the weighted analysis may be worse than for an unweighted analysis. Since the *t*-test is most valuable for its robustness in analysing CRTs with small numbers of clusters, we would not generally recommend use of the weighted *t*-test unless there are good prior estimates of ρ or σ_B^2. For larger numbers of clusters, the individual-level regression methods of Chapter 11 would usually be the preferred approach to gaining power and precision.

10.4 Statistical Inference Based on a Quasi-likelihood Approach

Section 10.3 provides straightforward inferential approaches to analysing the cluster-specific measures of Section 10.2.1. For the analysis of overall measures, as discussed in Section 10.2.2, weighted versions of the *t*-test may be employed, although these become somewhat more complicated. As an alternative, for rates and proportions, we can carry out popula-tion-averaged analyses using a *quasi-likelihood* approach. These methods have the advantages of being easy to implement and of directly handling binomial and Poisson responses, so that data transformation is rarely necessary.

A full explanation of quasi-likelihood theory is beyond the scope of this book. It is sufficient to note that it is a robust approach that involves making assumptions only about the mean-variance relationship, without specifying higher moments of the response distribution. We begin by fitting a standard regression model ignoring clustering, Poisson regression for rates or logistic regression for proportions. We know that the variance of the parameter for the intervention effect is *under-estimated* in these models, as between-cluster variability is not accounted for. We now proceed to multiply the variance by a *scale parameter* σ^2, which depends on the degree of clustering in the data.

For rates and proportions, the scale parameter is usually taken as the Pearson χ^2 goodness-of-fit statistic divided by its degrees of freedom. Suppose we are analysing rates. If d_{ij} denotes the number of events in the jth cluster in the ith treatment arm, then the fitted value of d_{ij} from the model is given by:

$$e_{ij} = y_{ij} \times r_i$$

where y_{ij} is the number of person-years in that cluster and r_i is the overall observed rate in that treatment arm. Then the scale parameter is given by:

$$\hat{\sigma}^2 = \frac{\sum_{i,j}(d_{ij}-e_{ij})^2/e_{ij}}{c_1+c_0-2}.$$

Note that $\hat{\sigma}^2$ will be close to 1 when the empirical variance estimates $(d_{ij}-e_{ij})^2$ are close to the variance e_{ij} assumed by the Poisson model, which will be the case when there is an absence of between-cluster variation.

The parameter estimate with its corrected standard error can be used to obtain a p-value and confidence interval that take account of clustering. Note that it is not possible to carry out likelihood ratio tests when the quasi-likelihood approach is used.

Example 10.7

In Example 10.5, we saw how the t-test could be used to carry out an unadjusted analysis of the effect of bednets in the Ghana bednet trial. Box 10.2 shows how the same data can be analysed using the quasi-likelihood approach.

We first use the *glm* command to carry out a Poisson regression on the cluster-level rates ignoring clustering. The same model fit can be obtained using the *poisson* command, but this does not allow us to estimate and apply a scale parameter. Note that the estimated rate ratio of 0.841 is identical to the population-averaged rate ratio based on the overall rates in the two treatment arms as shown in Table 10.2. However, the standard error, p-value and confidence interval take no account of clustering.

We note that the Pearson χ^2 goodness-of-fit statistic from this model is 152.06 on 94 df, giving a scale parameter of 1.62 as shown. Now using the *glm* command again, but with the *scale* option, we see that the standard error of the intervention

BOX 10.2

```
· use ghana.bednet.dta
. xi:poisson outcome i.agegp i.sex, exp(follyr) irr
```

Poisson regression					Number of obs = 26342	
					LR chi2(5) = 364.61	
					Prob > chi2 = 0.0000	
Log likelihood = -4709.4989					Pseudo R2 = 0.0373	

outcome	IRR	Std. Err.	z	P>|z|	[95% Conf. Interval]	
_Iagegp_1	.3958551	.0382054	-9.60	0.000	.3276301	.4782872
_Iagegp_2	.2988595	.030804	-11.72	0.000	.2441924	.3657649
_Iagegp_3	.1713254	.0255614	-11.82	0.000	.1278863	.2295195
_Iagegp_4	.1823218	.0415171	-7.47	0.000	.1166833	.2848843
_Isex_1	.9417309	.0643878	-0.88	0.380	.8236234	1.076775
follyr	(exposure)					

```
. predict fv
. collapse (mean) bednet (sum) fv outcome follyr, by(cluster)
. gen residr=outcome/fv
. gen residd=(outcome-fv)/follyr
. ttest residr, by(bednet)
```

Two-sample *t* test with equal variances

Group	Obs	Mean	Std. Err.	Std. Dev.	[95% Conf.	Interval]
0	48	1.090595	.0710939	.4925527	.9475728	1.233618
1	48	.9203973	.0502305	.3480069	.8193467	1.021448
combined	96	1.005496	.0441661	.4327381	.9178154	1.093177
diff		.1701979	.0870485		-.0026389	.3430346

```
     diff = mean(0) - mean(1)                          t =  1.9552
Ho: diff = 0                          degrees of freedom =      94

  Ha: diff < 0              Ha: diff != 0              Ha: diff > 0
Pr(T < t) = 0.9732  Pr(|T| > |t|) = 0.0535     Pr(T > t) = 0.0268
. ttest residd, by(bednet)
```

Two-sample *t* test with equal variances

Group	Obs	Mean	Std. Err.	Std. Dev.	[95% Conf.	Interval]
0	48	.0023436	.0018249	.0126436	-.0013277	.0060149
1	48	-.0019204	.0013364	.0092586	-.0046088	.000768
combined	96	.0002116	.0011461	.0112291	-.0020636	.0024868
diff		.004264	.0022619		-.0002271	.0087551

```
     diff = mean(0) - mean(1)                          t =  1.8851
Ho: diff = 0                          degrees of freedom =      94

  Ha: diff < 0              Ha: diff != 0              Ha: diff > 0
Pr(T < t) = 0.9687  Pr(|T| > |t|) = 0.0625     Pr(T > t) = 0.0313
```

effect has been multiplied by $1.27 = \sqrt{1.62}$. The estimated rate ratio remains unchanged at 0.841, but the p-value has now increased to 0.047 and the 95% confidence interval for the rate ratio is (0.71, 1.00).

10.5 Adjusting for Covariates

In Section 10.2 and Section 10.3, we have shown how to obtain *unadjusted* point estimates and confidence intervals and to carry out significance tests by using simple methods based on analysis of cluster-level summaries using the t-test. As we shall see, this approach is most useful when we have small numbers of clusters, since then the regression methods of Chapter 11 cannot be relied upon to give robust results. When there are few clusters, however, it is quite common to find important imbalances between treatment arms in covariates that are predictive of the outcome of interest.

In this section, we describe a *two-stage* procedure that can be used to carry out an *adjusted* analysis based on cluster summaries. In the first stage, a standard regression analysis is carried out to obtain a *residual* for each cluster that is adjusted for the covariates of interest. These cluster residuals are then analysed using methods based on the t-test in the second stage of analysis.

10.5.1 Stage 1: Obtaining Covariate-adjusted Residuals

We now describe the two-stage method in more detail. In the first stage, we carry out a standard regression analysis of the outcome of interest, which incorporates all covariates *except the intervention effect*. At this stage, we ignore the effect of clustering, and so the regression methods used are *Poisson regression* for event rates, *logistic regression* for proportions and *linear regression* for means.

If all covariates are measured at cluster level, we can enter the data for each cluster as "grouped data". If there are individual-level covariates, however, it is simpler to enter one record of data for each individual.

After fitting the regression model, we compare fitted and observed values by computing a *residual* for each cluster. Depending on whether we wish to obtain a *ratio* or *difference* measure of intervention effect, this residual will either be based on the *ratio* of observed to predicted, or the *difference* between observed and predicted. If the intervention has no effect, then the residuals in the two treatment arms should be similar on average. If, however, there is an intervention effect, then the residuals in the two arms should differ systematically. In the second stage of analysis, we therefore compare the residuals between treatment arms using the methods described in previous sections.

We now describe the calculation of residuals in more detail for each type of outcome data.

10.5.1.1 Event Rates

We first fit the *Poisson regression* model to the data, *ignoring the intervention effect*. Using the notation of Section 9.3, we model the log-rate in the kth individual in the jth cluster in the ith treatment arm as:

$$\log(\lambda_{ijk}) = \alpha + \sum_l \gamma_l z_{ijkl}$$

where z_{ijkl} is the value of covariate z_l in this individual. Using the fitted model, the *expected* number of events e_{ij} in this cluster is computed as:

$$e_{ij} = \sum_k y_{ijk} \hat{\lambda}_{ijk} = \sum_k y_{ijk} \times \exp\left(\hat{\alpha} + \sum_l \hat{\gamma}_l z_{ijkl}\right)$$

If we wish to estimate the *rate ratio*, we compute the *ratio-residual* R_r for each cluster as:

$$R_{rij} = \frac{d_{ij}}{e_{ij}}$$

where d_{ij} is the *observed* number of events in this cluster.

If we wish to estimate the *rate difference*, we compute the *difference-residual* R_d for each cluster as:

$$R_{dij} = \frac{d_{ij} - e_{ij}}{y_{ij}}$$

where y_{ij} is the total person-years of observation in this cluster.

10.5.1.2 Proportions

We first fit the *logistic regression* model to the data, *ignoring the intervention effect*. The log-odds for the kth individual in the jth cluster in the ith treatment arm is modelled as:

$$\log\left(\frac{\pi_{ijk}}{1 - \pi_{ijk}}\right) = \alpha + \sum_l \gamma_l z_{ijkl}$$

where z_{ijkl} is the value of covariate z_l in this individual. Using the fitted model, the *expected* number of events in the jth cluster is computed as:

$$e_{ij} = \sum_k \hat{\pi}_{ijk} = \sum_k \left[\frac{\exp\left(\hat{\alpha} + \sum_l \hat{\gamma}_l z_{ijkl}\right)}{1 + \exp\left(\hat{\alpha} + \sum_l \hat{\gamma}_l z_{ijkl}\right)}\right]$$

If we wish to estimate the *risk ratio*, we compute the *ratio-residual* R_r for each cluster as:

$$R_{rij} = \frac{d_{ij}}{e_{ij}}$$

where d_{ij} is the *observed* number of events in this cluster.

If we wish to estimate the *risk difference*, we compute the *difference-residual* R_d for each cluster as:

$$R_{dij} = \frac{d_{ij} - e_{ij}}{m_{ij}}$$

where m_{ij} is the sample size (number of individuals) in this cluster.

10.5.1.3 Means

We first fit the linear regression model to the data, *ignoring the intervention effect*. The expected value (mean) of the outcome variable x for the kth individual in the jth cluster in the ith treatment arm is modelled as:

$$\mu_{ijk} = \alpha + \sum_l \gamma_l z_{ijkl}$$

where z_{ijkl} is the value of covariate z_l in this individual. Using the fitted model, the *expected* mean value of x in this cluster is computed as:

$$\bar{e}_{ij} = \frac{1}{m_{ij}} \sum_k e_{ijk} = \frac{1}{m_{ij}} \sum_k \left(\hat{\alpha} + \sum_l \hat{\gamma}_l z_{ijkl} \right)$$

where m_{ij} is the sample size (number of individuals) in this cluster. The difference-residual is then computed as:

$$R_{dij} = \bar{x}_{ij} - \bar{e}_{ij}$$

10.5.2 Stage 2: Using the Covariate-adjusted Residuals

In the second stage of analysis, the covariate-adjusted residuals take the place of the cluster-level summaries in the procedures documented in Section 10.2 and Section 10.3. The methods are briefly summarised below for ratio and difference measures of intervention effect.

10.5.2.1 Ratio Measures of Effect

A point-estimate of the intervention effect is obtained as:

$$\text{Adjusted rate ratio or risk ratio} = \frac{\bar{R}_{r1}}{\bar{R}_{r0}}$$

where $\bar{R}_{ri}$ is the arithmetic mean of the ratio-residuals for the clusters in the ith treatment arm. For proportions, note that using this two-stage approach we obtain a *risk ratio* rather than *odds ratio* even though logistic regression is used to obtain the *expected values*.

The unpaired t-test can be applied to the cluster-level residuals, R_{rij} to test the significance of the difference between treatment arms. From Equation 10.5, an approximate 95% confidence interval for the adjusted rate or risk ratio can be obtained using the error factor:

$$EF = \exp\left(t_{v,0.025} \times \sqrt{V}\right)$$

where

$$V = \frac{s_1^2}{c_1 \bar{R}_{r1}^2} + \frac{s_0^2}{c_0 \bar{R}_{r0}^2}$$

In this equation, s_i^2 is the empirical variance of the observed cluster-level residuals in the ith treatment arm.

Alternatively, if the ratio-residuals are positively skewed, a logarithmic transformation may be applied as described in Section 10.3.4.

10.5.2.2 Difference Measures of Effect

A point-estimate of the intervention effect is obtained as:

$$\text{Adjusted rate difference, risk difference or mean difference} = \bar{R}_{d1} - \bar{R}_{d0}$$

where $\bar{R}_{di}$ is the arithmetic mean of the difference-residuals for the clusters in the ith treatment arm.

The unpaired t-test can be applied to the cluster-level residuals, R_{dij} to test the significance of the difference between treatment arms. A 95% confidence interval for the adjusted rate, risk or mean difference can be obtained as:

$$(\bar{R}_{d1} - \bar{R}_{d0}) \pm t_{v,0.025} \times s \sqrt{\frac{1}{c_1} + \frac{1}{c_0}}$$

where s^2 is the pooled variance estimate based on the cluster-level residuals in each treatment arm:

$$s^2 = \frac{\sum_{i,j}(R_{dij} - \bar{R}_{di})^2}{c_1 + c_0 - 2}$$

When the above two-stage procedures are used to adjust for cluster-level covariates, an adjustment should be made to the degrees of freedom of the *t* distribution used for statistical inference. Because information on between-cluster variability is used to fit regression parameters for these cluster-level covariates, as well as to make inferences about the intervention effect, we reduce the degrees of freedom from $v = c_1 + c_0 - 2$ to $v' = c_1 + c_0 - 2 - p$, where *p* is the number of parameters corresponding to the cluster-level covariates in the regression model. No such adjustment is needed for individual-level covariates.

10.5.3 Case Study

Example 10.8

In the Ghana bednet trial, the unadjusted analysis based on the *t*-test gave an estimated rate ratio of $RR = 0.859$ with a 95% confidence interval of (0.721, 1.023) and $p = 0.091$.

All-cause mortality rates were strongly age-related, and there was a slight imbalance in age between treatment arms, with mean ages at enrolment of 25.1 months and 25.5 months among children in the bednet and control arms, respectively. Further analyses were therefore carried out adjusting for age-group (6–11 months, 1 year, 2 years, 3 years, 4 years) and sex.

Table 10.4 shows the means and standard deviations of the ratio-residuals and difference-residuals obtained from the Poisson regression of mortality on age-group and sex, by treatment arm. The means of the ratio-residuals in the bednet and control arms were 0.920 and 1.091, respectively, giving an *adjusted rate ratio* of:

$$RR_{adj} = \frac{0.920}{1.091} = 0.844$$

TABLE 10.4

Residuals from Poisson Regression of Ghana Bednet Trial Mortality Data Adjusted for Age-group and Sex

	Intervention Arm	Control Arm	Effect Estimates
Number of clusters	48	48	
Analyses based on ratio-residuals			
Mean of cluster residuals	0.920	1.091	
SD of cluster residuals	0.348	0.493	
Adjusted rate ratio			0.844
95% CI			(0.713, 0.999)
*Analyses based on difference-residuals**			
Mean of cluster residuals	−1.92	2.34	
SD of cluster residuals	9.26	12.64	
Adjusted rate difference			−4.26
95% CI			(−8.76, 0.23)

*Shown per 1000 person-years.

a slightly greater effect than the unadjusted *RR* of 0.859 based on cluster summaries. An unpaired *t*-test on the cluster residuals gives $t = 1.955$ on 94 df, and a two-sided *p*-value of 0.054. This compares with the unadjusted *p*-value of 0.091, indicating that adjustment for age-group and sex has strengthened the evidence for a treatment effect. As in the unadjusted analysis, the distributions of residuals in the two treatment arms were only slightly skewed, and logarithmic transformation was not appropriate.

To obtain a confidence interval, we compute:

$$V = \frac{0.348^2}{48 \times 0.920^2} + \frac{0.493^2}{48 \times 1.091^2} = 0.00723$$

giving the error factor:

$$EF = \exp(1.986 \times \sqrt{0.00723}) = 1.184$$

Dividing and multiplying the point estimate by 1.184, this gives an approximate 95% confidence interval for the adjusted rate ratio of (0.713, 0.999).

For completeness, using the difference-residuals we obtain an *adjusted rate difference* of: $RD_{adj} = -1.92 - 2.34 = -4.26$ per 1000 person-years.

This compares with an unadjusted rate difference based on cluster summaries of −3.95 per 1000 person-years. The pooled standard deviation is $s = 11.08$, and a 95% confidence interval for the adjusted rate difference is obtained as:

$$-4.26 \pm 1.986 \times 11.08 \times \sqrt{\frac{1}{48} + \frac{1}{48}} = -4.26 \pm 4.49$$

or (−8.76, 0.23) per 1000 person-years.

Box 10.3 shows how this analysis can be carried out in Stata. The *predict* and *collapse* commands are used following Poisson regression to obtain observed and expected numbers of events in each cluster. The *generate* command is used to compute ratio and difference residuals and the *t-test* command to compare these residuals across treatment arms.

BOX 10.3

```
. use ghana.bednet.dta
. collapse (mean) bednet (sum) outcome follyr, by(cluster)
. gen ly=log(follyr)
. glm outcome bednet, f(poisson) l(log) offset(ly)
Generalised linear models              No. of obs      =        96
Optimisation      : ML                 Residual df     =        94
                                       Scale parameter =         1
Deviance          = 156.3093118        (1/df) Deviance  =  1.662865
Pearson           = 152.0580843        (1/df) Pearson   =  1.617639
Variance function : V(u)  = u          [Poisson]
Link function     : g(u)  = ln(u)      [Log]

                                       AIC             =   5.57401
Log likelihood    = -265.552465        BIC             = -272.7394
```

(continued)

BOX 10.3   (CONTINUED)

```
                           OIM
   outcome|    Coef.  Std. Err.     z     P>|z|  [95% Conf. Interval]
   bednet| -.172759  .0685161    -2.52  0.012   -.307048    -.03847
    _cons| -3.577404 .0465746   -76.81  0.000   -3.668689  -3.486119
      ly|  (offset)
```

. glm outcome bednet, f(poisson) l(log) offset(ly) eform

```
                           OIM
   outcome|    IRR Std. Err.       z    P>|z|  [95% Conf. Interval]
   bednet|  .8413404 .0576453    -2.52  0.012   .7356153   .9622606
      ly|  (offset)
```

. glm outcome bednet, f(poisson) l(log) offset(ly) scale(x2)

```
Generalised linear models              No. of obs      =       96
Optimisation        : ML               Residual df     =       94
                                       Scale parameter =        1
Deviance           = 156.3093118       (1/df) Deviance = 1.662865
Pearson            = 152.0580843       (1/df) Pearson  = 1.617639
Variance function : V(u) = u           [Poisson]
Link function     : g(u) = ln(u)       [Log]
                                       AIC             =  5.57401
Log likelihood    = -265.552465        BIC             = -272.7394
```

```
                           OIM
   outcome|    Coef.  Std. Err.     z     P>|z|  [95% Conf. Interval]
   bednet| -.172759  .0871431    -1.98  0.047   -.3435564  -.0019616
    _cons| -3.577404 .0592366   -60.39  0.000   -3.693506  -3.461302
      ly|  (offset)
```

(Standard errors scaled using square root of Pearson X2-based dispersion)

. glm outcome bednet, f(poisson) l(log) offset(ly) scale(x2) eform

```
                           OIM
   outcome|    IRR Std. Err.       z    P>|z|  [95% Conf. Interval]
   bednet| .8413404  .073317    -1.98  0.047   .7092435   .9980404
      ly|  (offset)
```

(Standard errors scaled using square root of Pearson X2-based dispersion)

10.6 Nonparametric Methods

10.6.1 Introduction

The methods presented in Section 10.3 and Section 10.5 are based on use of the *t* distribution. Their validity depends on the assumption that the cluster-level summaries, unadjusted or adjusted, are normally distributed. As we have indicated, simulation studies have shown that these methods are remarkably robust to departures from this assumption, particularly when there are equal numbers of clusters in each treatment arm. This robustness results essentially from the *central limit theorem*, which ensures that the sampling distribution of the *mean* of cluster summaries is approximately normal, even if the distribution of the cluster summaries is markedly non-normal.

Clearly, however, there are limits to this robustness. In particular, when there are small numbers of clusters in each treatment arm, the above methods will be less robust to non-normality of the underlying distribution of cluster summaries. Unfortunately, when there are so few values in each treatment arm, this is also a situation where it is very difficult to make a reliable *assessment* of whether the distribution is non-normal.

In these circumstances, it may be advisable to adopt a nonparametric procedure that does not rely on the assumption of normality and that is resistant to outliers. This might be done either to supplement or replace inference based on the *t* distribution. We present some simple nonparametric approaches below. The main advantage of these methods is that they should provide valid *p*-values irrespective of the underlying distributional form. Disadvantages are that they are somewhat less powerful than the parametric methods when the distributional assumptions underlying those methods are valid, and that the main emphasis is on significance testing while obtaining nonparametric confidence intervals is less straightforward.

10.6.2 Rank Sum Test

Wilcoxon's *rank sum test* is the best known nonparametric alternative to the unpaired *t*-test. The cluster summaries from the two treatment arms under comparison are pooled and ranked, and the sum of the ranks in the intervention arm is compared with its sampling distribution under the null hypothesis to obtain a *p*-value. In practice, a normal approximation to the sampling distribution is often used.

Let T_i be the sum of the ranks in the ith treatment arm. Then we compute the test statistic:

$$z = \frac{T_1 - c_1(c_1 + c_0 + 1)/2}{\sqrt{c_1 c_0 (c_1 + c_0 + 1)/12}} \tag{10.10}$$

and refer this to tables of the standard normal distribution. If there are fewer than about 15 clusters per treatment arm, it is advisable to use exact percentage points for z which are available in published tables.

The null hypothesis is that the two sets of observations are sampled from the same underlying distribution, and the rank sum test is sensitive to a *shift* in one distribution compared to the other. If the mean rank for the intervention clusters is significantly higher than that for the control clusters, this provides evidence that the distribution of cluster summaries in the intervention arm is shifted to the right.

Note that, while the rank sum test will be more robust than the t-test for small numbers of clusters, it may have lower power. In particular, however large the difference between treatment arms, it is impossible to obtain a two-sided p-value of less than 0.05 unless we have at least four clusters per arm in an unmatched CRT.

Example 10.9

Figure 10.1 shows that the distributions of cluster-level rates in the Ghana bednet trial were reasonably symmetric. Also, there was a fairly large number of clusters $(c = 48)$ in each treatment arm in this trial, and we can therefore expect the t-test to perform robustly under these circumstances.

However, we demonstrate the use of the *rank sum test* to analyse these data. Table 10.5 shows the results of the test for the unadjusted analysis, based on cluster-level rates, and for the adjusted analysis, based on ratio-residuals (the ratio of observed to expected events in each cluster).

In the unadjusted analysis, the sum of ranks in the intervention arm was 2076, less than the 2328 expected in each arm under the null hypothesis. The test-statistic was computed from Equation 10.10 as:

$$z = \frac{2076 - 2328}{\sqrt{18,624}} = -1.847$$

Referring this to tables of the standard normal distribution, we obtain a two-sided $p = 0.065$, slightly lower than the p-value of 0.091 obtained using the t-test.

Using the ratio-residuals R_i, we obtain $p = 0.052$, very similar to the p-value of 0.054 from the adjusted t-test.

These results can be obtained using the *ranksum* command in Stata, as shown in Box 10.4.

10.6.3 Permutation Tests

In practice, the rank sum test often loses surprisingly little power compared with the corresponding parametric test. However, a more powerful alternative is available which retains the robustness of nonparametric methods. The *permutation test* is based on the observation that if the intervention has no effect, then randomly permuting the allocation of clusters between treatment arms should have no systematic effect on the observed effect measure.

TABLE 10.5

Results of the Rank Sum Test for Effects of the Intervention on Child Mortality in the Ghana Bednet Trial, Compared with Results of the *t*-test

	Intervention Arm	Control Arm	*p*-value
Number of clusters	48	48	
Unadjusted analysis			
Rank sum	2076	2580	
Expected rank sum	2328	2328	
Rank sum test			0.065
t-test			0.091
*Adjusted analysis**			
Rank sum	2063	2593	
Expected rank sum	2328	2328	
Rank sum test			0.052
t-test			0.054

*Based on ratio-residuals from a Poisson regression of child mortality on age-group and sex.

BOX 10.4

```
. ranksum r, by(bednet)
Two-sample Wilcoxon rank-sum (Mann-Whitney) test

        bednet |      obs       rank sum        expected
  -------------+-----------------------------------------
             0 |       48           2580            2328
             1 |       48           2076            2328
  -------------+-----------------------------------------
      combined |       96           4656            4656

unadjusted variance  18624.00
adjustment for ties      0.00
                     ---------
adjusted variance    18624.00

Ho: r(bednet==0) = r(bednet==1)
           z =  1.847
    Prob > |z| = 0.0648

. ranksum residr, by(bednet)
Two-sample Wilcoxon rank-sum (Mann-Whitney) test

        bednet |      obs       rank sum        expected
  -------------+-----------------------------------------
             0 |       48           2593            2328
             1 |       48           2063            2328
  -------------+-----------------------------------------
      combined |       96           4656            4656

unadjusted variance  18624.00
adjustment for ties      0.00
                     ---------
adjusted variance    18624.00

Ho: residr(bednet==0) = residr(bednet==1)
           z =  1.942
    Prob > |z| = 0.0522
```

In the simplest case of an unpaired CRT with two treatment arms, there are

$$^{c_1+c_0}C_{c_1} = \frac{(c_1+c_0)!}{c_1!c_0!}$$

ways of selecting which c_1 clusters will be allocated to the intervention arm and, if *unrestricted randomisation* is used, all of these permutations are equally likely. The permutation test proceeds by computing the observed intervention effect measure (for example, the rate ratio or rate difference) for each of these permutations. If the null hypothesis is true, and there is no intervention effect, then the observed effect measure can be regarded as having been randomly selected from this permutation distribution. Thus, a p-value is obtained as the proportion of all permutations giving an effect measure at least as extreme as the one observed.

For large numbers of clusters, the number of permutations may become too large for this procedure to be computationally feasible. In this case, we may instead select a random sample of permutations and work with this in place of the full permutation distribution. A sample of 5000 permutations should generally be sufficient; for example, a p-value of around 0.05 would be estimated to within about 0.006 of the true value based on the full permutation distribution.

Note also that, as for the rank sum test, at least four clusters per arm are needed to obtain a significant result (two-sided $p < 0.05$) using the permutation test. It may be shown that the rank sum is in fact the permutation test based on ranks rather than the original observations.

Example 10.10

In the Ghana bednet trial there were a total of 96 clusters, with 48 in each treatment arm. The total number of permutations was:

$$^{96}C_{48} = \frac{96!}{48! \times 48!} = 6.44 \times 10^{27}$$

which is an extremely large number. Rather than computing the test statistic for all possible permutations we select a random sample of 5000 permutations. For each of these permutations, we compute the rate difference based on the means of cluster rates in the two arms. This can be readily done using the *permute* command in Stata, as shown in Box 10.5.

The permutation distribution based on this sample of 5000 is shown in Figure 10.2. Note that it is very close to a normal distribution, which is not surprising given the relatively large number of clusters. The Stata output in Box 10.5 indicates that 448 of the 5000 permutations gave a rate difference further from zero than the observed difference of -3.95 per 1000 person-years, so that the two-sided p-value is given by:

$$p = \frac{448}{5000} = 0.090$$

and this is in close agreement with the result of the unpaired t-test ($p = 0.091$).

BOX 10.5

```
permute r d=(r(mu_2)-r(mu_1)), saving(permute5) reps(5000) :
ttest r, by(bednet)
```

Monte Carlo permutation results   Number of obs = 96

command   : ttest r, by(bednet)

d   : r(mu_2)-r(mu_1)

permute var: r

T	T(obs)	c	n	p=c/n	SE(p)	[95% Conf.	Interval]
d	-.0039509	448	5000	0.0896	0.0040	.0818248	.0978581

Note: Confidence interval is with respect to p=c/n.
Note: c = #{|T| >= |T(obs)|}

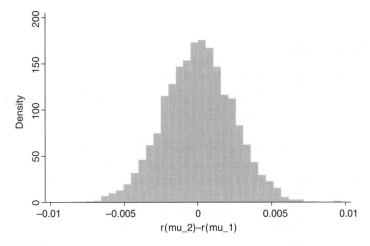

FIGURE 10.2

Histogram showing permutation distribution of rate difference based on mortality data from Ghana bednet trial (random sample of 5000 permutations).

A further application of this procedure is to allow for the use of *restricted randomisation* in the design of a CRT. It is common to ignore this feature of the design during the analysis, but use of the permutation test based on the restricted set of possible treatment allocations allows investigators to check the validity of their inferences.

In this case, the permutation distribution is derived by selecting all permutations that satisfy the pre-defined balance criteria, and evaluating the observed value of the test statistic against this distribution. When there are a very large number of acceptable permutations, this may again be achieved by sampling from the permutation distribution.

Example 10.11

Previously in this chapter we have analysed the SHARE trial of sexual health education ignoring the restricted randomisation that was used in the design of this trial. The approach to randomisation was described in Example 6.3. Briefly, the allocation of the 25 schools was restricted to achieve balance across geographical clusters, ethnic background of the students and a balance score based on 12 other variables.

In analysing this trial, the investigators computed the test statistic ($D =$ difference in mean outcome between arms) based on the observed data and evaluated this against the permutation distribution of test statistics obtained from a total of 20,000 allocations that could have been selected. A confidence interval for Δ (the true difference between means) was also obtained by testing the hypothesis $\Delta = K$ for different values of K and finding the values for which the two-sided p-value would be 0.05.

For the knowledge score among male students discussed in Example 10.6, they reported a p-value of 0.003 and a 95% confidence interval for the mean difference of (0.2, 1.2). These compare with $p < 0.001$ and a 95% confidence interval of (0.30, 0.94) obtained in Example 10.6.

10.7 Analysing for Effect Modification

In most randomised controlled trials, the primary objective is to measure the overall effect of an intervention in a defined study population. In some cases, however, a secondary objective is to examine whether the effect of the intervention differs between subgroups of individuals defined by values of a specified covariate. If it does vary, we say that the covariate is an *effect modifier* or, equivalently, that there is *interaction* between the intervention effect and the covariate. It is well known that in most trials the power to detect such interactions is low, and thus important interactions will often go unreported. When investigating an interaction of interest, it is best to report a *confidence interval* for the interaction effect, which will show how much precision was available for its assessment.

Similar subgroup analyses may also be of interest in CRTs. As for individually randomised trials, the power of such analyses is often low and cautious interpretation is needed. The cost and logistical challenges involved in CRTs mean that it is often difficult to recruit sufficient clusters to adequately address the primary objective of the trial, let alone to permit subgroup analyses to be carried out with adequate power.

In CRTs, it is helpful to distinguish between effect modification by *cluster-level* covariates and *individual-level* covariates. For a cluster-level covariate, we can simply carry out separate analyses for the relevant subgroups of clusters. For example, if we have 20 clusters overall (10 in each study arm) and wish to examine whether the effect of intervention is the same in the 10 urban clusters and the 10 rural clusters, we can carry out two separate analyses to obtain estimates of effect in these two strata, with appropriate confidence intervals and p-values. To examine whether any differences in effect may be due to chance, we can perform an *analysis of variance* on the 20 cluster-level summaries, with terms for intervention effect, urban/rural stratum and the interaction between them. More generally, for example if we wish to examine effect modification by a quantitative cluster-level variable, we can use linear regression of cluster-level summaries for this purpose.

More often, we wish to examine for effect modification by an individual-level covariate. For example, we may wish to compare the effect of the intervention in males and females. As before, we can obtain subgroup-specific estimates of intervention effect by carrying out a separate analysis in each subgroup using the methods discussed earlier in this chapter. However, comparison of these effect measures needs to take into account the correlations that occur because they are obtained from the same set of clusters.

For binary covariates, where we wish to compare intervention effects in two subgroups, a simple method of analysis is available (Cheung et al. 2008). For simplicity we present this for event rates, but the extension to other types of endpoints is obvious. Suppose the observed rate in the kth subgroup ($k=0$ or 1) in the jth cluster in the ith treatment arm is denoted as r_{ijk}. If the *rate difference* is the effect measure of interest, we can estimate the rate differences in the two subgroups (for example males and females) as:

$$\hat{\lambda}_{11} - \hat{\lambda}_{01} = \bar{r}_{11} - \bar{r}_{01} = \sum_j \frac{r_{1j1}}{c_1} - \sum_j \frac{r_{0j1}}{c_0}$$

and

$$\hat{\lambda}_{10} - \hat{\lambda}_{00} = \bar{r}_{10} - \bar{r}_{00} = \sum_j \frac{r_{1j0}}{c_1} - \sum_j \frac{r_{0j0}}{c_0}$$

respectively. Then we note that the interaction effect can be estimated by

$$(\hat{\lambda}_{11} - \hat{\lambda}_{01}) - (\hat{\lambda}_{10} - \hat{\lambda}_{00}) = (\hat{\lambda}_{11} - \hat{\lambda}_{10}) - (\hat{\lambda}_{01} - \hat{\lambda}_{00}) = (\bar{r}_{11} - \bar{r}_{10}) - (\bar{r}_{01} - \bar{r}_{00})$$

$$= \sum_j \frac{r_{1j1} - r_{1j0}}{c_1} - \sum_j \frac{r_{0j1} - r_{0j0}}{c_0}$$

In other words, we can compute the difference in rates between males and females in each cluster and then compare the mean difference in the intervention and control arms.

A test for interaction can then be carried out by performing an unpaired t-test on the cluster-level differences between the two subgroups, and this also provides a confidence interval for the interaction effect. If instead the *rate ratio* is the effect measure of interest, and we wish to examine whether the relative effect of the intervention differs between males and females, we simply replace the cluster-level rates by log-rates.

Example 10.12

In Example 10.6, we analysed the effects of the Project SHARE intervention on knowledge of sexual health in boys and girls. Basing our analysis on means of cluster summaries (Table 10.3), the mean difference in knowledge score was 0.62 (95% CI: 0.30, 0.94) in boys and 0.37 (95% CI: –0.10, 0.83) in girls. We concluded that there was strong evidence of an intervention effect on knowledge among boys ($p < 0.001$) but not among girls ($p = 0.12$).

Computing the difference in mean scores between girls and boys in each school, and averaging across schools, we find that the mean difference was 0.96 (SD = 0.41) in control schools but only 0.71 (SD = 0.39) in intervention schools. Comparing these mean differences using the *t*-test, we obtain $t = 1.58$ with 23 df, giving $p = 0.13$. We conclude that while the observed effect of the intervention was greater in boys, this difference may have occurred by chance. Box 10.6 shows how the analyses of effects in boys and girls as well as the analysis for effect modification can be carried out in Stata.

BOX 10.6

```
. use share.dta

. gen male=1 if sex==1

. gen female=1 if sex==2

. gen mscore=kscore*male

. gen fscore=kscore*female

. collapse mscore fscore arm, by(school)

. ttest mscore, by(arm)

Two-sample t test with equal variances
-------------------------------------------------------------------------------
   Group |  Obs     Mean   Std. Err.  Std. Dev.  [95% Conf.  Interval]
---------+---------------------------------------------------------------------
       0 |   12  3.619255   .125265   .4339306   3.343549   3.894962
       1 |   13  4.240223  .0958151   .3454663    4.03146   4.448987
---------+---------------------------------------------------------------------
combined |   25  3.942159  .0992435   .4962177    3.73733   4.146987
---------+---------------------------------------------------------------------
    diff |        -.620968  .1562391             -.9441732  -.2977628
-------------------------------------------------------------------------------
    diff = mean(0) - mean(1)                              t =  -3.9745
Ho: diff = 0                            degrees of freedom =       23

    Ha: diff < 0              Ha: diff != 0                 Ha: diff > 0
Pr(T < t) = 0.0003     Pr(|T| > |t|) = 0.0006      Pr(T > t) = 0.9997

. ttest fscore, by(arm)

Two-sample t test with equal variances
-------------------------------------------------------------------------------
   Group |  Obs     Mean   Std. Err.  Std. Dev.  [95% Conf.  Interval]
---------+---------------------------------------------------------------------
       0 |   12  4.579741  .1585442   .5492131   4.230788   4.928694
       1 |   13  4.946484  .1603183   .5780358    4.59718   5.295787
---------+---------------------------------------------------------------------
combined |   25  4.770447  .1166674   .5833371   4.529658   5.011237
---------+---------------------------------------------------------------------
    diff |        -.3667428  .2259547             -.8341658   .1006801
-------------------------------------------------------------------------------
```

(continued)

BOX 10.6 (CONTINUED)

```
   diff = mean(0) - mean(1)                                    t =-1.6231
Ho: diff = 0                                   degrees of freedom =     23

   Ha: diff < 0                Ha: diff != 0                Ha: diff > 0
Pr(T < t) = 0.0591      Pr(|T| > |t|) = 0.1182      Pr(T > t) = 0.9409

. gen dscore=fscore-mscore

. ttest dscore, by(arm)
```

Two-sample *t* test with equal variances

Group	Obs	Mean	Std. Err.	Std. Dev.	[95% Conf.	Interval]
0	12	.9604858	.1183986	.4101449	.6998921	1.221079
1	13	.7062606	.1091896	.3936886	.4683569	.9441642
combined	25	.8282887	.0828009	.4140044	.6573961	.9991812
diff		.2542252	.1607859	-.0783859	.5868363	

```
   diff = mean(0) - mean(1)                                    t = 1.5811
Ho: diff = 0                                   degrees of freedom =     23

   Ha: diff < 0                Ha: diff != 0                Ha: diff > 0
Pr(T < t) = 0.9362      Pr(|T| > |t|) = 0.1275      Pr(T > t) = 0.0638
```

11

Regression Analysis Based on Individual-level Data

11.1 Introduction

In Chapter 10, we presented methods for the analysis of CRTs based on cluster-level summaries. We also discussed how these methods can be extended to adjust for covariates measured at either cluster level or individual level. As we noted, these methods have been shown to perform robustly over a wide range of circumstances. In particular, they provide reliable results when there are a relatively small number of clusters in each treatment arm, as is the case in many CRTs.

However, these cluster-level methods also have a number of important disadvantages:

- They are not the most *efficient* method of analysis, particularly when there is substantial variation in the sample size per cluster. This is because equal weight is given in the analysis to each cluster-level summary, regardless of whether it is based on a large or a small sample size. Greater power and smaller standard errors could be obtained by weighting the cluster summaries according to the amount of information provided by each cluster. While there are procedures such as the *weighted t-test* (see Section 10.3.5) that do this, they are not straightforward and lose the advantage of simplicity that the cluster-level methods provide.

- In a cluster-level analysis, the effects of the intervention and of other covariates are not analysed together in the same regression model. Rather we use a two-stage approach in which the cluster-level summaries at the second stage have already had the effects of other covariates removed. We might prefer an approach in which the joint effects of all risk factors, including both the intervention and other covariates, could be analysed together in the same model.

- Computationally, there is some loss of convenience in adopting a two-stage approach, although this is perhaps not a serious criticism given the robustness and conceptual simplicity of the two-stage methods.

In this chapter, we review a number of *regression models* than can be used to analyse CRTs. These are single-stage methods, which allow us to analyse the effects of the intervention and other covariates in the same model. They are extensions of simpler regression models that are well known in epidemiological research, but modified to allow for *intracluster correlation* or, equivalently, *between-cluster variation*. Despite their advantages, however, they do not perform reliably for the analysis of CRTs with less than around 15 clusters per arm, in the sense that significance tests and confidence intervals may not have the correct size and coverage.

A wide range of regression methods have been suggested for this purpose, but we will focus on two specific approaches that have received the widest attention and which have advantages over other methods.

Random effects models are presented in Section 11.2. In these models, we take account of between-cluster variation by assuming that there are cluster-level effects (over and above the random sampling variation within each cluster) which follow a specified probability distribution. The parameters of this distribution are estimated using *likelihood* methods at the same time as the intervention and covariate effects are estimated. These random effects models perform well for event rate data and quantitative outcomes, but are sometimes less satisfactory for analysing proportions.

An alternative is provided by *generalised estimating equations (GEE)*, which are discussed in Section 11.3. GEE analysis does not explicitly model the variation between clusters, but does take account of the *correlations* between observations within the same cluster. GEE provide a useful alternative to random effects models, particularly for *binary outcomes*, although they do not provide a full probability model for the data.

We illustrate both random effects models and GEE using the same case studies as in Chapter 10, and compare the results with those based on cluster-level summaries.

Section 11.4 summarises the methods presented in Chapters 10 and 11, and discusses the appropriate choice of method. In Section 11.5, we briefly discuss the use of individual-level regression to examine for *effect modification*.

Finally, in Section 11.6, more complex analyses are discussed briefly, including methods for CRTs in which there is more than one follow-up survey, and the analysis of event rates where each subject can experience repeated episodes of the outcome of interest.

11.2 Random Effects Models

In Section 9.3, we discussed how to identify the *parameters of interest* in a CRT, by writing down a *statistical model* for the outcome of interest. We presented several models, appropriate for different types of endpoints, which were all of the same general form:

$$\theta_{ijk} = \alpha + \beta_i + \sum_l \gamma_l z_{ijkl} + u_{ij} \tag{11.1}$$

In this equation, θ_{ijk} is a parameter related to the outcome of interest and refers to the kth individual in the jth cluster in the ith treatment arm. For event-rate data, for example, θ might be the logarithm of the rate in that individual. The parameter β_i represents the intervention effect (with $\beta_0 = 0$), the γ_l parameters represent the effects of a set of covariates, $z_1, z_2, \ldots z_L$, each of which may be measured at individual or cluster level, and α is an intercept term representing the expected outcome in individuals in the control arm and with zero values for all the covariates.

The term u_{ij} is a *random effect* relating to the jth cluster in the ith treatment arm, and this is the term in the model which takes account of *between-cluster variation*. As a result, all models of this form are known as *random effects models*. These effects are assumed to be sampled from a probability distribution, and the additional parameters associated with the random effects term have to be estimated when a random effects model is fitted. Because Equation 11.1 provides a full probability model for the data, it is possible to use *likelihood inference* to estimate the parameters associated with the random effects as well as the parameters representing the effects of the intervention and the covariates.

We shall now discuss the fitting of random effects models for event rates, means and proportions in turn.

11.2.1 Poisson and Cox Regressions with Random Effects

11.2.1.1 Poisson Regression with Random Effects

Poisson regression is the standard method for analysing event rate data in epidemiological studies. First consider a simple observational study, in which we wish to investigate the effects of a set of covariates $z_1, \ldots, z_L$ on the rate of an event of interest. The covariates may be quantitative variables or indicator variables representing the effects of grouped or categorical variables. The *Poisson regression model* states that for an individual or group of individuals with y_k person-years of follow-up and covariate values $z_{k1}, \ldots, z_{kL}$, the observed number of events d_k follows the *Poisson distribution* with mean:

$$E(d_k) = y_k \lambda_k$$

and a *log-linear model* is assumed for the *rate* λ_k:

$$\log(\lambda_k) = \alpha + \sum_l \beta_l z_{kl}$$

where the β_l are the *regression coefficients*.

Applying this model to a CRT, *with no allowance for clustering,* we assume that the number of events d_{ijk} in the kth individual or group of individuals in the jth cluster in the ith treatment arm follows the Poisson distribution with mean:

$$E(d_{ijk}) = y_{ijk}\lambda_{ijk}$$

and rate λ_{ijk} given by:

$$\log(\lambda_{ijk}) = \alpha + \beta_i + \sum_l \gamma_l z_{ijkl} \tag{11.2}$$

In this formulation, β_i represents the intervention effect while the γ_i represent the effects of other covariates. As we saw in Section 9.3.1, because this is a *log-linear model,* the parameter β_i represents the *rate ratio* for the ith treatment arm compared with the control arm ($i = 0$).

As it stands, this model makes no allowance for clustering, and assumes that all subjects with the same covariate values in all clusters in each treatment arm have the *same rate* of the outcome of interest. As we know, this is very unlikely to be the case, and there is likely to be additional *between-cluster variation.* This variation may be less if we have measured a range of important covariates that are predictive of risk, but adjusting for such covariates is unlikely to account completely for variations between clusters.

To account for such between-cluster variation, we modify Equation 11.2 as follows:

$$\log(\lambda_{ijk}) = \alpha + \beta_i + \sum_l \gamma_l z_{ijkl} + u_{ij} \tag{11.3}$$

In this *Poisson regression random effects model,* the log-rate is assumed to be reduced or increased by a random effect u_{ij}, which is assumed to be constant within each cluster. Equivalently, the model may be written in terms of the rate rather than the log-rate:

$$\lambda_{ijk} = \exp\left(\alpha + \beta_i + \sum_l \gamma_l z_{ijkl} \right) \times v_{ij}$$

where

$$v_{ij} = \exp(u_{ij})$$

To fit the Poisson regression random effects model to data, we need to make an assumption about the probability distribution of the random effects. The most common assumption is that the v_{ij} follow the *gamma distribution* with mean 1 and variance α', where we use the notation α' to distinguish this parameter from the intercept term α in the regression model. The assumed distribution for the random effect u_{ij} in Equation 11.3 is therefore the *log-gamma*.

The *gamma distribution* is a family of positively skewed distributions and is shown in Figure 11.1 for various values of α'. It is chosen for this purpose for two main reasons. First, rates are constrained to be positive and often have a positively skewed distribution. Second, if we assume that the random effects follow the gamma distribution, it may be shown that a simple analytical form exists for the probability distribution of the number of events. In fact, the combination of the Poisson distribution with gamma random effects implies that the numbers of events in clusters follow the *negative binomial distribution*. This facilitates model-fitting using likelihood inference. It should be noted, however, that in circumstances where a single individual may experience multiple episodes of the event of interest, this may introduce an additional level of correlation. We consider this scenario in Section 11.6.3.

Poisson regression random effects models can readily be fitted using Stata, as illustrated by Box 11.1.

Example 11.1

We return to the results of the Ghana bednet trial, previously analysed in Chapter 10 (Binka et al. 1996). We first review the results of the simple unadjusted analyses presented in Example 10.3 and Example 10.5. In this CRT, all-cause child mortality was compared in 48 clusters provided with insecticide-impregnated bednets and 48 control clusters. The mortality rate ratio in the intervention arm compared with

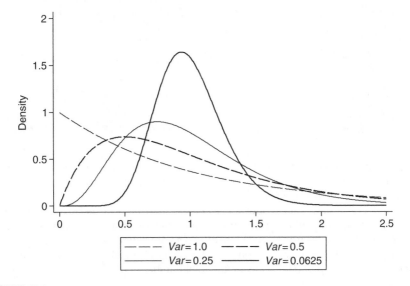

FIGURE 11.1
Illustrating the shape of the gamma distribution with mean 1 and different values of the variance α'.

BOX 11.1

```
. xi:poisson outcome i.bednet, exp(follyr) irr

Poisson regression                      Number of obs    =      26342
                                        LR chi2(1)       =       6.38
                                        Prob > chi2      =     0.0116
Log likelihood = -4888.6152             Pseudo R2        =     0.0007
------------------------------------------------------------------------
     outcome    IRR Std.  Err.    z    P>|z|  [95% Conf. Interval]
------------+-----------------------------------------------------------
 _ Ibednet _ 1   .8413404 .0576453  -2.52  0.012  .7356154      .9622607
      follyr  (exposure)
------------------------------------------------------------------------

. xi:xtpoisson outcome i.bednet, exp(follyr) irr i(cluster) re

Random-effects Poisson regression       Number of obs    =      26342
Group variable: cluster                 Number of groups =         96

Random effects u _ i ~ Gamma            Obs per group: min =        138
                                                       avg =      274.4
                                                       max =        439

                                        Wald chi2(1)     =       3.70
Log likelihood  = -4882.7073            Prob > chi2      =     0.0544
------------------------------------------------------------------------
     outcome    IRR Std.  Err.    z    P>|z|  [95% Conf. Interval]
------------+-----------------------------------------------------------
 _ Ibednet _ 1   .8472471 .0729997  -1.92  0.054  .7155989     1.003114
      follyr  (exposure)
------------+-----------------------------------------------------------
   /lnalpha   -2.764239 .4069338           -3.561814     -1.966663
------------+-----------------------------------------------------------
      alpha    .0630241 .0256466            .0283873       .139923
------------------------------------------------------------------------
Likelihood-ratio test of alpha = 0: chibar2(01) = 11.82 Prob >= chibar2 = 0.000

. est store A

. xi:xtpoisson outcome, exp(follyr) irr i(cluster) re

. est store B

. lrtest A B

Likelihood-ratio test                   LR chi2(1)       =       3.61
(Assumption: B nested in A)             Prob > chi2      =     0.0574
```

the control arm, based on individual-level data, was 0.841. The rate ratio based on cluster summaries was 0.859 with a 95% CI of (0.721, 1.023). The unpaired *t*-test gave a two-sided *p*-value of 0.091.

Box 11.1 shows Stata output for a Poisson regression of mortality on treatment arm, ignoring all other covariates. Note that identical results are obtained in these analyses regardless of whether the data are entered as *individual records* (showing the outcome and person-years for each individual in each cluster) or as cluster-level *grouped data* (showing the total number of deaths and total number of person-years per cluster).

In the first part of the output, clustering is ignored. In this standard *Poisson regression* analysis, the estimated rate ratio is 0.841, and note that this is *identical* to the simple rate ratio based on individual-level data. The 95% confidence interval for this rate ratio is (0.736, 0.962) and a likelihood ratio test of the null hypothesis of no treatment effect gives a χ^2 of 6.38 on 1df, and a p-value of 0.012. It is important to note that this analysis is *invalid* since it ignores the effects of the clustered design. For this reason, we would expect the p-value to be too small and the confidence interval too narrow.

To take account of clustering, we now repeat the analysis using a *Poisson regression random effects* model. The results are shown in the second part of the output. The estimated rate ratio now becomes 0.847 with a 95% CI of (0.716, 1.003). The Wald test, obtained by comparing the estimated regression coefficient with its standard error, gives a p-value of 0.054, as shown in the output. However, it is preferable to use a likelihood ratio test, obtained by comparing the likelihoods of random effects models with and without the intervention effect, and this gives $p = 0.057$. In any case, it is clear that the evidence of a treatment effect is much weaker than was suggested by the incorrect analysis that took no account of clustering, and the 95% confidence interval includes the null value.

We note also that the output provides a significance test of the null hypothesis that the parameter α' is zero. This is a formal test of clustering, and gives $p<0.001$. There is therefore very strong evidence of between-cluster variability in mortality, over and above the random variability consistent with the Poisson distribution. Even when this test is non-significant, however, we recommend using the random effects model. A nonsignificant result does *not* prove that there is no clustering, and by using the random effects model we ensure that we take account of any clustering that may be present. If there is little clustering, the estimate, confidence interval and p-value will be very similar to the results of the analysis ignoring clustering.

It may be helpful to get some idea of the meaning of the estimated α' parameter, which is 0.063 in this analysis. Since α' corresponds to the variance of the cluster-level v_{ij} multiplying factors, we can conclude that the true rate in individual clusters would vary roughly between the values:

$$\hat{\lambda}_{ij} \times \left(1 \pm 1.96 \times \sqrt{0.063}\right)$$

or from $(\hat{\lambda} \times 0.51)$ to $(\lambda \times 1.49)$ and note that this is quite a wide level of variability. Also, note from Figure 11.1 that an α' of 0.063 corresponds to a gamma distribution that is very nearly symmetric.

We now move on to analyses adjusted for covariates. Box 11.2 shows the Stata output for the analysis *adjusted* for age-group (coded 0: 6–11 months, 1: 12–23 months, 2: 24–35 months, 3: 36–47 months, 4: 48–59 months) and sex (coded 0: males, 1: females). To carry out this analysis, the data have to be entered either as *individual records* or as *grouped data* with one record for each age/sex group in each cluster, and again the results are identical whichever approach is taken.

The output shows an adjusted rate ratio for the intervention effect of 0.837 with a 95% CI of (0.710, 0.988). The likelihood ratio test, obtained by comparing likelihoods between the random effects models with and without the intervention effect, but including the effects of age-group and sex, gives a p-value of 0.038,

BOX 11.2

```
. xi:xtpoisson outcome i.bednet i.agegp i.sex, exp(follyr) irr i(cluster) re

Random-effects Poisson regression        Number of obs        =      26342
Group variable: cluster                  Number of groups     =         96

Random effects u _ i ~ Gamma             Obs per group: min   =        138
                                                        avg   =      274.4
                                                        max   =        439

                                         Wald chi2(6)          =     324.58
Log likelihood  =   -4701.0646           Prob > chi2           =     0.0000
```

outcome	IRR Std. Err.		z	P>|z|	[95% Conf.	Interval]
_Ibednet _ 1	.8374889	.070685	-2.10	0.036	.7098012	.9881467
_Iagegp _ 1	.3969492	.0383497	-9.56	0.000	.3284728	.4797008
_Iagegp _ 2	.2990543	.0308447	-11.70	0.000	.2443186	.3660527
_Iagegp _ 3	.1715907	.0256085	-11.81	0.000	.1280734	.2298946
_Iagegp _ 4	.1827192	.0416134	-7.46	0.000	.1169304	.2855229
_Isex _ 1	.9422119	.0644793	-0.87	0.384	.8239436	1.077456
follyr	(exposure)					
/lnalpha	-2.881458	.4360814			-3.736162	-2.026755
alpha	.056053	.0244437			.0238454	.1317625

```
Likelihood-ratio test of alpha=0: chibar2(01) = 9.80 Prob>=chibar2 =   0.001

. est store C

. xi:xtpoisson outcome i.agegp i.sex, exp(follyr) irr i(cluster) re

. est store D

. lrtest C D

Likelihood-ratio test                    LR chi2(1)    =       4.30
(Assumption: D nested in C)              Prob > chi2   =     0.0381
```

very similar to the Wald test for the intervention effect. The estimate of α' is 0.056, slightly lower than in the unadjusted analysis, presumably because some of the between-cluster variation is accounted for by cluster variations in age/sex distribution, but nevertheless the clustering (between-cluster variation) remains highly significant, with $p = 0.001$.

The results of the adjusted and unadjusted analyses are shown in Table 11.1. The point estimates, confidence intervals and p-values given by the cluster-level analysis and regression analysis are all fairly similar, and in both cases the evidence of an intervention effect is strengthened after adjusting for age and sex. Note however, that the Poisson regression random effects model provides a somewhat smaller p-value and narrower confidence interval for the rate ratio. This is likely because the regression analysis makes more efficient use of the data, giving more weight to clusters that provide more information because of a larger sample size.

A further advantage of the regression analysis is that we obtain estimates of the effects of age and sex in the same model output (see Box 11.2). We note that there

TABLE 11.1

Summary of Unadjusted and Adjusted Analyses of the Ghana Bednet Trial Using Cluster-level Summaries and Poisson Regression Random Effects Models

	Cluster-level Analysis	**Poisson Regression Random Effects Model**
Unadjusted Analysis		
Rate ratio	0.859	0.847
95% CI	(0.721, 1.023)	(0.716, 1.003)
p-value	0.091	0.057
*Adjusted Analysis**		
Adjusted rate ratio	0.844	0.837
95% CI	(0.713, 0.999)	(0.710, 0.988)
p-value	0.054	0.038

*Adjusted for age-group and sex.

was a clear downward trend in mortality with increasing age, but no difference in mortality between boys and girls.

The regression analysis can readily be extended to incorporate further variables in the model, for example to adjust for additional covariates or to test for *interactions* between the intervention effect and covariates.

In the above analysis, we adjusted for age at enrolment. This analysis could be further refined by dividing up the observation time for each child into several age-bands, for example using the *stsplit* command in Stata, and adjusting instead for *current age*. In Example 11.2, we discuss how this may alternatively be done by using *Cox regression* with the time variable defined as current age.

11.2.1.2 Cox Regression with Random Effects

Up to this point, we have used Poisson models to handle count data and to compare incidence rates between intervention and control arms. *Survival analysis* techniques, which model the time until an event occurs, can yield greater power to detect an intervention effect on disease occurrence. For each study participant, the outcome consists of the length of time from the start of observation until the earliest of occurrence of the event or censoring of information, where censoring is usually due to either loss to follow-up or study termination.

Accounting for within-cluster correlation can be handled with a random effects model in a manner similar to that of the Poisson regression model discussed above, with participants in a cluster sharing the same underlying risk multiplier v_{ij}, usually also taken to follow a gamma distribution. Such a survival model is also known as a *shared frailty* model. Although parametric models can be used, in public health applications the *Cox proportional hazards model* is the most common, as it does not require specification of the shape of the baseline hazard function and hence has an added measure of robustness. A full discussion of survival models is beyond the scope of this book, as they are not often employed in CRTs, but the following example gives a flavour of how they can be used in this context.

Example 11.2

Continuing with the analysis of the Ghana bednet trial, we first model the time from entry to death or censoring. Ignoring clustering, and fitting a standard Cox model (Box 11.3), we obtain an estimated hazard ratio of 0.842 with 95% confidence interval (0.736, 0.963) and a *p*-value of 0.012, all very similar to the Poisson regression results. We now proceed to allow for clustering by using the *shared* frailty option. This gives an estimated hazard ratio of 0.848 with 95% confidence interval (0.717, 1.002) and *p*-value 0.053, again very similar to the results of the Poisson regression random effects model.

To adjust for age, we can either incorporate terms for age at enrolment in the regression model (as in Example 11.1), or redefine age as our time variable as shown in Box 11.3. In this case, we have *staggered entry times* with each child entering follow-up at their age at enrolment. Adjusting sex by incorporating an additional term in the Cox regression model, the shared frailty model gives an adjusted hazard ratio of 0.836 with 95% confidence interval (0.709, 0.985) and *p*-value 0.032, again very similar to the results of the Poisson regression random effects model.

11.2.2 Mixed Effects Linear Regression

We turn now to the analysis of *quantitative* outcome variables. The standard method for analysing risk factors that influence the *mean* of such a variable is *linear regression*. Suppose x_k is the observed value of the outcome for the kth individual, and that there is a set of measured covariates $z_{k1}, \ldots, z_{kL}$ as before. Then the *linear regression model* assumes that x_k is normally distributed with mean μ_k and variance σ^2, where μ_k is given by:

$$E(x_k) = \mu_k = \alpha + \sum_l \beta_l z_{kl}$$

The corresponding model for a CRT, where *no allowance is made for clustering* is given by:

$$\mu_{ijk} = \alpha + \beta_i + \sum_l \gamma_l z_{ijkl}$$

where μ_{ijk} is the mean for the kth individual in the jth cluster in the ith treatment arm, β_i represents the intervention effect and the γ_l represent the effects of the covariates. Note that, in contrast to Section 11.2.1, this model is written in terms of μ_k rather than $\log(\mu_k)$. It is therefore an *additive* model, providing an estimate of the *difference of means* between treatment arms, whereas *Poisson regression* is a *multiplicative* model which provides estimates of the *rate ratio*.

BOX 11.3

```
stset follyr, fail(outcome)
```

```
-----------------------------------------------------------------
   26342   total obs.
       0   exclusions
-----------------------------------------------------------------
   26342   obs. remaining, representing
     857   failures in single record/single failure data
33335.92   total analysis time at risk, at risk from t   =       0
                          earliest observed entry t   =       0
                            last observed exit t   =       2
```

```
. stcox bednet
```

```
            failure _d:   outcome
      analysis time _t:   follyr
```

Cox regression -- Breslow method for ties

```
No. of subjects   =       26342     Number of obs      =     26342
No. of failures   =         857
Time at risk      =   33335.9203
                                    LR chi2(1)         =      6.33
Log likelihood    =   -8490.1856    Prob > chi2        =    0.0119
```

_t	Haz. Ratio	Std. Err.	z	P>|z|	[95% Conf. Interval]	
bednet	.8418857	.0576827	-2.51	0.012	.736092	.9628844

```
. stcox bednet, shared(cluster)
```

```
            failure _d:   outcome
      analysis time _t:   follyr
```

Cox regression --
```
      Breslow method for ties     Number of obs      =     26342
      Gamma shared frailty         Number of groups   =        96
Group variable: cluster
```

```
No. of subjects   =       26342     Obs per group: min  =       138
No. of failures   =         857                     avg  =  274.3958
Time at risk      =   33335.9203                     max  =       439
                                    Wald chi2(1)        =      3.73
Log likelihood    =   -8484.7665    Prob > chi2         =    0.0533
```

_t	Haz. Ratio	Std. Err.	z	P>|z|	[95% Conf. Interval]	
bednet	.8479882	.0723588	-1.93	0.053	.7173924	1.002358
theta	.0598043	.025127				

Likelihood-ratio test of theta=0: chibar2(01) = 10.84 Prob>=chibar2 = 0.000

(continued)

BOX 11.3   (CONTINUED)

```
. gen enter=agemn/12

. gen exit=enter+follyr

. stset exit, fail(outcome) enter(enter)
--------------------------------------------------------------------
    26342  total obs.
        0  exclusions
--------------------------------------------------------------------
    26342  obs. remaining, representing
      857  failures in single record/single failure data
 33335.92  total analysis time at risk, at risk from t     =          0
                            earliest observed entry t      =   .5010267
                               last observed exit t        =   4.997947

. stcox bednet sex, shared(cluster)

              failure _d:   outcome
        analysis time _t:   exit
        enter on or after:  time enter


Cox regression --
          Breslow method for ties        Number of obs    =      26342
          Gamma shared frailty           Number of groups =         96
Group variable: cluster


No. of subjects    =          26342   Obs per group: min  =        138
No. of failures    =            857                  avg  =   274.3958
Time at risk       =       33335.9203                max  =        439
                                       Wald chi2(2)        =       5.33
Log likelihood     =      -7629.1174   Prob > chi2         =     0.0695

--------------------------------------------------------------------
    _t | Haz. Ratio  Std. Err.     z    P>|z|   [95% Conf. Interval]
-------+------------------------------------------------------------
 bednet |   .835537   .0701266   -2.14  0.032    .708801    .9849338
    sex |  .9433124   .0645482   -0.85  0.394    .8249169      1.0787
-------+------------------------------------------------------------
  theta |  .0542289   .0241792
--------------------------------------------------------------------
Likelihood-ratio test of theta=0: chibar2(01) = 9.24 Prob>=chibar2 = 0.001
```

To take account of between-cluster variation, we introduce an additional random effects term as follows:

$$\mu_{ijk} = \alpha + \beta_i + \sum_l \gamma_l z_{ijkl} + u_{ij} \tag{11.4}$$

It is usual to assume that the random effect u_{ij} corresponding to the *j*th cluster in the *i*th treatment arm is normally distributed with mean 0 and variance σ_{Bt}^2.

Equation 11.4 is known as the *mixed effects linear regression* model because it has both *fixed effects*, indicated by the parameters α, $β_i$ and $γ_l$, as well as the random effects represented by u_{ij}. Note that the model assumes that the observed value x_{ijk} is given by:

$$x_{ijk} = \mu_{ijk} + v_{ijk} = \alpha + \beta_i + \sum_l \gamma_l z_{ijk} + u_{ij} + v_{ijk}$$

where v_{ijk} represents individual-level departure from the mean, with variance σ_W^2, and u_{ij} represents the cluster-level variation, with variance σ_{Bi}^2. Note that both these variance components need to be estimated from the data. Because x_{ijk} is the sum of two normally distributed variables, u_{ij} and v_{ijk}, it follows that x_{ijk} is also normally distributed. Hence, standard statistical packages such as Stata can be used to obtain estimates of the parameters and to carry out significance tests, as illustrated below.

Example 11.3

In Chapter 10, we analysed the results of the SHARE trial of sexual health education in Scotland (Wight et al. 2002). We used the *t*-test to analyse cluster-level means of a sexual health knowledge score, and found that the mean score was increased in the intervention arm in both girls and boys, but that the increase was only statistically significant in boys. We now reanalyse the data for girls using linear regression based on *individual-level data*.

Box 11.4 shows Stata output for the unadjusted analysis, beginning with an analysis *ignoring clustering*. Regression of the knowledge score on treatment arm gives an estimated mean difference of 0.50 (95% CI: 0.33, 0.67) and a *t*-statistic of 5.85 on 2956 df giving $p < 0.001$. The results of this linear regression analysis are *identical* to carrying out an *unpaired t-test* for the difference between treatment arms. Note that the difference in mean scores is highly significant, but this analysis is *invalid* since it ignores between-cluster variation.

We next fit a *mixed effects linear regression model*, defining the 25 schools as clusters. The mean difference is slightly lower at 0.40, but the *standard error* for the intervention effect increases substantially from 0.09 to 0.23. Consequently the 95% confidence interval (−0.05, 0.84) is much wider and includes the null value. The *z*-statistic for the regression coefficient is also smaller at 1.76, giving a non-significant *p*-value of 0.079. The regression output also shows estimates of σ_W (2.28, shown as *sigma_e*) and σ_B (0.52, shown as *sigma_u* and assumed equal in the two treatment arms).

The results of this analysis are quite similar to those obtained in a cluster-level analysis, where the estimated mean difference was 0.37 with a 95% CI of (−0.10, 0.83) and a *p*-value of 0.12.

We now extend the analysis to adjust for the social class of the parents (Box 11.5). The categories correspond to the Registrar General's classification of social class based on occupation (coded 10: I (highest), 20: II, 31: III non-manual, 32: III manual, 40: IV, 50: V (lowest), 99: not coded; based on highest social class of mother or father). Adding this covariate to the *mixed effects linear regression*

BOX 11.4

. xi:regress kscore i.arm if sex==2

```
                                          Number of obs  =      2958
    Source │    SS         df       MS     F( 1,  2956)  =     34.28
  ─────────┼──────────────────────────────  Prob > F      =    0.0000
     Model │ 184.519686     1   184.519686  R-squared     =    0.0115
  Residual │ 15912.6514   2956   5.38317029  Adj R-squared =    0.0111
  ─────────┼──────────────────────────────  Root MSE      =    2.3202
     Total │ 16097.1711   2957   5.44375078
```

```
  ─────────────────────────────────────────────────────────────────────
    kscore │    Coef.   Std. Err.      t    P>|t|    [95% Conf. Interval]
  ─────────┼─────────────────────────────────────────────────────────────
   _Iarm_1 │  .4995307  .0853218     5.85   0.000    .3322346    .6668268
      cons │  4.609939  .0605352    76.15   0.000    4.491243    4.728634
  ─────────────────────────────────────────────────────────────────────
```

. xi:xtreg kscore i.arm if sex==2, re i(school)

```
Random-effects GLS regression              Number of obs   =      2958
Group variable: school                     Number of groups =       25

R-sq: within  = 0.0000                     Obs per group: min =       39
      between = 0.1028                                     avg =    118.3
      overall = 0.0115                                     max =      212

Random effects u_i ~ Gaussian              Wald chi2(1)  =       3.08
corr(u_i, X)          = 0 (assumed)        Prob > chi2   =     0.0792
```

```
  ─────────────────────────────────────────────────────────────────────
    kscore │    Coef.   Std. Err.      z    P>|z|    [95% Conf. Interval]
  ─────────┼─────────────────────────────────────────────────────────────
   _Iarm_1 │  .3955563  .2253205     1.76   0.079   -.0460637    .8371763
      cons │  4.585929  .161633     28.37   0.000    4.269134    4.902724
  ─────────┼─────────────────────────────────────────────────────────────
   sigma_u │  .51782483
   sigma_e │  2.2811432
       rho │  .04900484  (fraction of variance due to u_i)
  ─────────────────────────────────────────────────────────────────────
```

model, we note that the estimated mean difference remains similar at 0.41. This reflects the close similarity in social class distribution between the two treatment arms, and this was ensured by the use of *restricted randomisation* in this trial (see Section 6.2). The intervention effect is therefore not *confounded* by social class and the point estimate remains similar after adjustment. However, there is a considerable decrease in the *standard error* of the intervention effect, from 0.23 to 0.17. Consequently the 95% confidence interval (0.07, 0.75) is narrower and the z-statistic larger ($z = 2.37$) with $p = 0.018$. The reason for this is that the estimate of the between-cluster standard deviation σ_B has decreased from 0.52 to 0.37, and this is because some of the between-school variation in knowledge score was due to differences in the social class distribution. Note from the regression output that knowledge score was strongly associated with social class, with lower scores among girls with lower parental social class.

BOX 11.5

```
. xi:xtreg kscore i.arm i.scpar if sex==2, re i(school)
```

```
Random-effects GLS regression          Number of obs    =    2900
Group variable: school                 Number of groups =      25

R-sq:  within   = 0.0134               Obs per group: min =     39
       between  = 0.2261                            avg =   116.0
       overall  = 0.0302                            max =     208
Random effects u_i ~ Gaussian          Wald chi2(7)     =   49.21
corr(u_i, X)        = 0 (assumed)       Prob > chi2      = 0.0000
```

kscore	Coef.	Std. Err.	z	P>|z|	[95% Conf.	Interval]
_Iarm_1	.4099191	.1733004	2.37	0.018	.0702566	.7495815
_Iscpar_20	-.4088257	.1542639	-2.65	0.008	-.7111774	-.106474
_Iscpar_31	-.4686595	.1649056	-2.84	0.004	-.7918685	-.1454505
_Iscpar_32	-.4692181	.1810306	-2.59	0.010	-.8240315	-.1144047
_Iscpar_40	-.8171368	.2125908	-3.84	0.000	-1.233807	-.4004666
_Iscpar_50	-1.170468	.2881637	-4.06	0.000	-1.735258	-.6056776
_Iscpar_99	-1.228288	.2170693	-5.66	0.000	-1.653736	-.80284
_cons	5.104777	.1821015	28.03	0.000	4.747865	5.46169
sigma_u	.37222004					
sigma_e	2.267726					
rho	.0262345	(fraction of variance due to u_i)				

This emphasises the point that adjustment for covariates when analysing a CRT is not necessary only when there is *covariate imbalance* between treatment arms, but may also be of value in reducing the level of between-cluster variation in the outcome of interest.

11.2.3 Logistic Regression with Random Effects

Finally, we consider the analysis of *binary* outcome variables. The standard method for analysing risk factors that influence the *proportion* with such an outcome is *logistic regression*. Suppose π_k is the true probability of the outcome for the kth individual, and that there is a set of measured covariates $z_{k1}, \ldots, z_{kL}$ as before. Then the *logistic regression model* assumes that

$$\text{logit}(\pi_k) = \log\left(\frac{\pi_k}{1 - \pi_k}\right) = \alpha + \sum_l \beta_l z_{kl} \tag{11.5}$$

More generally, if there is a group of individuals of size n_k sharing the same covariate values, then the observed number d_k with the binary outcome of interest is assumed to follow the *binomial distribution* with mean:

$$E(d_k) = n_k \pi_k$$

where π_k is given by Equation 11.5.

The corresponding model for a CRT, where *no allowance is made for clustering*, is given by:

$$\text{logit}(\pi_{ijk}) = \log\left(\frac{\pi_{ijk}}{1 - \pi_{ijk}}\right) = \alpha + \beta_i + \sum_l \gamma_l z_{ijkl}$$

where π_{ijk} is the true probability for the kth individual in the jth cluster in the ith treatment arm, β_i represents the intervention effect and the γ_l represent the effects of the covariates. As for event-rates, the logarithm on the left-hand side of the equation means that this is a *multiplicative* model, this time in the *odds* of the outcome of interest.

To take account of between-cluster variation, we introduce an additional random effects term as follows:

$$\log\left(\frac{\pi_{ijk}}{1 - \pi_{ijk}}\right) = \alpha + \beta_i + \sum_l \gamma_l z_{ijkl} + u_{ij} \qquad (11.6)$$

It is usual to assume that the random effect u_{ij} corresponding to the jth cluster in the ith treatment arm is normally distributed with mean 0 and variance σ_{B}^2. This model is known as a *logistic regression random effects model*.

In contrast to the *Poisson regression random effects model* (with gamma random effects) and *mixed effects linear regression model* (with normal random effects), the combination of *binomial* variation within clusters and *normal* variation between clusters does not provide a simple composite distribution with a likelihood that can be written down in analytical form. Numerical methods therefore have to be used to maximise the likelihood and to obtain parameter estimates, confidence intervals and significance tests for this model. The numerical procedure used for this purpose is known as *quadrature* and involves approximating the normal distribution (a continuous bell-shaped curve) by a series of vertical "slices". After fitting the model, it is important to evaluate whether the model fit is reliable by carrying out a procedure known as a *quadrature check*, which involves comparing the results obtained as the number of slices is varied. The usual advice is to be cautious about the model fit if there is more than a 1% relative difference in the likelihood or any of the parameter estimates when the number of slices is varied. This can readily be assessed in Stata by using the *quadchk* command. Fortunately, recent versions of Stata use a method known as *adaptive quadrature* and experience shows that this method usually provides an acceptable fit.

Finally, we recall from Section 9.3.2 that the estimate of the parameter β_i obtained from a logistic regression random effects model yields a *cluster-specific* estimate of the intervention effect. More specifically, $\exp(\hat{\beta}_i)$ estimates the *cluster-specific odds ratio* of the outcome of interest in the ith treatment arm compared with the control arm ($i = 0$).

Example 11.4

We return to the results of the SHARE trial of sexual health education and analyse two *binary* outcomes that were recorded at the follow-up survey 2 years after baseline (Wight et al. 2002). One of the behavioural outcomes of the trial was *reported sexual debut*, defined as onset of sexual activity after the first year of the in-school programme, and this was assessed among students who were not sexually active at baseline.

In Example 10.4 and Example 10.6, we saw that the proportion of boys reporting sexual debut was approximately 24% in both arms, with no significant difference on cluster-level analysis. Box 11.6 shows the corresponding individual-level analysis. *Ignoring clustering*, and carrying out a standard logistic regression analysis, we obtain an estimated odds ratio of 0.98, a 95% CI of (0.81, 1.18) and a *p*-value of 0.83.

Repeating this analysis using a *logistic regression random effects model*, we see that the estimated odds ratio becomes 0.97. Note that this is slightly further from one than the population-averaged odds ratio of 0.98. Due to between-cluster variation, the standard error of the estimate is increased and the 95% CI of (0.69, 1.36) is now much wider. The output also provides an estimate of the between-cluster standard deviation, $\hat{\sigma}_B = 0.35$ (shown as *sigma_u*). Note that this is assumed equal in both arms, and refers to the standard deviation of the u_{ij} in Equation 11.6 which are measured on the log-odds scale.

When a *quadrature check* is performed on this analysis, we see that the *relative differences* are all extremely small, indicating that the quadrature has achieved an acceptable fit.

We now turn to an outcome for which there was some evidence of intervention effect. When sexually active students who reported more than one partner were asked whether they regretted their first sexual intercourse with their most recent partner, the proportion of boys reporting regret was 19.4% in the control arm but only 9.6% in the intervention arm, and cluster-level analysis showed this effect to be statistically significant. The output for the individual-level analysis is shown in Box 11.7.

Logistic regression analysis ignoring clustering gives an estimated odds ratio of 0.44 with a 95% CI of (0.23, 0.84) and a *p*-value (likelihood ratio test) of 0.011. Taking clustering account, we now fit a *logistic regression random effects model*. The estimated odds ratio is almost unchanged at 0.44 and there is only a slight increase in the width of the 95% confidence interval which becomes (0.22, 0.88) with a *p*-value (likelihood ratio test) of 0.025. The likelihood ratio test for the null hypothesis $\sigma_B = 0$ (or equivalently $\rho = 0$) gives $p = 0.34$ indicating no clear evidence of clustering in these data. Despite this, we would prefer to use a method of analysis that takes account of any clustering that may be present, and note that the point estimate of the between-cluster standard deviation was $\hat{\sigma}_B = 0.24$. As before, the quadrature check indicates that the quadrature has achieved an acceptable fit. Finally, we adjust this analysis for the effect of parental social class as in Example 11.3. The output shows that social class had an appreciable effect on this outcome, with boys with parents in "lower" social classes reporting greater regret. However adjusting for this variable had little effect on the intervention effect with an adjusted odds ratio of 0.43 (95% CI: 0.22, 0.83) and a similar *p*-value of 0.016. Note that the estimated between-cluster standard deviation after adjusting for social class is close to zero ($\hat{\sigma}_B = 0.001$).

BOX 11.6

```
. xi:logit debut i.arm if sex==1, or

Logistic regression                              Number of obs =    2363
                                                 LR chi2(1)    =    0.04
                                                 Prob > chi2   = 0.8323
Log likelihood = -1295.0815                      Pseudo R2     = 0.0000
```

debut	Odds Ratio	Std. Err.	z	P>|z|	[95% Conf.	Interval]
_Iarm_1	.9796929	.0949029	-0.21	0.832	.810278	1.184529

```
. xi:xtlogit debut i.arm if sex==1, or re i(school)

Random-effects logistic regression           Number of obs    =    2363
Group variable: school                       Number of groups =      25

Random effects u_i ~ Gaussian                Obs per group: min =     25
                                                            avg =   94.5
                                                            max =    184

                                             Wald chi2(1)     =    0.04
Log likelihood  = -1282.9297                 Prob > chi2      = 0.8440
```

debut	OR	Std. Err.	z	P>|z|	[95% Conf.	Interval]
_Iarm_1	.9662634	.1685609	-0.20	0.844	.6864465	1.360142
/lnsig2u	-2.09282	.4292696			-2.934173	-1.251467
sigma_u	.3511964	.075379			.2305964	.5348691
rho	.0361358	.0149515			.0159061	.0800024

```
Likelihood-ratio test of rho=0: chibar2(01) = 24.30 Prob >= chibar2   =   0.000

. quadchk
```

Quadrature check

	Fitted quadrature 12 points	Comparison quadrature 8 points	Comparison quadrature 16 points	
Log	-1282.9297	-1282.9297	-1282.9297	
likelihood		-2.356e-07	1.326e-10	Difference
		1.837e-10	-1.033e-13	Relative difference
debut:	-.03431876	-.03431777	-.03431779	
_Iarm_1		9.915e-07	9.770e-07	Difference
		-.00002889	-.00002847	Relative difference

(continued)

BOX 11.6 (CONTINUED)

```
debut:      -1.144755   -1.144756   -1.1447559
_ cons                  -9.591e-07  -9.079e-07   Difference
                         8.378e-07   7.931e-07   Relative difference
lnsig2u:    -2.0928195  -2.0928168  -2.0928166
_ cons                   2.725e-06   2.899e-06   Difference
                        -1.302e-06  -1.385e-06   Relative difference
```

BOX 11.7

```
. xi:logit regret i.arm if sex==1, or

Logistic regression                          Number of obs =      327
                                             LR chi2(1)    =     6.49
                                             Prob > chi2   =   0.0108
Log likelihood = -133.14599                  Pseudo R2     =   0.0238
```

regret	Odds Ratio	Std. Err.	z	P>|z|	[95% Conf.	Interval]
_Iarm_1	.4385403	.1463116	-2.47	0.013	.228045	.843332

```
. xi:xtlogit regret i.arm if sex==1, or re i(school)

Random-effects logistic regression           Number of obs    =      327
Group variable: school                        Number of groups =       25

Random effects u_i ~ Gaussian                 Obs per group: min =       4
                                                             avg =    13.1
                                                             max =      27

                                              Wald chi2(1)     =     5.44
Log likelihood = -133.06127                   Prob > chi2      =   0.0197
```

regret	OR	Std. Err.	z	P>|z|	[95% Conf.	Interval]
_Iarm_1	.4408574	.1547969	-2.33	0.020	.2215227	.8773602
/lnsig2u	-2.852804	2.682119			-8.109661	2.404052
sigma_u	.2401714	.3220842			.0173384	3.32685
rho	.0172312	.0454198			.0000914	.7708655

```
Likelihood-ratio test of rho=0: chibar2(01) =0.17 Prob >=chibar2   =  0.340

. est store A

. xi:xtlogit regret if sex==1, or re i(school)

. est store B

. lrtest A B
```

(continued)

BOX 11.7   (CONTINUED)

```
Likelihood-ratio test                              LR chi2(1)  =    5.00
(Assumption: B nested in A)                        Prob > chi2 = 0.0254

. xi:xtlogit regret i.arm if sex==1, or re i(school)

. quadchk
```

                             Quadrature check

	Fitted quadrature 12 points	Comparison quadrature 8 points	Comparison quadrature 16 points	
Log	-133.06127	-133.06127	-133.06127	
likelihood		-1.373e-11	5.684e-14	Difference
		1.032e-13	-4.272e-16	Relative difference
regret:	-.81903387	-.81903387	-.81903387	
_Iarm_1		-2.215e-09	-2.480e-09	Difference
		2.704e-09	3.028e-09	Relative difference
regret:	-1.4556454	-1.4556454	-1.4556454	
_cons		1.398e-08	1.520e-08	Difference
		-9.603e-09	-1.044e-08	Relative difference
lnsig2u:	-2.8528045	-2.8528052	-2.8528052	
_cons		-7.339e-07	-7.713e-07	Difference
		2.573e-07	2.704e-07	Relative difference

```
. xi:xtlogit regret i.arm i.scpar if sex==1, or re i(school)
Random-effects logistic regression   Number of obs      =       320
Group variable: school               Number of groups   =        25

Random effects u_i ~ Gaussian        Obs per group: min =         4
                                                    avg =      12.8
                                                    max =        27

                                     Wald chi2(7) =       10.30
Log likelihood = -129.42177          Prob > chi2  =      0.1720
```

regret	OR	Std. Err.	z	P>|z|	[95% Conf.	Interval]
_Iarm_1	.4277396	.1452156	-2.50	0.012	.2198874	.8320674
_Iscpar_20	4.136403	4.411967	1.33	0.183	.511346	33.46037
_Iscpar_31	3.955363	4.275245	1.27	0.203	.4754947	32.90236
_Iscpar_32	5.221391	5.659457	1.52	0.127	.6239793	43.69203
_Iscpar_40	5.829939	6.850436	1.50	0.134	.5827262	58.32617
_Iscpar_50	7.31255	9.000824	1.62	0.106	.6551601	81.61882
_Iscpar_99	2.017352	2.408433	0.59	0.557	.1943423	20.94093
/lnsig2u	-13.65277	694.4192			-1374.689	1347.384
sigma_u	.0010848	.3766436			3.1e-299	3.8e+292
rho	3.58e-07	.0002484			0	.

(continued)

BOX 11.7 (CONTINUED)

```
Likelihood-ratio test of rho=0: chibar2(01) = 2.5e-06 Prob >=
  chibar2 = 0.499
. est store C
. xi:xtlogit regret i.scpar if sex==1, or re i(school)
. est store D
. lrtest C D
Likelihood-ratio test                        LR chi2(1)  =    5.86
(Assumption: D nested in C)                  Prob > chi2 = 0.0155
```

11.3 Generalised Estimating Equations

In the previous section, we considered the use of regression methods incorporating additional model terms that explicitly encapsulate the random variability between clusters. These *random effects* models seem to work well for quantitative data and event rates, providing there are a sufficiently large number of clusters in each treatment arm. They do not always work as well for binary data because, as we have noted in Section 11.2.3, the *logistic regression random effects* model relies on numerical quadrature to approximate the normal distribution and consequently may not always provide reliable results.

GEE provide an alternative method of individual-level regression modelling and make allowance for clustering without incorporating additional terms in the model. They do this by assuming that observations in the same cluster are *correlated* and using the data to estimate the strength of the correlation. As for random effects models, GEE only works reliably when there are a sufficiently large number of clusters in each treatment arm.

We begin by discussing the use of GEE for the analysis of *binary* outcomes, since random effects models do not always work well for such data.

11.3.1 GEE Models for Binary Data

The basic regression model for GEE is identical to that for a standard logistic regression model ignoring clustering:

$$\text{logit}(\pi_{ijk}) = \log\left(\frac{\pi_{ijk}}{1 - \pi_{ijk}}\right) = \alpha + \beta_i + \sum_l \gamma_l z_{ijkl} \tag{11.7}$$

However, while standard logistic regression assumes that the observed outcomes are binomially distributed and *statistically independent*, GEE assumes that observations within the same cluster may be *correlated*. For the analysis of CRTs, it is usual to assume that the correlation matrix is *exchangeable*, meaning that observations on individuals in different clusters are *uncorrelated*, while observations on individuals in the same cluster all have the same correlation coefficient ρ. In this book, we shall only consider GEE models with an exchangeable correlation matrix, as this is usually the most relevant correlation structure for individuals living within the same community, or patients within the same medical practice.

The observed data are used to estimate the value of ρ, and this is used to obtain estimates of the regression coefficients and their standard errors that are adjusted for the correlations in the data. If $\hat{\rho}$ is large, less weight will be given to each individual in large clusters, since the outcomes within a cluster will tend to be similar. Conversely, if $\hat{\rho}$ is close to zero, this means that there is little clustering and all individuals will be given similar weight in the analysis.

Because no *random effect* is assumed for each cluster in Equation 11.7, the logarithm of the regression coefficient β_i must be interpreted as a *population-average* odds ratio, as discussed in Section 9.3.2.

It is important to note that, while GEE models do make allowance for within-cluster correlation, they do not correspond to a full probability model for the data. For this reason, we cannot define the *likelihood* of the data and so we cannot obtain *maximum likelihood estimators* of the parameters or carry out *likelihood ratio tests*. Instead, GEE uses an iterative *generalised least squares* method to estimate the parameters together with *robust standard errors* obtained using a *sandwich variance* estimator. The *Wald* test, obtained by computing $z = \hat{\beta} / SE(\hat{\beta})$ and referring z to tables of the standard normal distribution can be used for hypothesis testing. The corresponding Wald-based 95% confidence interval is obtained as $\hat{\beta} \pm 1.96 SE(\hat{\beta})$.

When the number of clusters is small, the increased variability of the GEE sandwich variance estimator can substantially inflate the Type I error. Pan and Wall (2002) show how to account for this by referring to a t distribution instead of the standard normal distribution. The calculation of the degrees of freedom, however, requires extra matrix calculations that have not yet been implemented in any statistical package.

Example 11.5

When analysing the effect of the SHARE trial intervention on reported sexual debut among boys in Example 11.4, we found that there was no significant intervention effect. The estimated odds ratio was 0.97, with a 95% CI of (0.69, 1.36) and a p-value of 0.84.

Box 11.8 shows the equivalent analysis using GEE, with an exchangeable correlation matrix and robust standard errors. The estimated odds ratio is 0.95, with a 95% CI of (0.67, 1.33) and a p-value from the Wald test of 0.76, quite similar to the results of the random effects regression.

This analysis is readily adjusted for the effects of individual-level or cluster-level covariates. Box 11.8 shows that after adjustment for parental social class, the

BOX 11.8

```
. xi:xtlogit debut i.arm if sex==1, or pa i(school) robust
```

GEE population-averaged model		Number of obs	=	2363
Group variable:	school	Number of groups	=	25
		Obs per group: min	=	25
Link:	logit	avg	=	94.5
Family:	binomial	max	=	184
Correlation:	exchangeable	Wald chi2(1)	=	0.09
		Prob > chi2	=	0.7591
Scale parameter:	1			

(Std. Err. adjusted for clustering on school)

debut	Odds Ratio	Semi-robust Std. Err.	z	P>|z|	[95% Conf.	Interval]
_Iarm_1	.9480567	.1649073	-0.31	0.759	.6741774	1.333197

```
. xi:xtlogit debut i.arm i.scpar if sex==1, or pa i(school) robust
```

GEE population-averaged model		Number of obs	=	2319
Group variable:	school	Number of groups	=	25
		Obs per group: min	=	24
Link:	logit	avg	=	92.8
Family:	binomial	max	=	177
Correlation:	exchangeable	Wald chi2(7)	=	10.96
		Prob > chi2	=	0.1404
Scale parameter:	1			

(Std. Err. adjusted for clustering on school)

debut	Odds Ratio	Semi-robust Std. Err.	z	P>|z|	[95% Conf.	Interval]
_Iarm_1	.8961	.1444368	-0.68	0.496	.6533661	1.229013
_Iscpar_20	1.326639	.2059096	1.82	0.069	.9786705	1.798328
_Iscpar_31	1.565618	.2808851	2.50	0.012	1.101471	2.225351
_Iscpar_32	1.490818	.3057023	1.95	0.051	.9974241	2.228277
_Iscpar_40	1.112707	.2504164	0.47	0.635	.7158411	1.729598
_Iscpar_50	1.305916	.4412843	0.79	0.430	.673417	2.532481
_Iscpar_99	1.574411	.3354362	2.13	0.033	1.036968	2.390402

estimated intervention effect is increased slightly, with an adjusted odds ratio of 0.90, a 95% CI of (0.65, 1.23) and *p*-value of 0.50, but the effect is still far from being statistically significant.

11.3.2 GEE for Other Types of Outcome

GEE models may also be fitted for event-rates data and quantitative outcomes. In both cases, we assume an *exchangeable* correlation matrix and obtain *robust* standard errors. We also use the *Wald* test to carry out significance tests.

Example 11.6

We recall our analysis of the sexual health knowledge score among girls in the SHARE trial, as shown in Table 11.2.

Fitting a GEE model with exchangeable correlation matrix and robust standard errors, we obtain an estimated mean difference of 0.41 with a 95% CI of (0.01, 0.81) and a *p*-value of 0.045. Adjusting for parental social class, the estimated mean difference remains unchanged at 0.41 but the 95% CI (0.06, 0.77) is narrower, and the *p*-value smaller at 0.022.

Comparing the methods applied in Table 11.2, we note that mixed effects linear regression and GEE give very similar results, with an unadjusted effect of borderline significance. On adjustment for parental social class, the point estimate of the intervention effect remains similar, but the standard error of the estimate is reduced and the evidence of an effect became stronger, with a narrower

TABLE 11.2

Summary of Unadjusted and Adjusted Analyses of the Sexual Health Knowledge Score Among Girls in the Share Trial Using Cluster-level Summaries and Individual-level Regression Analysis

	Unadjusted Analysis	Adjusted Analysis*
Cluster-level Analysis		
Mean difference	0.37	0.37
95% CI	(−0.10, 0.83)	(−0.06, 0.79)
p-value	0.12	0.085
Linear Regression Unadjusted for Clustering		
Mean difference	0.50	0.49
95% CI	(0.33, 0.67)	(0.32, 0.66)
p-value	<0.001	<0.001
Mixed Effects Linear Regression		
Mean difference	0.40	0.41
95% CI	(−0.05, 0.84)	(0.07, 0.75)
p-value	0.079	0.018
Generalised Estimating Equations		
Mean difference	0.41	0.41
95% CI	(0.01, 0.81)	(0.06, 0.77)
p-value	0.045	0.022

*Adjusted for parental social class.

confidence interval and smaller *p*-value. For comparison, a linear regression analysis ignoring clustering gives a highly significant result, but is clearly *invalid* as between-cluster variability is not taken into account.

A cluster-level analysis based on means of the knowledge score for all the girls in each school (or of the residuals from a regression of score on parental social class, in an adjusted analysis) gives broadly similar results to the individual-level regression analysis. However, standard errors are somewhat larger and the evidence of an effect is weaker, with *p*-values above 0.05. As discussed in Section 11.1, the individual-level regression methods make more efficient use of the data, for example giving more weight to schools with larger numbers of students. This may explain the lower standard error in these analyses. However, the number of clusters is relatively small in this trial, and GEE and mixed effects linear regression may not perform reliably in such situations, with departures from nominal Type I error rates. It may therefore be appropriate to place more reliance on the cluster-level analysis in this study.

11.4 Choice of Analytical Method

In Chapter 10 and Chapter 11, we have presented several alternative statistical methods for the analysis of unmatched CRTs, of different levels of complexity. In this section, we attempt to give some guidance as to which of these methods should be used depending on the characteristics of the trial (Table 11.3).

11.4.1 Small Numbers of Clusters

If there is a small number of clusters per treatment arm, say less than 15, the individual-level regression methods may not be reliable. The GEE approach

TABLE 11.3

Choice of Statistical Methods for Analysis of Unmatched CRTs

	Less than 15 Clusters per Treatment Arm	More than 15 Clusters per Treatment Arm
Event rates	Unpaired *t*-test	Poisson regression random effects model
	Rank sum test	GEE
Proportions	Unpaired *t*-test	Logistic regression random effects model*
	Rank sum test	GEE
Means of quantitative outcomes	Unpaired *t*-test	Mixed effects linear regression
	Rank sum test	GEE

*Quadrature check should be carried out to evaluate reliability of results.

tends to have inflated Type I error in such situations (Bellamy et al. 2000), while the distributional assumptions of random effects models can be difficult to verify without large numbers of clusters. We therefore recommend use of the cluster-level methods of Chapter 10 for such trials.

Point estimates of the intervention effect can be obtained using either individual-level data or cluster summaries. Approximate confidence intervals can be obtained from cluster summaries using the *t* distribution as described in Section 10.3. Hypothesis tests can be carried out using the unpaired *t*-test, which has been shown to be highly robust even for small numbers of clusters. If the cluster summaries appear to have a highly non-normal distribution, we can consider using a logarithmic transformation before analysis to provide a more symmetric distribution. Alternatively, or if the logarithmic transformation is ineffective, we may use a nonparametric procedure such as the rank sum test as a check on the *p*-value provided by the *t*-test. This is particularly advisable in trials with very few clusters, say six or less per treatment arm.

11.4.2 Larger Numbers of Clusters

For trials with larger numbers of clusters, say 15 or more per arm, the individual-level regression methods seem to perform reliably, and are likely to be preferred because of their greater convenience when analysing the effects of individual-level covariates. They should also be statistically more efficient than the cluster-level methods since they use optimal weights for each cluster in order to minimise the standard errors of parameter estimates.

For such trials, we recommend the use of either random effects regression or GEE with an exchangeable correlation matrix and robust standard errors. There is little to choose between these methods, which usually give very similar results. Random effects regression corresponds to a full probability model for the data and therefore has the advantage of allowing use of the likelihood ratio test, which is the preferred approach to statistical inference. However, this comes at the cost of making more stringent model assumptions, for example that cluster-level rates follow the gamma distribution. GEE avoids such assumptions and may thus be regarded as more robust.

For binary outcomes, we have noted that the logistic regression random effects model does not always provide reliable results, because of the use of quadrature to approximate the normal distribution (although the use of *adaptive quadrature* may largely obviate this problem). If using this method, we therefore recommend carrying out a quadrature check for the main analysis. If this check fails, we prefer the use of GEE for such outcomes.

If *restricted randomisation* is used, the above methods can still be applied. However, it may be advisable to check the robustness of the main findings by also carrying out a permutation test that takes into account the randomisation scheme.

11.5 Analysing for Effect Modification

As noted in Section 10.7, we may sometimes wish to examine whether the effect of an intervention differs between subgroups of clusters or individuals. One advantage of methods based on individual-level regression is that *interaction* terms can readily be incorporated in the model to examine the evidence for effect modification. Care is needed in applying this method to examine for interaction with cluster-level covariates, especially when the number of clusters is small, since this relies on between-cluster comparisons. The method should generally work well for individual-level covariates, however.

Example 11.7

In Example 10.12 we compared the effects of the Project SHARE intervention on sexual health knowledge in boys and girls. This analysis is repeated in Box 11.9 using mixed effects linear regression as in Example 11.3. In this analysis, we note from the interaction term that the estimated difference in intervention effect between girls and boys is –0.20 with a 95% CI of (–0.44, 0.04). Although the effect is greater among boys, the Wald test for the interaction indicates that this difference could easily have occurred by chance ($z = -1.62$, $p = 0.10$). These results are broadly similar to those based on analysis of cluster-level summaries in Example 10.12.

BOX 11.9

```
. use share.dta

. xi:xtreg kscore i.arm*i.sex, re i(school)

Random-effects GLS regression        Number of obs        =      5501
Group variable: school               Number of groups     =        25

R-sq:  within  = 0.0363              Obs per group: min    =        66
       between = 0.2250                             avg    =     220.0
       overall = 0.0499                             max    =       382

Random effects u_i ~ Gaussian       Wald chi2(3)          =    215.05
corr(u_i, X)      = 0 (assumed)      Prob > chi2           =    0.0000
```

kscore	Coef.	Std. Err.	z	P>|z|	[95% Conf. Interval]	
_Iarm_1	.6194901	.1794795	3.45	0.001	.2677169	.9712634
_Isex_2	.9739854	.0860921	11.31	0.000	.805248	1.142723
IarmXsex~2	-.2003517	.1233793	-1.62	0.104	-.4421706	.0414672
_cons	3.611875	.1275317	28.32	0.000	3.361917	3.861833
sigma_u	.38277533					
sigma_e	2.2744745					
rho	.02754207	(fraction of variance due to u_i)				

11.6 More Complex Analyses

In Sections 11.2 through 11.4, we focused on the simplest type of analysis where there is only one measure of the outcome, recorded at a single follow-up survey or over a single period of time. In some RCTs, there are repeated surveys of the trial population, and we briefly discuss appropriate analyses taking into account these study designs.

11.6.1 Controlling for Baseline Values

In some CRTs, data are collected on baseline values of the main endpoints. This is most common for endpoints that can be measured in a single cross-sectional survey, for example the mean of a quantitative variable or the prevalence of a binary variable. Occasionally, baseline data are also available for endpoints that require measurement over time, for example the incidence of a disease event, although this is less common since it requires an extended follow-up period prior to intervention and this adds to the duration and cost of a study.

We may wish to adjust estimated intervention effects for baseline values, for two reasons:

- To control for any baseline imbalances in the endpoint of interest between treatment arms. Such imbalances are not unlikely, especially when the number of clusters is small, and call into question the credibility of the trial results if they are not adjusted for.

- To reduce between-cluster variation in the endpoint and thus to increase the power and precision of the study. If baseline values of the endpoint are predictive of the follow-up values, it is likely that some of the variation in the endpoint between clusters will be explained by the baseline differences.

We note that when baseline data are available before randomisation, a highly restricted randomisation can be implemented that assures balance between treatment arms with respect to the baseline data. For logistical reasons related to study schedules and budgets, however, this is not always possible.

Depending on the study design, we may have baseline and follow-up data on the *same* individuals if we use a cohort design, or on *different* individuals if we use a repeated cross-sectional design. With a repeated cross-sectional design we can clearly only adjust for the baseline value of the endpoint at the *cluster* level. With a cohort design, however, we are able to adjust for the baseline value in the *same* individual.

Two alternative analytical approaches can be used to adjust for baseline values. We can either analyse the *change* in the endpoint of interest (either at cluster or individual level), or we can adjust for the baseline value as a *covariate* in the regression analysis. While analysis of *change* is superficially an attractive approach, we generally favour adjustment for baseline as a *covariate*, and this is mainly because of the phenomenon of *regression to the mean*. Because of random variation in measured endpoints, within individuals or clusters, those with low observed values at baseline are expected to show an increase in observed value at follow-up even in the absence of any true change, while those with high observed values at baseline are expected to show a decrease. To control for this effect, it is recommended to adjust for the baseline value *even if* the change from baseline to follow-up value is analysed.

As an example, suppose we measure a quantitative variable x at baseline and follow-up in a CRT with a cohort design. Let x_{ijk0} and x_{ijk1} be the observed values at baseline and follow-up in the kth individual in the jth cluster in the ith treatment arm. If we fit the baseline value as a covariate we obtain the linear regression model:

$$E(x_{ijk1}) = \alpha + \beta_i + \gamma x_{ijk0}$$

where, for simplicity, we ignore any other covariates. It follows that the expected value of the *change* $z_{ijk} = x_{ijk1} - x_{ijk0}$ is given by:

$$E(z_{ijk}) = \alpha + \beta_i + (\gamma - 1)x_{ijk0}$$

This confirms that, unless $\gamma = 1$, adjustment for the baseline value is still called for when *change* is analysed.

In a repeated cross-sectional design, we can use similar regression models but the baseline covariate has to be a cluster-level summary.

11.6.2 Repeated Measures during Follow-up

In the examples we have discussed previously, data on the outcome of interest during follow-up were available at only one time-point or during one time period. In some trials, however, outcome data are collected at several consecutive follow-up surveys, or over several periods of time.

As an example, suppose repeated cross-sectional surveys are carried out annually for 3 years in each cluster. The most common reason for adopting such a design is to evaluate whether the effect of intervention varies over time. For example, where treatment for a condition is delivered at one time-point, we may wish to determine whether the beneficial effects of the treatment decrease over time. Conversely, where an intervention is sustained over time, as may be the case with long-term treatment, repeated doses of a vaccine or a population-based health education programme, we may wish to examine whether the cumulative effect of the intervention leads to a steadily increasing effect.

In cohort studies that involve repeated household visits, the marginal cost of taking additional measurements of the outcome may be minimal. For example, if child growth is of interest, taking repeated measures of length and height will increase the power to detect growth differentials over time.

There are two main approaches to the analysis of data from such a trial. One is to carry out a *separate* analysis of the intervention effect at each time-point, using any of the methods of Chapter 10 and Chapter 11. The intervention impact after 1 year is based on comparison of the outcome of interest in the intervention and control clusters at the 1-year survey. Similarly, the impact after 2 years is based on comparison of intervention and control clusters at the 2-year survey, and so on. At each time-point, adjustment for baseline values can be made if appropriate.

As an illustration, suppose that the outcome is binary, e.g., whether or not a child is stunted at the time of measurement, and that a separate random effects logistic regression analysis is carried out at each time-point, giving rise to the following estimates of the odds ratio associated with a nutritional intervention:

| Year 1: | OR = 0.60 | 95% CI: 0.41–0.89 | SE(log OR) = 0.20 |
| Year 2: | OR = 0.30 | 95% CI: 0.17–0.54 | SE(log OR) = 0.30 |

where the standard errors are adjusted for between-cluster variation.

If we wish to test whether the effect of intervention increased over time, we might consider carrying out an approximate z-test as:

$$z = \frac{\log(0.60) - \log(0.30)}{\sqrt{0.20^2 + 0.30^2}} = 1.92$$

giving a p-value of 0.055. However, this procedure ignores the fact that the two odds ratios are estimated based on the *same* set of clusters, and that observations on the same cluster at consecutive surveys will usually be *correlated*. Similarly, if the study were individually randomised and the same children were measured at each of the two rounds of data collection, there would be within-child correlation that would need to be addressed. Only if separate sets of children were measured at the two rounds in an individually randomised study could one use the above z-test with confidence.

A more powerful test of the hypothesis can be obtained if these correlations are taken into account. This can be done most conveniently if individual-level regression analysis is used. Adding a suffix t to represent the time-point, all the data from the 1-year and 2-year follow-up surveys can be handled with one model as follows:

$$\text{logit}(\pi_{ijkt}) = \log\left(\frac{\pi_{ijkt}}{1 - \pi_{ijkt}}\right) = \alpha + \beta_i + \delta_t + \eta_{it} + \sum_l \gamma_l z_{ijklt} \qquad (11.8)$$

where $\beta_0 = 0$, $t = 0$ for the first round and $t = 1$ for the second round, $\delta_0 = 0$ and $\eta_{i0} = 0$. Here, η_{it} is the interaction term that estimates, for the ith treatment arm, the differential effect of the ith treatment arm relative to the control arm ($i = 0$) across the two survey rounds. In a software package, Equation 11.8 would be fitted by including covariates for treatment arm, time point and the product of these two.

Similarly, if there are several time-points, $t = 0, ..., T$, we can test for, say, a linear trend in the effects of a treatment over time by fitting the model:

$$\text{logit}(\pi_{ijkt}) = \log\left(\frac{\pi_{ijkt}}{1 - \pi_{ijkt}}\right) = \alpha + \beta_i + \delta_t + \eta_i t + \sum_l \gamma_l z_{ijklt} \qquad (11.9)$$

with η_i tracking the linear interaction effect.

Note that for both the models in Equation 11.8 and Equation 11.9, we need to account for within-cluster correlation and, if the same individuals are measured more than once, within-individual correlation over time. This is readily accomplished by adding in random effects terms, producing a mixed model. A random cluster-level intercept u_{ij} will account for within-cluster correlation, also handling the correlation within clusters over time, and a random intercept v_{ijk} can be added to account for within-individual correlation over time. Special software may be needed to accommodate estimation of more than one random effects distribution. In Stata, one can fit such models by installing the freeware third-party routine *glamm*, an acronym for Generalised Linear Latent And Mixed Models, described on the website http://www.gllamm.org.

11.6.3 Repeated Episodes

In some trials in which the outcome is an *event rate*, we can assume that each individual will experience at most one occurrence of the event of interest. This is clearly the case for studies of mortality, but is also approximately the case for studies of other rare outcomes. In such cases, no additional statistical complications are introduced by the continuous follow-up of the same individuals over time.

In other trials, however, the outcome is a relatively common event, and repeated episodes in the same individual may be observed quite frequently. In trials of interventions against childhood diarrhoea, for example, it is likely that some children will experience multiple, separate episodes of diarrhoea over a 2- or 3-year follow-up period. Because children vary in their exposures and susceptibility, there will be within-child correlation of episodes. Accounting for this additional layer of correlation requires a three-level multilevel model, with the episode, the child, and the cluster constituting the three levels.

From a theoretical standpoint, as the number of clusters increases, accounting for the cluster-level variability also accounts for any lower levels of correlation that exist within each cluster. We usually have only a small number of clusters, however, and explicit modelling of the relevant levels of correlation will, in general, result in greater power and precision.

In Section 11.2.1, the *negative binomial distribution* was used to model the varying Poisson counts across clusters. Similarly, we can use the negative binomial as a model for the number of episodes experienced by an individual, where each individual's intrinsic incidence rate follows a *gamma distribution*. To handle the additional between-cluster variability, another random effect w_{ij} can be added, which is used to specify variation in the gamma distribution between clusters. In Stata, the distribution of w_{ij} is based on the *beta* distribution.

Example 11.8

A phase III CRT of a *Streptococcus pneumoniae* vaccine was conducted among American Indians living in 38 geographically defined clusters in the USA (Moulton et al. 2001; O'Brien et al. 2003). Infants in 19 randomly selected clusters were offered the seven-valent pneumococcal conjugate vaccine (PnCRM7), while those in the other 19 clusters were offered, as a comparator, a meningococcal C conjugate vaccine (MnCC). The primary endpoint was invasive pneumococcal disease, but here we examine a secondary endpoint that consisted of all episodes of bacterial pneumonia documented in hospital visits. This secondary endpoint was determined by randomly sampling the hospital charts of a subset of infants in the study area who had participated in the trial.

Table 11.4 shows the number of episodes of bacterial pneumonia per child in each trial arm. The results of fitting a Poisson regression random effects model

TABLE 11.4

Summary of Bacterial Pneumonia Episodes among Infants in the American Indian *S. pneumoniae* Vaccine Trial

	Vaccine Group	
	MnCC	PnCRM7
Number of Episodes per Infant	**Number of Infants**	
0	185	176
1	43	32
2	6	3
3	4	0
Total infants	238	211
Total episodes	67	38

TABLE 11.5

Summary of Poisson (Two-level: Accounts for Intracluster Correlation) and Negative Binomial (Three-level: Accounts for Intracluster and Intra-individual Correlation) Random Effects Models Fitted to Data from Infants in the American Indian *S. Pneumoniae* Vaccine Trial

Result	Poisson Regression Random Effects Model	Negative Binomial Regression Random Effects Model
Rate ratio (PnCRM7/MnCC)	0.617	0.661
95% CI	(0.394, 0.967)	(0.423, 1.031)
p-value	0.035	0.068

that accounts for cluster-level variation, and a negative binomial random effects regression model that accounts for both cluster- and infant-level variation, are shown in Table 11.5. The results are quite close to each other, with the negative binomial model yielding a slightly larger rate ratio, indicating slightly lower efficacy. This may be due to the greater reduction of multiple episodes than single episodes in the PnCRM7 arm. Under the negative binomial model, because of positive within-infant correlation, those with larger numbers of events are downweighted so that, for example, two episodes in one infant have less influence in the analysis than one episode in each of two infants.

12

Analysis of Trials with More Complex Designs

12.1 Introduction

In Chapter 10 and Chapter 11, we have focused on the analysis of CRTs with the simplest possible study design, in which there are two treatment arms and no matching or stratification. We now consider the analysis of trials with more complex designs.

In Section 12.2, we discuss the analysis of pair-matched trials. Many published CRTs have used this design although, as we have seen in Section 5.6, it is not always the most efficient choice. Analytical methods are available that take account of the matched design. As for unmatched studies, these include methods based on cluster-level summaries, which can be extended to take account of covariates. As we shall see, methods based on individual-level regression are generally not suitable for the analysis of pair-matched studies.

As we saw in Chapter 5, stratified trials avoid some of the limitations of pair-matched trials and are often likely to be the design of choice. In Section 12.3, we show how cluster-level and individual-level methods of analysis can be extended for use with stratified CRTs.

Finally, in Section 12.4, we consider the analysis of CRTs with other designs, including unmatched trials with more than two treatment arms, factorial trials and stepped-wedge trials.

12.2 Analysis of Pair-matched Trials

12.2.1 Introduction

In a pair-matched trial, clusters are first arranged into pairs that are matched on factors expected to be correlated with the outcome of interest, and then randomly allocated between the two treatment arms. If the matching is effective, the between-cluster variation within matched pairs (in the absence of intervention) is smaller than the variation between all the clusters. Accounting for the matching in this situation yields effect estimates with a smaller variance. However, this benefit has to be set against the loss in precision and power due to the reduction in degrees of freedom associated with a matched analysis.

Section 5.6 discusses the option of using a paired-matched design but then *breaking the matching* for the analysis, and sets out the advantages and disadvantages of this approach. If this method is adopted, we can use the full range of analytical methods presented in Chapter 10 and Chapter 11. In the present chapter, we shall focus on methods that preserve the matching and that take account of the reduced variance that this achieves.

12.2.2 Analysis Based on Cluster-level Summaries

We first consider how to obtain point estimates, confidence intervals and significance tests for pair-matched trials where no adjustment is made for potential confounders.

Extending the notation of previous chapters, suppose r_{ij} is the observed rate of an outcome of interest in the jth matched pair ($j = 1, \ldots, c$) and the ith treatment arm ($i = 1$: intervention; $i = 0$: control). Then each matched pair provides an independent estimate of the rate difference or rate ratio:

$$\text{Estimated rate difference from jth matched pair} = r_{1j} - r_{0j}$$

$$\text{Estimated rate ratio from jth matched pair} = \frac{r_{1j}}{r_{0j}} \tag{12.1}$$

If we wish to obtain an overall estimate of the *rate difference*, the simplest approach is to compute the unweighted mean of the pair-wise rate differences, as follows:

$$\text{Estimated rate difference} = \frac{1}{c}\sum_j (r_{1j} - r_{0j}) = \bar{r}_1 - \bar{r}_0 \tag{12.2}$$

so that the point estimate in this case is identical to that obtained from an unmatched analysis.

Clearly, if the sample size or event rate varies substantially between clusters, some matched pairs may provide much more information than others about the size of the rate difference. This might suggest that a *weighted* average across matched pairs would provide a more precise estimate of the rate difference. The optimal weights, however, depend on the variances of the pair-specific estimates, and these depend not only on sample sizes and rates but also on the degree of between-cluster variation within each matched pair. Estimation of these optimal weights is therefore relatively complex, and this detracts from what is otherwise a very simple method of analysis.

If we wish to estimate the *rate ratio*, θ, we could take the unweighted mean of the pair-wise rate ratios obtained from Equation 12.1. Since ratios often have a skewed distribution, however, it may be more appropriate to take logarithms and to work in terms of the log(rate ratios). If we write $l_{ij} = \log(r_{ij})$, then the unweighted mean of the log(rate ratios) is given by:

$$\frac{1}{c}\sum_j \log \hat{\theta}_j = \frac{1}{c}\sum_j \log\left(\frac{r_{1j}}{r_{0j}}\right) = \frac{1}{c}\sum_j (l_{1j} - l_{0j}) = \bar{l}_1 - \bar{l}_0 \qquad (12.3)$$

Note that taking logarithms has reduced this estimate to a difference of means of the same form as the rate difference in Equation 12.2. To obtain our overall estimate of the rate ratio, we then take antilogarithms of this expression as follows:

$$Estimated\ rate\ ratio = \hat{\theta} = \exp(\bar{l}_1 - \bar{l}_0) = \left[\prod_j \left(\frac{r_{1j}}{r_{0j}}\right)\right]^{1/c}$$

and note that this is the *geometric mean* of the pair-wise rate ratios.

For binary outcomes, similar expressions can be obtained for the *risk difference* or *risk ratio*, while for quantitative outcomes the *mean difference* is likely to be the effect measure of interest.

We illustrate the derivation of significance tests and confidence intervals for *rate ratios*. Extensions to other types of effect measure are obvious.

If we write:

$$h_j = l_{1j} - l_{0j} = \log(\hat{\theta}_j) \qquad (12.4)$$

as the observed difference in log-rates in the *j*th matched pair, we can test the null hypothesis that the true rate ratio is 1, corresponding to a log(rate ratio) of zero, by carrying out a *paired t-test* on these pair-wise differences as:

$$t_m = \frac{\bar{h}}{\sqrt{\dfrac{s_m^2}{c}}} \qquad (12.5)$$

where $\bar{h}$ is the mean of the differences across matched pairs and s_m^2 is the empirical variance of these differences:

$$s_m^2 = \frac{1}{c-1}\sum_j (h_j - \bar{h})^2$$

The computed value of t_m from Equation 12.5 is referred to tables of the *t* distribution with $\upsilon = (c-1)$ degrees of freedom.

A 95% confidence interval for the log(rate ratio) can be obtained as:

$$\bar{h} \pm t_{\upsilon,0.025} \times \frac{s_m}{\sqrt{c}}$$

and the corresponding confidence limits for the rate ratio can be found either by taking anti-logarithms of the above expression:

$$\exp\left(\overline{h} \pm t_{v,0.025} \times \frac{s_m}{\sqrt{c}}\right)$$

or, equivalently, by multiplying and dividing the estimated ratio ratio $\exp(\overline{h})$ by the error factor:

$$EF = \exp\left(t_{v,0.025} \times \frac{s_m}{\sqrt{c}}\right)$$

Strictly, the *t-test* relies on the assumption that the log(rate ratios) are normally distributed. The test has been shown to be robust to departures from this assumption, however, especially for large numbers of matched pairs. When there are a small number of matched pairs, it may be advisable to additionally carry out a nonparametric test, for example the *signed rank test*. Note, however, that at least six pairs are needed to achieve a significant result (two-sided $p < 0.05$) when using such a nonparametric test.

Example 12.1

We return to the analysis of the Mwanza STD treatment trial, previously discussed in Example 5.3. In this CRT in Tanzania, the cumulative incidence of HIV infection was compared in six matched pairs of communities which were randomised to receive improved STD treatment services or to act as control communities (Grosskurth et al. 1995). The results are shown in Table 12.1.

TABLE 12.1

Cumulative HIV Incidence Observed over 2 Years of Follow-up in the Mwanza Trial of STD Treatment for HIV Prevention

Matched pair	Intervention	Control	Crude Risk Ratio	Adjusted Risk Ratio[†]
1	5/568 (0.9%)	10/702 (1.4%)	0.62	0.55
2	4/766 (0.5%)	7/833 (0.8%)	0.62	0.61
3	17/650 (2.6%)	20/630 (3.2%)	0.82	1.04
4	13/734 (1.8%)	23/760 (3.0%)	0.59	0.52
5	4/732 (0.5%)	12/782 (1.5%)	0.36	0.44
6	5/699 (0.7%)	10/693 (1.4%)	0.50	0.66
Overall	48/4149 (1.2%)	82/4400 (1.9%)		
Means of cluster summaries	1.18%	1.91%	0.57* (0.42, 0.76)	0.61* (0.45, 0.83)

*Geometric mean with 95% CI.
[†] Adjusted for age-group, sex and community HIV prevalence at baseline.

Although there were substantial differences in HIV incidence between matched pairs, the incidence was consistently lower in the intervention community than the control community in each of the six pairs, with observed risk ratios ranging from 0.36 to 0.82. Using these data, an overall estimate of the risk difference can be obtained as:

$$Estimated\ risk\ difference = 0.0118 - 0.0191 = -0.0073$$

or an absolute reduction in cumulative incidence of about 0.7%. Note that this estimate is very similar to the risk difference based on the overall proportions in the two arms (1.2%–1.9%). However, this will not always be the case, especially when there is a substantial difference in sample size between clusters.

In this trial, the *protective efficacy* afforded by the intervention is likely to be of more interest, and this is computed from the *risk ratio* as $(1-RR) \times 100\%$. Taking logarithms of the pair-wise risk ratios, we find that $\bar{h} = -0.570$ and $s_m = 0.280$. The estimated risk ratio is therefore given by:

$$Estimated\ risk\ ratio = \exp(-0.570) = 0.57$$

and a 95% CI is given by:

$$\exp\left(-0.570 \pm 2.57 \times 0.280/\sqrt{6}\right) = (0.42,\ 0.76)$$

This corresponds to a protective efficacy of 43% (95% CI: 24%, 58%).

If a formal significance test is required, we can compute:

$$t_m = \frac{-0.570}{0.280/\sqrt{6}} = -4.99$$

and referring this to tables of the t distribution with 5 df, we obtain a two-sided p-value of 0.004, indicating very strong evidence against the null hypothesis.

If we are concerned about the robustness of the *paired t-test* with six matched pairs, we may wish to supplement this with a nonparametric test. With six pairs, a two-sided p-value less than 0.05 is only achieved if the risk ratios are consistently below or above 1. This was the case in the Mwanza trial, and both the *signed rank test* and the *sign test* give a two-sided p-value of 0.03.

12.2.3 Adjusting for Covariates

In a pair-matched CRT, we aim to match the clusters on one or more factors that are expected to be correlated with the outcome of interest. If close matching is achieved, we can assume that the two treatment arms will be similar with respect to those matching factors. There are likely to be other potential confounding factors, however, that are not so well balanced between arms, especially if the number of matched pairs is small. We may therefore wish to adjust for these covariates in the analysis.

Even if a covariate shows overall balance between treatment arms, there are still likely to be differences between the clusters within each matched pair. These differences will serve to inflate the observed between-cluster variation. By adjusting for the covariate, we hope to reduce this variability and hence improve the power and precision of the trial.

Covariate adjustment can be achieved through a two-stage procedure similar to that described in Section 10.4. For rates, the first stage involves fitting a *Poisson regression* model to the data, including terms for the matched pairs and for the covariates of interest but *ignoring the intervention effect*. Using similar notation to that of Section 10.4.1, the log-rate in the kth individual in the jth matched pair and the ith treatment arm is modelled as:

$$\log(\lambda_{ijk}) = \alpha_j + \sum_l \gamma_l z_{ijkl}$$

where z_{ijkl} is the value of covariate z_l in this individual, and α_j represents the overall log-rate in the jth matched pair for zero values of the covariates. Using the fitted model, the *expected* number of events in this cluster is computed as:

$$e_{ij} = \sum_k y_{ijk} \hat{\lambda}_{ijk} = \sum_k y_{ijk} \times \exp\left(\hat{\alpha}_j + \sum_l \hat{\gamma}_l z_{ijkl} \right)$$

We now compare the observed and expected numbers of events in the two clusters in each matched pair. Note first that the observed and expected numbers should add up to the same total:

$$e_{1j} + e_{0j} = d_{1j} + d_{0j}$$

If the intervention has a protective effect, however, then d_{1j} will tend to be less than e_{1j} while d_{0j} will tend to exceed e_{0j}.

If we wish to work in terms of the *rate ratio*, we can proceed to compute the *adjusted rate ratio* in each matched pair:

$$\hat{\theta}'_j = \frac{d_{1j}/e_{1j}}{d_{0j}/e_{0j}}$$

If we take logarithms and write

$$h_j = \log(\hat{\theta}'_j)$$

we can then apply the methods of the previous section to obtain estimates, confidence intervals and significance tests for the adjusted rate ratio. Similar methods can be employed for binary or quantitative outcomes.

Example 12.2

In the Mwanza STD treatment trial, we have seen that the unadjusted risk ratio was 0.57 (95% CI: 0.42, 0.76). We now examine the effect of adjusting for covariates.

HIV prevalence in this study population showed substantial variation by age and sex, and it was anticipated that HIV incidence might also show such variation. Even though the overall age/sex distributions of the two treatment arms were similar, variations between communities in the same matched pair could increase between-cluster variation leading to lower precision. It was therefore decided to adjust for these two individual-level covariates.

There were substantial differences between communities in the baseline prevalence of HIV infection. Moreover, the overall baseline prevalence of 3.8% in the intervention arm was somewhat lower than the 4.4% prevalence in the control arm. Although this is a relatively small difference, and is subject to random error as only a sample of 1000 adults were tested in each community, this may give rise to concern that some or all of the observed difference in HIV *incidence* may be due to differences between communities in exposure to HIV. Note that the primary outcome in this trial, HIV incidence, can only be assessed in those who were HIV-negative at baseline, and so it is not possible to adjust for baseline HIV status as an *individual-level* covariate. Instead, the baseline prevalence in each community was entered into the first stage of the analysis as a cluster-level covariate.

Box 12.1 shows Stata output for the unadjusted and adjusted analyses of these data. In the first stage of the adjusted analysis, a *logistic regression* analysis is

BOX 12.1

```
. use mwanza.stdtrial.dta

. xi: logistic hiv i.pair i.agegp i.sex hivbase
```

Logistic regression				Number of obs =	8549
				LR chi2(10) =	39.10
				Prob > chi2 =	0.0000
Log likelihood = -653.64071				Pseudo R2 =	0.0290

hiv	Odds Ratio	Std. Err.	z	P>|z|	[95% Conf. Interval]	
_Ipair_2	.6968391	.3047773	-0.83	0.409	.2956934	1.64219
_Ipair_3	1.558383	.8867615	0.78	0.436	.5108785	4.753687
_Ipair_4	1.766484	.6146626	1.64	0.102	.8931557	3.493754
_Ipair_5	.8499273	.3102041	-0.45	0.656	.4156355	1.738005
_Ipair_6	.9371934	.3444539	-0.18	0.860	.4560165	1.926096
_Iagegp_2	1.043767	.2293906	0.19	0.845	.6784739	1.605734
_Iagegp_3	.9802907	.2472384	-0.08	0.937	.5979625	1.607074
_Iagegp_4	.8195215	.222742	-0.73	0.464	.4810695	1.396088
_Isex_2	.7365977	.1312974	-1.72	0.086	.5194037	1.044614
hivbase	1.121573	.1228919	1.05	0.295	.9048163	1.390255

```
. predic fv
. gen n=1
. collapse (sum) hiv n fv (mean) pair arm, by(community)
. gen logprev1=log(hiv/n) if arm==1
. gen logprev0=log(hiv/n) if arm==0
. gen logadj1=log(hiv/fv) if arm==1
. gen logadj0=log(hiv/fv) if arm==0
. collapse (sum) logprev1 logprev0 logadj1 logadj0, by(pair)
. ttest logprev1=logprev0
```

(continued)

BOX 12.1 (CONTINUED)

```
Paired t test
-------------------------------------------------------------------------
 Variable | Obs        Mean  Std. Err. Std. Dev. [95% Conf. Interval]
----------+--------------------------------------------------------------
 logprev1 |   6   -4.635765  .2684075  .6574614  -5.325728   -3.945801
 logprev0 |   6   -4.065613  .2071424  .5073933  -4.598089   -3.533136
----------+--------------------------------------------------------------
     diff |   6    -.570152  .1141297  .2795596  -.8635319   -.2767722
-------------------------------------------------------------------------
    mean(diff) = mean(logprev1 - logprev0)                 t = -4.9956
Ho: mean(diff) = 0                            degrees of freedom =      5

Ha: mean(diff) < 0        Ha: mean(diff) != 0        Ha: mean(diff) > 0
Pr(T < t) = 0.0021    Pr(|T| > |t|) = 0.0041    Pr(T > t) = 0.9979

. signtest logprev1=logprev0

Sign test

Two-sided test:
Ho: median of logprev1 - logprev0 = 0 vs.
Ha: median of logprev1 - logprev0 != 0
Pr(#positive >= 6 or #negative >= 6) =
   min(1, 2*Binomial(n = 6, x >= 6, p = 0.5)) = 0.0313

. ttest logadj1=logadj0
Paired t test
-------------------------------------------------------------------------
 Variable | Obs        Mean  Std. Err. Std. Dev. [95% Conf. Interval]
----------+--------------------------------------------------------------
  logadj1 |   6   -.2990392  .0756751  .1853654  -.4935682   -.1045102
  logadj0 |   6    .1933976  .0462103  .1131918   .0746101     .312185
----------+--------------------------------------------------------------
     diff |   6   -.4924367  .1199564   .293832  -.8007945    -.184079
-------------------------------------------------------------------------
    mean(diff) = mean(logadj1 - logadj0)                  t = -4.1051
Ho: mean(diff) = 0                            degrees of freedom =      5

Ha: mean(diff) < 0        Ha: mean(diff) != 0        Ha: mean(diff) > 0
Pr(T < t) = 0.0047    Pr(|T| > |t|) = 0.0093    Pr(T > t) = 0.9953

. signtest logadj1=logadj0

Two-sided test:
Ho: median of logadj1 - logadj0 = 0 vs.
Ha: median of logadj1 - logadj0 != 0
Pr(#positive >= 5 or #negative >= 5) =
   min(1, 2*Binomial(n = 6, x >= 5, p = 0.5)) = 0.2188
```

carried out with terms for the matched pair (six categories), age-group (four categories), sex (two categories) and baseline HIV prevalence (continuous). Using predicted values from this model, we can compute adjusted risk ratios for each matched pair, as shown in Table 12.1.

Taking logarithms of the adjusted risk ratios, we obtain $\bar{h} = -0.492$ and $s_m = 0.294$. The adjusted risk ratio is therefore given by:

$$Adjusted\ risk\ ratio = \exp(-0.492) = 0.61$$

and a 95% CI is given by:

$$\exp\left(-0.492 \pm 2.57 \times 0.294 \big/ \sqrt{6}\right) = (0.45, 0.83)$$

This corresponds to an adjusted protective efficacy of 39% (95% CI: 17%, 55%). A significance test of the null hypothesis of no intervention effect gives $t_m = -4.11$ on 5 df, corresponding to a two-sided p-value of 0.009.

Note that, after adjustment, only five of the six matched pairs give an estimated risk ratio below 1, the other being very close to 1 (Table 12.1). The *sign test* gives a two-sided p-value of 0.22. The *signed rank* test, which also takes into account the *sizes* of the risk ratios, gives an exact two-sided p-value of 0.062.

12.2.4 Regression Analysis Based on Individual-level Data

While we might prefer to use a regression-based method, to provide greater flexibility in modelling the effects of the intervention as well as cluster-level and individual-level covariates of interest, the options are limited for pair-matched trials. To see the reason for this, we consider a possible regression model for a binary outcome:

$$\text{logit}(\pi_{ijk}) = \log\left(\frac{\pi_{ijk}}{1 - \pi_{ijk}}\right) = \alpha_j + \beta_i + \sum_l \gamma_l z_{ijkl} + u_{ij} \qquad (12.6)$$

Note that this is identical to Equation 11.6 except for the fixed effects α_j representing the effects of the matched pairs. It is thanks to the incorporation of these effects that we hope that the variance of the cluster-specific random effects u_{ij} will be reduced compared with an unmatched design.

We might proceed to fit this model using *random effects logistic regression*, as explained in Section 11.2.3. However, logistic regression is an example of a *generalised linear model* which is fitted using the statistical method of *likelihood inference*. Such methods rely for their validity on large sample approximations. More specifically, they assume that the number of parameters to be estimated is very much smaller than the number of data points used to estimate them. In Equation 12.6, there is a separate parameter for each matched pair and, together with the additional parameters for the intervention and covariate effects, the number of parameters may approach the number of clusters. The regression analysis cannot be relied upon to give robust results under these conditions. Other regression methods for binary data, such as the use of GEE or robust (sandwich) standard errors, are similarly unreliable for the pair-matched design.

Similar concerns apply to regression methods for event rates, such as *random effects Poisson regression* as discussed in Section 11.2.1. We therefore recommend use of the *cluster-level* methods of previous sections, when analysing proportions or event rates in pair-matched trials.

For *quantitative* outcome variables, however, it *is* possible to carry out individual-level regression analysis since this does not depend on the approximate methods of likelihood inference. Providing the random effects in the model can be assumed to be normally distributed, valid estimates, confidence intervals and significant tests can be obtained that do not depend on large sample assumptions. The simplest form of the model would be:

$$x_{ijk} = \alpha_j + \beta_i + \sum_l \gamma_l z_{ijkl} + u_{ij} + v_{ijk}$$

In this model, the random effects u_{ij} and v_{ijk} are assumed to be normally distributed with mean zero and variances σ_B^2 and σ_W^2, where σ_B^2 represents between-cluster variation within matched pairs (after accounting for intervention and covariate effects) while σ_W^2 represents variation between individuals in the same cluster.

Note, however, that if the number of clusters is small, the dependence on assumptions of normality becomes critical, and so this method is unlikely to be as robust as the cluster-level methods even for quantitative outcomes. Careful consideration should be given to making a logarithmic transformation of the outcome variable if the data seem to have a positively skewed distribution, or if the differences between the clusters seem larger in matched pairs with larger mean values.

12.3 Analysis of Stratified Trials

12.3.1 Introduction

We have seen in Chapter 5 that the stratified design combines many of the best features of pair-matched and unmatched designs. By stratifying on factors that are correlated with the outcome of interest, the design helps to improve balance between treatment arms and to reduce between-cluster variability. But, unlike the pair-matched design, it does this without excessively reducing the degrees of freedom available when estimating intervention effects. As the advantages of this design become better recognised, it is likely that it will be used more frequently. In this section, we consider methods of analysis for such trials.

In many ways, the analytical choices are similar to those for pair-matched trials. However, the key difference is that we have some replication within each stratum, and this means that it is possible to obtain direct estimates of between-cluster variance (or equivalently the intracluster correlation coefficient) within strata. Replication also means that it is possible to examine whether the intervention effect varies between strata. This is not possible in a pair-matched trial because the pair-wise differences reflect both between-cluster variation and any variations in intervention effect, and it is not possible to separate these out.

12.3.2 Analysis Based on Cluster-level Summaries

Extending our notation to include a suffix for the stratum, suppose r_{sij} is the observed rate of an outcome of interest in the jth cluster in the ith treatment arm ($i = 1$: intervention; $i = 0$: control) in the sth stratum ($s = 1, ..., S$). Each stratum provides an independent estimate of the rate difference or rate ratio:

$$\text{Estimated rate difference from sth stratum} = \bar{r}_{s1} - \bar{r}_{s0} \qquad (12.7)$$

$$\text{Estimated rate ratio from sth stratum} = \frac{\bar{r}_{s1}}{\bar{r}_{s0}}$$

where $\bar{r}_{si}$ is the mean rate across clusters in the ith treatment arm in the sth stratum.

As in the previous section, we note that ratios often have a skewed distribution, and so it may be more appropriate to work in terms of the logarithms of the rates. If we write $l_{sij} = \log(r_{sij})$, then we can obtain an estimate of the log(rate ratio) from the sth stratum as:

$$\bar{l}_{s1} - \bar{l}_{s0} = \frac{1}{c_{s1}} \sum_j \log(r_{s1j}) - \frac{1}{c_{s0}} \sum_j \log(r_{s0j})$$

where c_{si} is the number of clusters in the ith treatment arm in the sth stratum. Note that taking logarithms has reduced this estimate to a difference of means of the same form as the rate difference in Equation 12.7. The corresponding estimate of the rate ratio is obtained by taking anti-logarithms of this expression, giving:

$$\text{Estimated rate ratio from sth stratum} = \hat{\theta}_s = \exp(\bar{l}_{s1} - \bar{l}_{s0}) = \frac{\bar{r}_{Gs1}}{\bar{r}_{Gs0}}$$

where $\bar{r}_{Gsi}$ is the geometric mean of the rates in the ith treatment arm in the sth stratum.

For binary outcomes, similar expressions can be obtained for the *risk difference* or *risk ratio*, while for quantitative outcomes the *mean difference* is likely to be the effect measure of interest.

We illustrate the derivation of significance tests and confidence intervals for *rate ratios*. Extensions to other types of effect are obvious.

If we write:

$$h_s = \bar{l}_{s1} - \bar{l}_{s0} = \log(\hat{\theta}_s)$$

as the observed difference in mean log-rates in the sth stratum, we can obtain an overall estimate of the log rate-ratio as a weighted average of the stratum-specific estimates:

$$\bar{h}_W = \frac{\sum_s w_s h_s}{\sum_s w_s} \tag{12.8}$$

Suppose the between-cluster variance in log-rates within each combination of stratum and treatment-arm may be assumed constant and equal to σ_S^2. Then the variance of each stratum-specific estimate, h_s, is given by:

$$Var(h_s) = Var(\bar{l}_{s1} - \bar{l}_{s0}) = \sigma_S^2 \left(\frac{1}{c_{s1}} + \frac{1}{c_{s0}} \right)$$

Then the optimal weights in Equation 12.8 are inversely proportional to the stratum-specific variances and are equal to:

$$w_s = \frac{1}{1/c_{s1} + 1/c_{s0}}$$

and with these weights, we obtain:

$$Var(\bar{h}_W) = \frac{\sigma_S^2}{\sum_s w_s}$$

We may estimate σ_S^2 by using the empirical variance of rates within each combination of stratum and treatment-arm, pooled over all these combinations:

$$\hat{\sigma}_S^2 = s^2 = \frac{\sum_{s,i,j} (l_{sij} - \bar{l}_{si})^2}{\upsilon}$$

where υ, the *degrees of freedom* of this estimate, is the total number of clusters minus the number of combinations:

$$\upsilon = \sum_{s,i} c_{si} - 2S$$

We may test the null hypothesis that the true rate ratio is 1 by carrying out a *stratified t-test* as follows:

$$t_S = \frac{\bar{h}_W}{s / \sqrt{\sum_s w_s}}$$

and referring the computed value of t_s to tables of the t distribution with υ degrees of freedom. A 95% CI for the rate ratio can be obtained as:

$$\exp\left(\bar{h}_W \pm t_{\upsilon, 0.025} \times \frac{s}{\sqrt{\sum_s w_s}} \right)$$

In many stratified trials, equal numbers of clusters are allocated to the two treatment arms within each stratum. In this special case, the computations become simpler. It may be shown that the weights are now proportional to the number of clusters in each stratum, so that Equation 12.8 reduces to:

$$\bar{h}_W = \frac{\sum_s c_s (\bar{l}_{s1} - \bar{l}_{s0})}{\sum_s c_s} = \frac{\sum_{s,j} l_{s1j}}{c} - \frac{\sum_{s,j} l_{s0j}}{c} = \bar{l}_1 - \bar{l}_0$$

where c_s clusters are allocated to each treatment arm in the sth stratum, and c is the total number allocated to each arm. In other words, the log(rate ratio) is estimated by the difference between the simple means of the log-rates in each treatment arm. The *stratified t-test* is then obtained as:

$$t_S = \frac{\bar{l}_1 - \bar{l}_0}{s\sqrt{2/c}}$$

and a 95% CI as:

$$\exp\left[(\bar{l}_1 - \bar{l}_0) \pm t_{\upsilon, 0.025} \times s\sqrt{2/c} \right]$$

The above methods for stratified trials are analogous to carrying out a *two-way analysis of variance* of the log-rates, the two factors being the stratum and the treatment arm. The variance estimate, s^2, is obtained from the residual mean square in an analysis of variance that incorporates stratum by treatment arm interactions.

Adjustment for covariates can be carried out with the usual two-stage analysis. At the first stage, a regression model is fitted which incorporates the stratum (as a fixed effect) and all covariates of interest but *not* the intervention effect. Fitted values from the regression model are used as in previous sections to compute a *residual* for each cluster. The residuals then replace the cluster-specific observations in the analysis. This procedure is illustrated in the numerical example that follows.

Example 12.3

We return to the stratified trial carried out in Mwanza Region, Tanzania to measure the impact of the *MEMA kwa Vijana* adolescent sexual health intervention, first described in Example 2.4 (Ross et al. 2007). In this trial, 20 rural communities were grouped into three strata that were expected to have a high risk (six communities), medium risk (eight communities) or low risk (six communities) of HIV and other STIs based on an initial community-based survey. Half the communities in each stratum were randomly selected to receive the intervention, the others acting as control communities. A cohort of students aged 14 years and over was recruited from the final three standards at the primary schools in each community, and followed up for 3 years to measure effects on knowledge, attitudes, reported sexual behaviour, HIV incidence, and the incidence and prevalence of other biomedical endpoints including STIs and pregnancy.

Table 12.2 shows the proportion of boys in each community who were recorded as having "good" knowledge of HIV acquisition at the final follow-up survey, meaning that they were able to respond correctly to all three test questions on this subject. Box 12.2 shows Stata output for the unadjusted analysis of these data.

The overall proportions of boys with good HIV knowledge were 65% in the intervention arm and 45% in the control arm. Although this difference was

TABLE 12.2

Proportion of Boys with Good Knowledge of HIV Acquisition in Trial of *MEMA kwa Vijana* Adolescent Sexual Health Intervention

Stratum	Intervention	Control
High risk	164/204 (80.4%)	110/226 (48.7%)
	141/206 (68.4%)	69/178 (38.8%)
	111/171 (64.9%)	65/171 (38.0%)
Medium risk	139/219 (63.5%)	87/194 (44.8%)
	172/237 (72.6%)	102/229 (44.5%)
	111/187 (59.4%)	84/243 (34.6%)
	115/207 (55.6%)	121/196 (61.7%)
Low risk	119/169 (70.4%)	101/226 (44.7%)
	157/219 (71.7%)	102/175 (58.3%)
	127/257 (49.4%)	67/186 (36.0%)
Overall	1356/2076 (65.3%)	908/2024 (44.9%)
Geometric mean of cluster summaries	65.0%	44.2%

BOX 12.2

```
. use mkvtrial.dta
. tab arm know, row
```

Intervention/ control group	know 0	1	Total
0	1,116	908	2,024
	55.14	44.86	100.00
1	720	1,356	2,076
	34.68	65.32	100.00
Total	1,836	2,264	4,100
	44.78	55.22	100.00

```
. gen n=1
. collapse (sum) know n, by(community arm stratum)
. gen pknow=know/n
. gen lpknow=log(pknow)
. help summ
. summarise lpknow if arm==1
```

Variable	Obs	Mean	Std. Dev.	Min	Max
lpknow	10	-.4302522	.1432081	-.704889	-.2182536

```
. gen l1=r(mean)
. summarise lpknow if arm==0
```

Variable	Obs	Mean	Std. Dev.	Min	Max
lpknow	10	-.8156558	.1943914	-1.062245	-.4823241

```
. gen l0=r(mean)
. gen rr=exp(l1-l0)
. xi:regress lpknow i.stratum*i.arm
```

Source	SS	df	MS			
Model	.792137123	5	.158427425	Number of obs	=	20
				F(5,14)	=	4.67
				Prob > F	=	0.0102
Residual	.475211696	14	.033943693	R-squared	=	0.6250
				Adj R-squared	=	0.4911
Total	1.26734882	19	.066702569	Root MSE	=	.18424

lpknow	Coef.	Std. Err.	t	P>|t|	[95% Conf. Interval]	
_Istratum_2	-.0000565	.1407142	-0.00	1.000	-.3018584	.3017455
_Istratum_3	-.0895754	.1504298	-0.60	0.561	-.4122153	.2330644
_Iarm_1	.3259305	.1504298	2.17	0.048	.0032906	.6485704
_IstrXar~2_1	-.0082456	.1989999	-0.04	0.968	-.435058	.4185668
_IstrXar~3_1	.2092378	.2127399	0.98	0.342	-.2470439	.6655194
cons	-.7887605	.1063699	-7.42	0.000	-1.016901	-.5606197

(*continued*)

> **BOX 12.2 (CONTINUED)**
>
> ```
> . gen sigma=e(rmse)
> . gen selogrr=sigma*sqrt(2/10)
> . gen t=log(rr)/selogrr
> . gen rrcil=rr/exp(invttail(14,0.025)*selogrr)
> . gen rrciu=rr*exp(invttail(14,0.025)*selogrr)
> . disp rr,rrcil,rrciu,t
> 1.4702076 1.2320586 1.7543892 4.6775799
> ```

substantial, there was also considerable variation between communities, the observed proportions ranging from 49 to 80% in the intervention arm, and from 35 to 62% in the control arm.

Noting that equal numbers of communities were allocated to the two treatment arms within each stratum, and taking logarithms of the proportions in each community, we obtain:

$$\text{Mean log-proportion in intervention arm} = \bar{l}_1 = -0.430$$

$$\text{Mean log-proportion in control arm} = \bar{l}_0 = -0.816$$

Taking anti-logarithms, the corresponding geometric means of the proportions in each arm were 65.0 and 44.2%, very similar to the overall proportions. The estimated risk ratio was obtained as:

$$\exp(\bar{h}_w) = \exp(\bar{l}_1 - \bar{l}_0) = \exp(-0.430 + 0.816) = 1.470$$

and this is equal to the ratio of the geometric means.

To carry out a significance test and compute a confidence interval, we need an estimate s^2 of the within-stratum between-cluster variance σ_s^2. This can be obtained as the residual mean square from a two-way analysis of variance of the log-proportions on stratum and treatment arm, including interaction terms, and is equal to $s^2 = 0.0339$.

The *stratified t-test* of the null hypothesis of no intervention effect is given by:

$$t_s = \frac{\bar{l}_1 - \bar{l}_0}{s\sqrt{2/c}} = \frac{-0.430 + 0.816}{0.184 \times \sqrt{2/10}} = \frac{0.386}{0.0824} = 4.68$$

and referring this to tables of the t distribution with 14 df, we obtain a two-sided $p < 0.001$, indicating very strong evidence against the null hypothesis.

A 95% CI for the risk ratio is obtained as:

$$\exp\left[(\bar{l}_1 - \bar{l}_0) \pm t_{v,0.025} \times s\sqrt{2/c}\right] = \exp(0.386 \pm 2.145 \times 0.0824) = (1.23, 1.75)$$

Baseline comparison of treatment arms suggested some imbalance in ethnic group and lifetime sexual partners at enrolment. A further analysis was therefore carried out to adjust for these covariates as well as age-group which was expected to be an important predictor of the outcome of interest, and this is shown in Box 12.3. Logistic regression of the knowledge outcome against stratum, age-group, ethnic group and lifetime partners was used to obtain the fitted value and hence the ratio-residual for each community. Replacing the logarithms of the observed proportions with the logarithms of the ratio-residuals, we estimate the adjusted risk ratio as:

$$\exp(\bar{h}_w) = \exp(\bar{l}_1 - \bar{l}_0) = \exp(0.155 + 0.211) = 1.442$$

Based on the residual mean square from the two-way analysis of variance, we obtain $s^2 = 0.0226$, and hence:

$$t_S = \frac{0.155 + 0.211}{0.150 \times \sqrt{2/10}} = \frac{0.366}{0.0672} = 5.44$$

and $p < 0.001$ as before. A 95% CI for the adjusted risk ratio is given by:

$$\exp(0.366 \pm 2.145 \times 0.0672) = (1.25, 1.67)$$

Note that while the risk ratio is reduced slightly following covariate adjustment, the estimate becomes somewhat more precise, presumably because some of the variation between clusters is accounted for by the effects of the covariates.

BOX 12.3

```
. use mkvtrial.dta

. xi:logistic know i.agegp i.ethnicgp i.lifepart i.stratum
Logistic regression                          Number of obs =     4100
                                             LR chi2(8)    =    76.55
                                             Prob > chi2   =   0.0000
Log likelihood = -2781.2466                  Pseudo R2     =   0.0136
-----------------------------------------------------------------------
      know │Odds Ratio Std. Err.     z   P>│z│  [95% Conf. Interval]
-----------------------------------------------------------------------
  _Iagegp_2 │ 1.039119  .086169   0.46 0.644   .8832413  1.222506
  _Iagegp_3 │ 1.335965 .0999312   3.87 0.000   1.153784  1.546912
_Iethnicgp_1 │ .5647307 .0453194  -7.12 0.000   .4825395  .6609216
_Ilifepart_1 │ 1.161596 .1123366   1.55 0.121   .9610291  1.404022
_Ilifepart_2 │ .9195933 .0954813  -0.81 0.419   .7502665  1.127135
_Ilifepart_3 │ .9505656 .0736716  -0.65 0.513   .8166039  1.106503
 _Istratum_2 │ 1.096657 .0847754   1.19 0.233    .942475  1.276061
 _Istratum_3 │ 1.210777 .1018536   2.27 0.023   1.026736  1.427806
-----------------------------------------------------------------------
. predict e

. collapse (sum) know e, by(community arm stratum)

. gen eknow=know/e

. gen leknow=log(eknow)

. summarise leknow if arm==1
```

(continued)

```
      Variable |     Obs          Mean    Std. Dev.           Min          Max
   -------------+------------------------------------------------------------
        leknow |      10      .1550984     .0905034     -.0147603     .3091297
   . gen l1=r(mean)

   . summarise leknow if arm==0

      Variable |     Obs          Mean    Std. Dev.           Min          Max
   -------------+------------------------------------------------------------
        leknow |      10     -.2109332     .1836578     -.4136048     .1640678
   . gen l0=r(mean)

   . gen rr=exp(l1-l0)

   . xi:regress leknow i.stratum*i.arm
```

Source	SS	df	MS		Number of obs	=	20
Model	.730611909	5	.146122382		F(5, 14)	=	6.46
					Prob > F	=	0.0026
Residual	.316573619	14	.022612401		R-squared	=	0.6977
					Adj R-squared	=	0.5897
Total	1.04718553	19	.055115028		Root MSE	=	.15037

leknow	Coef.	Std. Err.	t	P>|t|	[95% Conf. Interval]	
_Istratum_2	.0162503	.1148502	0.14	0.889	-.2300789	.2625795
_Istratum_3	-.1322486	.12278	-1.08	0.300	-.3955856	.1310883
_Iarm_1	.3096281	.12278	2.52	0.024	.0462911	.572965
_IstrXar~2_1	-.0243189	.1624227	-0.15	0.883	-.3726809	.3240432
_IstrXar~3_1	.2204371	.1736372	1.27	0.225	-.1519776	.5928518
_cons	-.1777588	.0868186	-2.05	0.060	-.3639661	.0084486

```
   . gen sigma=e(rmse)

   . gen selogrr=sigma*sqrt(2/10)

   . gen t=log(rr)/selogrr

   . gen rrcil=rr/exp(invttail(14,0.025)*selogrr)

   . gen rrciu=rr*exp(invttail(14,0.025)*selogrr)

   . disp rr,rrcil,rrciu,t
   1.4420009 1.2483168 1.6657363 5.4428992
```

12.3.3 Regression Analysis Based on Individual-level Data

As for unmatched studies, we might prefer individual-level regression methods for their greater convenience and flexibility. Possible methods include the GEE and random effects models discussed in Chapter 11, the only modification being that additional fixed effect parameters are included for the strata. For binary outcomes, for example, we could fit the random effects logistic regression model:

$$\text{logit}(\pi_{sijk}) = \log\left(\frac{\pi_{sijk}}{1-\pi_{sijk}}\right) = \alpha_s + \beta_i + \sum_l \gamma_l z_{sijkl} + u_{sij}$$

where α_s represents the stratum effect and u_{sij} is the random effect corresponding to the jth cluster in the ith treatment arm and sth stratum.

Note that this estimates an overall treatment effect, although the effect of the intervention may differ substantially across strata. When strata are formed according to a variable that may be of intrinsic interest, such as baseline HIV prevalence or predominant ethnic group, the stratum-specific risk ratios should be examined for qualitative differences. It may be of interest to formally test for differences in treatment effect across strata by incorporating appropriate interaction terms in the above model, although such tests will tend to have very low power due to limited numbers of clusters.

We noted in Section 12.2.4 that the fitting of individual-level regression models was problematic for pair-matched trials because the number of parameters to be estimated approached the number of cluster-level data points, thus violating the large sample assumptions underlying likelihood inference. Stratified trials fall between the extremes of unmatched and pair-matched trials in this regard, because there is replication within at least some of the strata, and only one parameter is fitted for each stratum rather than one for each matched pair.

In Section 11.4, we cautioned against the use of individual-level regression for unmatched trials with less than 15 clusters per arm. Furthermore research is needed on the performance of such methods for stratified trials, but it would seem prudent to apply somewhat more stringent criteria because of the additional parameters fitted. As a rough guideline, such methods might be considered for trials with more than 20 clusters per treatment arm. However, we recommend that additional analyses are carried out using cluster-level summaries, at least for the unadjusted analysis, to check that the conclusions are robust.

12.4 Analysis of Other Study Designs

We briefly discuss analysis methods for some of the other study designs considered in earlier chapters.

12.4.1 Trials with More than Two Treatment Arms

CRTs with a large number of treatment arms are very uncommon due to their cost and logistical complexity. Sometimes, however, two or three alternative interventions are compared with a single control arm.

The primary analysis in such trials will often focus on pair-wise comparisons between each intervention arm and the control arm. Clearly, any of the methods discussed in Chapters 10 through 12 can be used for such comparisons.

As usual when making *multiple comparisons* of this kind, the investigator needs to be aware that the more tests that are carried out, the higher the probability that some effects will be found statistically significant just by chance. One way of guarding against this is to carry out an overall test of the null hypothesis that there are *no differences* between any of the treatment arms. If this is non-significant, then significant effects seen for individual comparisons would need to be interpreted cautiously.

If conducting a cluster-level analysis, such an overall test would be conducted by performing a *one-way analysis of variance* and obtaining an F-test for differences between treatment arms. The unpaired t-test can be regarded as a special case of the F-test when there are only two arms. Similarly, in individual-level regression, it is possible to carry out a test of the null hypothesis:

$$H_0: \beta_i = 0, \quad \text{for all } i$$

For random effects models, this is done by performing a *likelihood ratio test* comparing the fit of nested models with and without these β_i parameters present. For GEE, it can be done by performing a Wald test of this null hypothesis, for example by using the *testparm* command in Stata.

If the treatment arms represent increasing intensities of exposure to intervention, it may be desired to examine the evidence of a *dose–response* effect. The above methods may readily be extended to allow for this. In cluster-level analysis this is done by replacing the one-way analysis of variance with linear regression on a variable representing the dose of intervention. Similarly, in individual-level regression, the β_i terms can be replaced by βx_i where x_i represents the dose for the ith treatment arm. This will provide a more powerful test than the overall test if there is a steady increase or decrease in the endpoint of interest between the ordered treatment arms.

12.4.2 Factorial Trials

In a two-way factorial design, we examine the joint effects of two interventions I_1 and I_2. In the simplest 2×2 design, each intervention is either absent or present, and we would wish to fit models of the form:

$$\mu = \alpha + \beta_1 x_1 + \beta_2 x_2 \qquad (12.9)$$

where μ is either the mean of a quantitative outcome; a risk or rate; or a log(risk), log(odds) or log(rate), depending on the endpoint and effect measure of interest. In Equation 12.9, x_1 and x_2 are indicator variables denoting the absence or presence of interventions I_1 and I_2, respectively.

In a cluster-level analysis, *linear regression* would be performed on the cluster summaries using the model shown in Equation 12.9. If we are willing to assume that the effects of the two interventions are *independent*, as discussed in Section 8.2.2, then no interaction terms are included in Equation 12.9 and the estimates of β_1 and β_2 represent the estimates of the two intervention effects. Note that each of these estimates can be thought of as the estimated effect of one intervention in a trial that is *stratified* on the presence of the other intervention. The assumption of independence can be evaluated by incorporating interaction terms in the regression model and carrying out a test for interaction, although this is generally likely to be of low power. If interactions are present, then each intervention effect has to be reported separately in the absence or presence of the other intervention. Extensions to individual-level regression are obvious, although large numbers of clusters would be needed for such methods to be robust.

12.4.3 Stepped Wedge Trials

In Section 8.2.4, we introduced the stepped wedge design, which is essentially a one-way crossover trial. The phased introduction of an intervention with randomised entry of clusters into intervention status may have political, ethical and logistical advantages over a standard parallel cluster randomised trial. The analysis of stepped wedge trials, however, requires more care due to the imbalance over most of the course of the study in the numbers of clusters in the treatment and control arms. Although possible, we are not aware of any multiple-arm stepped wedge trials, and so in this section we only address two-arm designs.

Most stepped wedge trials will be conducted over a relatively long interval of time, during which there may well be secular trends that can affect the outcomes of interest in the study clusters. This means that an analysis that just compares "after" to "before" within each cluster can be biased, as underlying rates of disease, say, may become higher or lower during the study. There are two main approaches to accounting for time-related trends: the *horizontal* approach, in which time effects are modelled explicitly, and the *vertical* approach, in which a conditional analysis is performed at each step and the results combined across steps.

Suppose we have event rate data for which a Poisson model would be appropriate. For simplicity, we illustrate the approaches with cluster-level data. The *horizontal* approach would employ the following type of model:

$$\log(\lambda_{jt}) = \alpha + \beta x_{jt} + \sum_{t=1}^{T} \gamma_t z_t + u_j$$

where $j = 1, \ldots, J$ indexes the clusters, $t = 1, \ldots, T$ indexes the steps, x_{jt} is an indicator variable that takes the value 0 when the jth cluster is in the control phase and 1 when it is in the intervention phase, and the z_t indicate the steps. Note that we do not need a subscript i for treatment arm, because all clusters receive both treatment conditions. In this model, β represents the treatment effect while the γ_t account for any time-specific effects. The u_j are cluster-level random effects that account for within-cluster correlation (Hussey and Hughes 2007). Unless there are a large number of clusters relative to the number of steps, however, estimation of all the γ_t will be problematic. In this case, one may instead estimate one parameter for every two or three steps, say, or else fit a curve, for example replacing γ_t by γt to fit a linear trend in the log-rate. If time effects change more rapidly or unpredictably, this approach may not be ideal.

The *vertical* approach analyses the data at each step, using all the data in time slice *t* as shown in Figure 8.3. Viewing all the individuals in the clusters in a particular time slice as the *risk set*, and conditioning on the total observed events in that slice, we can calculate the *conditional probability* that the observed events in that slice would occur in the intervention or control sets of clusters in which they did occur. This is done in the same manner as in the analysis of a matched case-control study, with the matching being on time in this situation. The analysis can be carried out with statistical routines for *conditional logistic regression* or *Cox proportional hazards regression*, but with one further modification: the within-cluster correlation needs to be accounted for. The addition of a random effect (frailty distribution) to the Cox model, the use of a robust variance estimator, or bootstrapping of entire cluster-level histories may be used to this end (Moulton et al. 2006, 2007). The conditional analysis eliminates the need to estimate any γ_t parameters; in fact, the analysis can be done with the time slice being as thin as one day, to perfectly account for any changes across time, which can happen due to extraneous happenings (e.g., an earthquake in the study region) or, say, weekend effects. For binary or continuous outcome data, a similar method can be used, estimating time-specific contrasts and combining across time by bootstrapping the clusters (Moulton and Zeger 1989).

Note that, using the vertical approach, information on the treatment effect comes only from time slices (or steps) where there are clusters in both the intervention and control phases, and relies on the randomisation scheme for the comparability of these two sets of clusters. In contrast, the horizontal approach makes some use of data from time periods at the start or end of the study when all the clusters are in either the control or intervention phase, since these data provide information on the u_j cluster-specific effects. By using "before" and "after" information on each cluster, the horizontal approach may provide greater power and precision, but it does so at the cost of additional assumptions about the constancy of the cluster effects which may not be appropriate, particularly if there is a lengthy period of follow-up.

With the additional complexities of analysis, interpretation and communication attendant on the stepped wedge design, it would be advisable to give careful consideration to the use of a standard, parallel-arms CRT before opting for this study design.

Part D

Miscellaneous Topics

13

Ethical Considerations

13.1 Introduction

The main focus of this book is on CRTs that involve the experimental study of interventions in human participants. The ethical requirements for clinical trials involving human subjects have received much attention during the past 30 or 40 years, and there are now internationally accepted guidelines setting out the minimal requirements that should be met by such studies (Council for International Organisations of Medical Sciences (in collaboration with WHO) 2002; International Conference on Harmonisation of Technical Requirements for Registration of Pharmaceuticals for Human Use 1996). During the planning of a CRT, investigators need to give careful consideration to how these requirements will be met, since cluster randomisation introduces a number of ethical complications that do not usually apply in individually randomised trials.

In Section 13.2, we briefly review the general ethical principles that apply to any randomised clinical trial involving human participants. The following sections focus on the application of these principles to CRTs. Section 13.3 considers special issues relating to risks and benefits of trial participation in the context of group allocation. The requirement for fully informed consent lies at the heart of accepted ethical guidelines for clinical trials, but this involves a number of specific issues in CRTs that are discussed in Section 13.4. Finally, Section 13.5 considers other ethical issues in CRTs, including scientific validity, phased intervention designs and trial monitoring.

13.2 General Principles

We briefly outline the key requirements that apply to any randomised clinical trial. These may be summarised under the headings *beneficence, equity* and *autonomy*.

13.2.1 Beneficence

The basic principles here are that risks to participants resulting from participation in the trial should be minimised, and that any such risks should be justified by the benefits of the research.

Application of this principle requires careful consideration of the potential adverse effects associated with the intervention or with trial participation, and ways in which these might be avoided or mitigated. In the case of new biomedical products, such as drugs and vaccines, this may include carrying out pre-clinical and animal studies as well as small-scale (Phases 1 and 2) trials to evaluate the safety of the new product. In the case of preventive interventions, such as health education programmes, there may be data from pilot studies or previous trials of comparable interventions. In many cases, it is not possible to completely avoid all adverse events, in which case the ethical review committee that considers the proposed research will wish to consider whether the frequency and severity of adverse effects is likely to be acceptable given the potential benefits resulting from the intervention and from the results of the trial.

The ethical case for carrying out a trial is clearest if it is possible to argue that there is *equipoise* between the arms of the trial, in other words that there is *genuine uncertainty* as to which arm will provide the best outcome taking into account all the risks and benefits resulting from allocation to this arm.

An important principle related to beneficence is that trial participants should not, as a result of taking part in the trial, be denied services or interventions to which they would normally have access.

Finally, it is difficult to make a convincing case that the benefits of a trial outweigh the risks if the design or conduct of the trial are flawed. Unless the *scientific validity* of the trial is assured, trial participants are subject to risk or inconvenience without the prospect that the study will provide useful evidence of intervention effectiveness that will guide future health policy to the benefit of patients or populations.

13.2.2 Equity

The principle of *equity* requires that study populations and participants should be selected fairly. This implies for example that participation should not favour particular socioeconomic groups, ethnic groups, age-groups or genders unless there is a sound medical or scientific justification.

A related principle is that trials of interventions should not generally be carried out in study populations where there is no reasonable prospect of the intervention being provided if it is shown to be effective. For example, investigators may seek to carry out a trial of a new drug in a developing country setting because of the logistical advantages of conducting the research in a stable or compliant population with a high incidence of the disease of interest. This would not be appropriate if the price or other characteristics of the drug mean that it is very unlikely to be made available in that country subsequent to the trial. Some caution is needed in making these judgements, however, as past experience has shown that prices of products sometimes decrease dramatically as they are rolled out on a large scale.

13.2.3 Autonomy

The principle of *autonomy* requires that participants are fully informed about the purpose and nature of the research, and are able to make a free choice as to whether to participate. To ensure autonomy, trials need to incorporate effective arrangements for *informed consent*. This requires that potential participants are given full information, in a form that they can understand, on the study methods (including randomisation and the use of placebos if appropriate), the procedures that they will be expected to follow, the possible risks and benefits from taking part in the trial, their right to withdraw at any time and provisions to ensure data confidentiality.

Informed consent is most often documented by means of a form signed by the participant. In some cases, and especially where participants are illiterate, the consent form may be signed by an independent witness who confirms by their signature that the study information has been read to and understood by the participant.

13.3 Ethical Issues in Group Allocation

Most individually randomised clinical trials involve new drugs or vaccines, and the potential for harm is usually well recognised by investigators and ethical review committees. By contrast, CRTs often involve public health interventions such as health education programmes where the potential for harm may be less obvious. Nevertheless, almost all such interventions may result in adverse effects, and it is important that these are considered carefully when the trial is designed and presented for ethical review.

This point is illustrated by two examples in sexual health. School-based programmes to promote adolescent sexual health have been widely promoted, and it is generally assumed that improved knowledge and skills will result in lower rates of risk behaviour, teenage pregnancy and STIs. However, some have argued that sex education programmes may result in increased sexual experimentation and promiscuity and have the opposite of the desired effect. Clearly, this possibility needs to be kept in mind when the intervention programme is developed and when its effects are evaluated. Similarly, condom social marketing aims at promoting condom use, especially in casual relationships, to protect against HIV and other STIs. It might, however, have the perverse effect of encouraging casual sexual relationships, and this might offset some or all of the protective effect of condom use.

We noted above that the principle of *beneficence* requires a careful assessment of the benefit/risk ratio in trial participants. This may be more problematic in a CRT, for example where entire communities are allocated to one intervention or another. For example, in a trial of mass administration of anti-helminthic drugs to reduce worm infections in young children, children from some socioeconomic backgrounds may be at much lower risk of helminth infections than others, and so the benefit/risk ratio may be much lower in these children.

In individually randomised trials, *inclusion criteria* may be applied to restrict recruitment to participants where the benefit/risk ratio is more likely to be favourable. For this reason, trials of new drugs or vaccines often exclude pregnant or lactating women, to avoid possible adverse effects on the women or their infants. It is sometimes feasible and appropriate to incorporate such *inclusion criteria* in CRTs also. For example, in a trial in which medical practices are randomised, and patients diagnosed with diabetes in the intervention arm are given a new experimental drug, this intervention might be restricted to exclude pregnant women just as in an individually randomised trial. However, this would not be possible with population-level interventions, such as mass-media health education programmes, where exclusion of individuals within communities is not feasible.

A further complication is that risks and benefits in some CRTs may occur in *different individuals*. In most individually randomised trials, we are interested in the trade-off between adverse effects and benefits in the same individual. However, we have seen that one of the reasons for adopting cluster randomisation is to capture the population-level effects of interventions against infectious diseases. A good example is provided by vaccines targeted at the gametocyte stage of the malaria parasite. Such *transmission-blocking vaccines* do not protect the individual vaccine recipient against infection or disease, but are intended to reduce the rate of *transmission* of infection to other members of the community. The most favourable benefit/risk ratio in this example would occur in an unvaccinated individual in a vaccinated community, since they would benefit from reduced malaria transmission resulting from other community members being vaccinated without being subject to any adverse effects of the vaccine. However, the full benefit of vaccination at population-level would only be seen if a large proportion of the population were vaccinated.

13.4 Informed Consent in Cluster Randomised Trials

Obtaining informed consent from participants or their representatives is a key ethical requirement in clinical trials. Where individual informed consent is not to be obtained, a clear case needs to be made and the independent ethics committee will wish to scrutinise this carefully before giving approval for the trial. An example is provided by trials of interventions in emergency trauma cases where patients may be unconscious and representatives may not always be available to give consent.

In most trials, individual participants are asked for their consent to be randomised to alternative treatment conditions and to undergo the planned study procedures set out in the trial protocol. In CRTs, however, treatment conditions are allocated not to individuals but to entire clusters and this therefore raises special considerations that do not apply in individually randomised trials. In the sections that follow, we discuss approaches that may be adopted to obtain consent to randomisation and participation, which may need to be considered separately in the case of CRTs.

Throughout the discussion, it is important to keep in mind the distinction between randomisation of a cluster, which occurs at the cluster level, and application of the treatment conditions, which may occur at the cluster level or at the individual level. The effects of some cluster-level interventions, such as radio transmissions or water fluoridation, are difficult for individuals to avoid. Others, such as provision of family planning services in a local clinic, or individual dosing with a micronutrient, are more easily declined by individuals.

13.4.1 Consent for Randomisation

Given that entire clusters are to be randomised to treatment arms, it is clearly not possible for individuals to decide separately whether or not to consent to randomisation. In essence, a decision has to be made at group level on behalf of the whole cluster.

In some CRTs with small clusters, such as trials where households are randomised, it may be feasible to seek consent from *all* individual members of the household before that household is accepted for recruitment to the trial. Where this is possible, this would usually be the preferred approach, although even this may be problematic in cultural settings where it is the norm for heads of household to make important decisions on behalf of other family members.

In CRTs with larger clusters, however, it will generally not be feasible to obtain separate consent from all individuals in the cluster prior to randomisation. We consider two simple examples.

Example 13.1

Consider a CRT in which large rural communities are to be randomised to different interventions designed to reduce malaria transmission. If there are many thousands of individuals living in each community, it will be difficult or impossible to obtain informed consent for randomisation in advance from every member of the community. In addition, if this approach were attempted, perfect consensus would be needed in order for a cluster to be recruited, and this would not be achieved if even one individual out of, say, 20,000 did not wish to give their consent. Clearly, if this form of consent were insisted on, no CRTs with large clusters could be carried out.

Example 13.2

A further example is provided by a CRT in which medical practices are randomised to arms providing different treatment regimens for new patients presenting with a certain condition during the defined study period. Since the identity of these patients will not be known at the time when randomisation is to be carried out, it will not be possible to seek their consent in advance of randomisation.

Given these practical constraints, it is generally accepted that CRTs may need to rely on some form of group-level consent to randomisation. Investigators need to give careful attention to the question of who should provide this consent for each cluster. A case justifying this choice needs to be made in the submission to the independent ethics committee, which will need to be convinced that the person or persons chosen can genuinely represent the interests of the cluster members. The submission should also define how consent will be documented, whether through verbal agreement, a signed statement or some other mechanism.

We briefly discuss some alternatives.

13.4.1.1 Political Authorities

This is a common choice in CRTs where large geographical units are randomised, especially when the clusters coincide with administrative units such as cities or districts. In many cases, the trial will need to be *approved* by such authorities in any case, but this does not necessarily mean that this can be regarded as an adequate form of group-level consent. The extent to which the authorities can genuinely *represent* the community may depend partly on whether it is elected through some kind of democratic process, although even this clearly does not imply that all members of the community would consider that the authorities legitimately represent their interests, particularly where there are factional or ethnic differences.

13.4.1.2 Village Heads

In some CRTs in developing countries, villages are the level of randomisation and *village heads* are asked to consent for their villages to participate in the trial, sometimes taking part in a formal randomisation ceremony so that they can be assured of the fairness of the allocation (see Chapter 6). In rural populations in such settings there is often a strong sense of community, and it is often well-accepted by local communities that village heads or groups of village elders should take major decisions on behalf of the community. Preferably this should be done after consultation with community members, and trial investigators may be able to assist with this process, for example by making available information materials or videos that can be presented at village meetings.

Example 13.3

In the Ghana Vitamin A Supplementation Trial, first considered in Example 3.4, periodic vitamin A supplements or placebo were delivered to children living in

185 arbitrary geographical zones (Ghana VAST Study Team 1993). The trial was explained in detail to the district authorities and to the paramount chiefs of the 10 chiefdoms making up the study area, all of whom gave their approval for the trial. Meetings were also held in each of the chiefdoms, to which chiefs, elders and all compound members were invited. The design of the trial was explained and open lotteries conducted to randomly allocate the clusters to the intervention and control arms.

13.4.1.3 Community Representatives

Alternatively, there may be an individual or group of individuals from the community that can formally represent community members. This may be an existing group or could be established specifically for the purposes of the trial. For example, in a trial of an HIV prevention programme among female sex workers, women working in each community might be asked to select one or more of their peers to represent them, either informally or through some kind of formal mechanism.

In conventional clinical trials, as well as CRTs, there is now increasing experience of approaches to setting up *community advisory boards* to represent the interests of the study population. These same approaches could be used to establish representative groups who could be asked to provide consent on behalf of their communities, and these groups could then continue in existence to facilitate a two-way flow of information during the conduct of the trial.

Example 13.4

In the *Thibela TB* trial, previously discussed in Example 4.9, 15 gold mines in South Africa have been randomised to intervention or control conditions. The intervention involves providing all miners with 6 months of isoniazid preventive therapy aimed at preventing TB, after initial screening to detect and treat active TB disease. As well as seeking the approval of the mine companies, the investigators considered that it was important to obtain the agreement of the workers' representatives, in this case the trade unions. This is especially important in settings where there may be a lack of trust between community members and employers or the authorities, as might be expected to be the case in South Africa following the experiences of the apartheid era.

13.4.1.4 Medical Practitioners

In trials in which medical practices are randomised to alternative interventions, it is most often the medical practitioners themselves who provide consent for the participation of their practices. Since it is generally the responsibility of clinicians to put the medical interests of their patients above all other considerations, this may be an appropriate choice, although there may be some conflict of interest if some or all of the practitioners are also involved in the trial as investigators. Where there are patient groups, as exist for some specific diseases, investigators might consider also involving them in the consent process.

It should be clear from the above discussion that different approaches will be appropriate in different settings. In the UK, guidelines produced by the Medical Research Council recommend that a *Cluster Representation Mechanism* (CRM) should be established for this purpose (Medical Research Council 2002). The CRM is expected to represent the interests of cluster members in providing consent for the trial and for the randomisation process, but is also expected to be kept informed of developments during the conduct of the trial, and to have the right to withdraw a cluster if this seems to be in its best interests.

Even though consent may be provided at cluster level, it is usually desirable to ensure that community members are well informed about the purposes and methods of the trial. This will help to ensure that they are in a position to make their views known, for example through the CRM, or to opt out of the intervention if this is provided to individuals.

13.4.2 Consent for Participation

While allocation at cluster level in a CRT often precludes seeking informed consent from all individuals prior to randomisation, it is often possible and appropriate to obtain individual consent at other stages of the research process.

In some trials, the intervention is allocated at cluster level, but still provided to individuals. In general, individuals can at this stage be given the choice of opting out of receiving the intervention. We give three examples.

Example 13.5

In the Ghana Vitamin A Supplementation Trial, discussed in Example 13.3, periodic vitamin A supplements or placebo were delivered to children living in 185 arbitrary geographical zones. While allocation to vitamin A or placebo occurred at zone level, mainly for reasons of logistical convenience, individual parents could opt for their children not to receive the intervention. Since the trial was placebo-controlled, and parents were blind to whether their children would receive the active produce or placebo, it is likely that any selection bias due to non-participation would apply equally in both treatment arms, thus preserving the internal validity of the trial in this case.

Example 13.6

In the CRT of bednets in The Gambia, first discussed in Example 4.1, villages were randomised to receive insecticide-impregnated bednets or to act as control villages (D'Alessandro et al. 1995). While individual subjects in the intervention villages could opt out of receiving or using the impregnated nets, this trial was not placebo-controlled and so there was no intervention for the control villagers to opt out of.

Example 13.7

In a CRT in which medical practices are randomised to apply a new treatment regimen or the current regimen to patients with a defined condition, patients in intervention practices would generally be given the opportunity to opt out of receiving the new treatment.

In Example 13.6 and Example 13.7, there are parallels with the so-called *randomised consent design* proposed by Zelen for standard individually-randomised trials (Zelen 1979, 1990). In this design, intended mainly for trials in which an experimental treatment is compared with current standard of care, only subjects randomly allocated to receive the experimental treatment are asked for their consent to participate. Those declining the experimental treatment are given the current standard of care. When using this design, it is important to apply an *intent-to-treat analysis* to avoid selection bias due to differential take-up of the new and current treatments. Thus, if a substantial proportion of subjects decline the experimental treatment, any effect of the treatment will be diluted.

Similar considerations apply in CRTs in which individuals are able to opt out of intervention in one arm but not the other. To avoid selection bias, it is important to collect outcome data from *all* subjects, irrespective of whether they chose to receive or use the intervention. However, interpretation of the estimated population-level effects of the intervention should take account of the degree of uptake of the intervention.

Even in trials where individual consent for intervention is requested, there are often clear limits to the ability of individuals to genuinely opt out. In trials of infectious disease interventions, for example, we have seen in Section 3.3 that an important rationale for cluster randomisation is to capture the population-level effects of an intervention. These often include secondary effects on community members who do not themselves access the intervention. In trials of impregnated bednets, for example, those not sleeping under nets may still be partially protected if the overall density of malarial vectors or transmission intensity of malaria in the village are decreased. And in trials of school-based sexual health education programmes, parents may choose to exclude their children from these classes, but these children are still likely to be exposed to any effects of the intervention on knowledge, attitudes or behaviour through their everyday contact with other students who have received the intervention, as well as to changes that may occur in peer-norms in the wider community.

Whether or not individuals are asked for consent to receive the intervention, most CRTs involve data collection from individual cluster-members, or a sample of those members, in order to evaluate the impact of the intervention. In general, these individuals must be asked for their informed consent to participate in such surveys. In non-blind trials, there is again a risk that non-participation may differ between the treatment arms. For example, individuals in control clusters might be less willing to contribute to the research if they have not received any intervention during the trial. Such differential non-participation may clearly lead to selection bias, and when reporting such trials investigators need to give accurate information on participation rates and, if possible, the characteristics of participants and non-participants.

Many CRTs involve interventions among adolescents, young children, infants or others who may not be able legally to provide informed consent on their own behalf. As in individually randomised trials, investigators need to give careful attention to the informed consent process in such trials. Age limits for legal consent vary between countries, but parents or guardians would normally be asked to provide formal informed consent on behalf of children. As a general rule, however, children who are old enough to make an informed decision should also be asked for their assent and this should be documented.

13.5 Other Ethical Issues

13.5.1 Scientific Validity

In Section 13.2.1, we noted that it is difficult to argue that a trial is ethical if its design or conduct are scientifically flawed. This is of special concern for CRTs, because the correct methods for their design and analysis are less well known than those for standard clinical trials.

One of the most common errors in CRTs in the published literature is that they have been under-powered because the design effect associated with cluster randomisation has not been appreciated or the level of between-cluster variability has been under-estimated and hence insufficient clusters have been randomised. In other CRTs, invalid methods of analysis have been used, for example methods that take no account of between-cluster variation or which are not robust when the number of clusters is small.

We consider that scientific rigour is a prerequisite for a trial to be ethical, and hope that the methods of design and analysis set out in this book will help investigators to ensure the scientific validity of CRTs they undertake.

13.5.2 Phased Intervention Designs

A key ethical concern during the design stage of some CRTs has been that equipoise between the treatment arms is difficult to defend. A good example is provided by the Gambia Hepatitis Intervention Study discussed in Example 8.4. The primary objective of this trial was to evaluate the long-term effect of infant hepatitis B vaccination against liver cancer. Trials in industrialised countries had already established the short-term efficacy of the vaccine in protecting against hepatitis B viral infection and carriage, and it would therefore be difficult to argue the case for equipoise. On the other hand, the vaccine was at that time very expensive, and there was little immediate prospect of its widespread provision in developing countries.

In Section 8.2.4, we have seen that phased intervention designs such as the *stepped wedge design* have sometimes been used to address such ethical concerns. In practice, most interventions have to be introduced in a phased manner for logistical or other reasons. By randomising the order of implementation in different communities, investigators can obtain a valid measure of the effects of an intervention, while ensuring that all the communities can benefit from the intervention by the end of trial.

13.5.3 Trial Monitoring

Effective trial monitoring is essential to ensure that any adverse effects of the intervention are quickly recognised, or to avoid prolonged recruitment or follow-up when the trial has already established clear evidence of benefit or harm. This requirement applies also to CRTs, and is discussed further in Chapter 14.

13.6 Conclusion

The general ethical principles that should underpin all trials of health interventions are now well-recognised and investigators have ready access to internationally agreed published guidelines. However, the interpretation of these general principles in the context of a specific trial is often controversial, and the ethics of particular studies have sometimes generated heated debate.

An issue that has received much attention in recent years, applying to individually randomised trials as well as CRTs, concerns the appropriate standard of care that should be provided to trial participants in resource-poor settings where local health services may not be adequate. In trials of HIV preventive interventions, for example, there has been widespread discussion of whether participants who become HIV infected during the trial, or who are screened out because they are HIV-positive at baseline, should be assured of effective antiretroviral therapy by the trial investigators (UNAIDS/WHO 2007).

The single most important measure to protect the ethical standards of trials is that they must be considered and approved by an effective and independent ethics committee within the country where the research is to be conducted. Such a committee is generally best placed to make an informed decision as to what is appropriate and ethically acceptable in the local context. In practice, many committees are insufficiently resourced or constituted to perform this function adequately, and the strengthening of national and local ethics committees is an important priority for health research.

14

Data Monitoring

14.1 Introduction

It is increasingly common for randomised controlled trials to be overseen by Data Monitoring Committees (DMCs), whose main tasks are to monitor the accumulating study data to ensure the safety of participants, to review study progress and to make recommendations to the investigators, sponsors and funding agencies regarding the continuation, modification or termination of the trial. Not all trials need to have a DMC, and they are most common for trials of new investigational products such as drugs and vaccines, and where definitive evidence of efficacy and safety is needed to guide regulatory decisions or health policy. Such committees are given a variety of names, including Data Monitoring and Ethics Committee (DMEC) or Data Safety and Monitoring Board (DSMB), but we shall use the term DMC here.

While there is considerable experience with the use and operation of DMCs in individually randomised trials, this is less the case with CRTs. Where CRTs do incorporate DMCs, these generally function in a similar way to DMCs in individually randomised trials. In this chapter, our main focus is on aspects of the operation of DMCs that are particular to the CRT design. The reader is referred to an excellent textbook for general information on DMCs (Ellenberg et al. 2003).

In Section 14.2, we briefly review the general responsibilities of DMCs, and go on to consider when a DMC may be necessary for a CRT. We then discuss the role of a DMC in monitoring for adverse events, efficacy and adequacy of sample size. In some cases, a DMC may also play a part in assessing the comparability of treatment arms and in reviewing and approving the analytical plan, and these roles are also explored.

Most DMCs carry out some form of interim analysis, possibly on repeated occasions, and Section 14.3 discusses the timing of analyses, stopping rules for CRTs and the dangers of premature trial termination.

14.2 Data Monitoring Committees

14.2.1 Review of DMC Responsibilities

The main responsibilities of a DMC have been clearly summarised as follows (Ellenberg et al. 2003):

The purpose of DMCs is to protect the safety of trial participants, the credibility of the study and the validity of study results.

The specific roles of a DMC vary from trial to trial, and are generally set out in a *DMC Charter* which spells out the composition and functioning of the DMC and provides detailed terms of reference. Some common roles are as follows:

- To review and comment on the study protocol. In the case of a CRT, the DMC will wish to assure itself that proper account has been taken of the special design features of such trials and in particular that sample size calculations and the analytical plan have allowed for between-cluster variability.

- To ensure that procedures are in place so that the trial is carried out to a high standard. This might include reviewing quality control procedures as well as the arrangements for the trial to be evaluated at regular intervals by clinical trial monitors. The DMC may also wish to review reports and data relating to the quality of trial implementation.

- To review the progress of the trial against protocol targets. This might include reviewing recruitment rates, retention of study participants at follow-up visits, withdrawal of participants from the study treatment, adherence to treatment and other key performance indicators. In the case of a CRT, the DMC will wish to ensure that the target number of clusters has been enrolled, and to monitor whether any clusters are lost to follow-up.

- To monitor data on adverse events. This may include unblinded analyses to explore whether there is an excess rate of events in one or more of the treatment arms.

- To monitor accumulating data concerning efficacy for the primary endpoint, in order to decide whether the trial should be continued, terminated or modified.

- Based on accumulating data on the primary endpoint as well as on recruitment and retention rates, to determine whether the sample size will be sufficient to answer the main study questions. In the case of a CRT, this may involve reviewing whether protocol assumptions concerning between-cluster variability are supported by the data.

- To serve as an endpoints adjudication committee, deciding, in a masked fashion, which events qualify as meeting stated endpoint definitions for the primary analysis.
- Following each meeting of the DMC, to provide a report to the investigators, sponsor or funding agency making recommendations regarding the continuation, termination or modification of the trial. The recommendations of the DMC should also take into account available data from other related studies.

Guidelines for the membership of DMCs are provided by Ellenberg et al. (2003). For a CRT, it is important that at least one member of the committee is familiar with the special aspects of the CRT design so that that the committee is equipped to interpret data from the trial appropriately and to advise the investigators on design and analysis issues.

14.2.2 When Are DMCs Necessary for CRTs?

Not all CRTs need to have a formally constituted DMC, and it is important for the investigators to consider at an early stage whether it is appropriate to establish a DMC for any particular trial. DMC arrangements should be clearly set out in the trial protocol, and it will usually be appropriate for them to be described and justified in the funding proposal so that the funding agency can satisfy itself that suitable arrangements for trial monitoring will be put in place.

It is impossible to give hard and fast rules as to when it is appropriate for a DMC to be set up, but we give some guidelines that may be helpful with special reference to CRTs.

14.2.2.1 Likelihood of Adverse Events

One of the main purposes of a DMC is to protect the safety of participants. This includes monitoring accumulating data from the trial with respect to the frequency and severity of adverse events, particularly those that may be attributable to the intervention under study. If the intervention is such that it can reasonably be assumed that significant adverse events related to the intervention are highly unlikely, it may be decided that there is no need for a DMC to monitor for adverse events. The case for this must be considered carefully for each individual trial. It is often impossible to rule out the potential for adverse events, as discussed in Section 13.3.

14.2.2.2 Seriousness or Severity of Outcome Measures

It is more likely that a DMC will be needed if the trial seeks to measure effects on efficacy or safety outcomes that are judged to be of a serious nature. Some examples might include trials looking at the effect of an intervention on mortality, incidence of HIV infection, recovery from a life-threatening disease following treatment or adverse events resulting in hospitalisation. Given the cost and complexity of carrying out CRTs, it is not surprising that they are often done to look at effects on important public health problems, and so it is often the case that the outcomes of CRTs are of a serious nature, although this is not invariably the case.

DMCs may be called for when there are serious or severe outcomes for three main reasons. First, to protect the trial participants since periodic review of the data may allow recruitment or follow-up to be terminated early, so that participants are protected against harm. Second, so that the results can be reported as early as possible when conclusive evidence of benefit or harm is available, thus increasing the rate at which findings can be taken up for the benefit of the wider population. Third, because it is particularly important for the development of evidence-based health policy that the findings of trials of interventions against important health problems are conducted rigorously and that they are able to provide credible and convincing results, and this can be facilitated by an effective DMC.

14.2.2.3 Timing of Data Collection

The timing of data collection may vary substantially between CRTs depending on the particular details of the study design. In studies where there is a baseline survey and then a single follow-up survey, there may be little scope for the DMC to carry out an interim analysis of the primary endpoint, unless recruitment of clusters to the trial is phased and takes place over a prolonged period. Conversely, if recording of the endpoint takes place continuously over time, or if there is a series of follow-up surveys, interim analysis is likely to be much more useful. Similar principles apply to the collection of data on adverse events, although it is more common for these to be recorded continuously.

Example 14.1

In the Mwanza STD treatment trial, previously discussed in Example 5.3, a baseline survey was carried out in a randomly selected cohort of 1000 adults from each of the 12 study communities which were arranged in six matched pairs (Grosskurth et al. 1995). Immediately following the baseline survey, the intervention was introduced in a randomly chosen community in each pair, and a single follow-up survey of the study cohort was carried out 2 years later. There was no interim survey, and data from the final survey only became available after all communities had been entered into the trial for at least 1 year. Furthermore, the intervention involved the provision of improved STD treatment services at existing health units, based on WHO-recommended guidelines, and serious adverse events associated with this intervention seemed unlikely. For these reasons, it was not considered that a DMC was required in this trial.

Example 14.2

In the Lombok vaccine-probe study for determination of the burden of *Haemophilus influenzae* type b (Hib) vaccine-preventable disease, 818 hamlets on the island of

Lombok, Indonesia were randomised to receive either the standard diphtheria, tetanus, pertussis (DTP) vaccine, or a DTP-PRP-T (Hib conjugate) vaccine (Gessner et al. 2005). Although no new investigational product was deployed, a DMC was constituted which gave advice on numerous aspects of the study, and carried out quarterly review of data on mortality and convulsions following vaccination. The DMC also proved useful in protecting the investigators and the integrity of the study when local concerns arose about a potential vaccine-related elevation in mortality rates.

14.2.3 Monitoring for Adverse Events

One of the main functions of a DMC is to protect the safety of the participants. This includes monitoring for adverse events. In preparing the trial protocol, investigators need to consider carefully what adverse events might occur and how any adverse events, either expected or unexpected, will be recorded and reported. This may include systematic questioning about side effects, clinical examinations or laboratory analyses during scheduled follow-up visits, as well as recording of adverse events occurring continuously during follow-up, for example hospital admissions, deaths or illnesses resulting in additional clinic visits.

In a standard clinical trial, it is generally the case that adverse events are measured in the same participants who have received the intervention and who are being followed for efficacy. In a CRT, however, adverse events are sometimes measured in a wider study population than those who are being followed for efficacy. In some trials, for example, the intervention is delivered at the community level but a randomly selected *sample* of the population is selected and followed up to measure efficacy. It may, however, be considered important to record adverse events in the entire community, especially if it is desired to capture the occurrence of rare but serious side effects.

Some CRTs are carried out to study behavioural or other interventions aimed at *prevention* of infection or disease. It is important to recognise that such interventions may sometimes have unanticipated harmful effects, and to seek ways of identifying and recording any such effects. Some examples include:

- There is clear evidence that male circumcision is partially protective against sexually transmitted HIV infection. In a trial of a community-wide intervention to promote and provide male circumcision, men undergoing the procedure may consider that they are at reduced risk and consequently engage in riskier sexual behaviour, a phenomenon known as *behavioural disinhibition* or *risk compensation*. It would therefore be important in such a trial to monitor for any such increases in risky behaviour.

- In a trial of a vaccine against acute respiratory infections in young children, mothers may consider that their children are protected, leading to a delay in treatment-seeking if they become ill. This may occur even in a placebo-controlled trial.

- In a trial of a community-based intervention to promote voluntary testing and counselling (VCT) for HIV infection, subjects diagnosed as HIV-positive may experience social stigma resulting in unintended adverse consequences such as marital break-up, domestic violence or loss of employment.

As in individually randomised trials, it may be difficult to attribute adverse events to the intervention, especially if they are non-specific. DMCs monitoring for adverse events may therefore wish to see rates of adverse events analysed by treatment arm, so as to determine whether there is an excess rate of events in the intervention arm. In trials measuring effects on *cause-specific mortality* in developing countries, where reliable systems for diagnosing and registering the exact cause of death may not be available, DMCs may ask to see a secondary analysis of all-cause mortality rates to ensure that there is no excess in the intervention arm.

14.2.4 Monitoring for Efficacy

One of the most important tasks of most DMCs is to carry out *interim analyses* during the course of the trial, based on accumulating data on efficacy, to determine whether there is sufficient evidence to recommend early termination of the trial. This could be because:

- There is already clear evidence that the intervention is beneficial.
- There is already clear evidence that the intervention is either harmful or has little or no effect.
- It is clear that the trial will be unable to adequately measure the effect of the intervention, for example because the incidence of the outcome is too low or because the recruitment or retention rate is inadequate.

As we have seen, it may or may not be appropriate for interim analyses to be carried out during a CRT, depending for example on the study design and timing of data collection. In Section 14.3, we discuss issues in the conduct of interim analyses in CRTs.

14.2.5 Monitoring Adequacy of Sample Size

A further task of a DMC is to keep under review the assumptions regarding sample size requirements set forward in the trial protocol, to evaluate whether the trial will be able to achieve its primary and secondary objectives if it continues as planned.

In an individually randomised trial, the DMC will wish to review whether the recruitment and retention rates are on target, so that the planned sample size can be achieved. It will also wish to see data on the primary endpoint to check the validity of the sample size assumptions. For example, for a quantitative outcome, the mean and standard deviation of the outcome variable can be compared with the values assumed in the trial protocol. Similarly, the prevalence or incidence of a binary outcome can be examined.

It is quite common for the incidence of an outcome in a trial to be less than expected at the time of study design. This can occur for several reasons. First, the study population enrolled in the trial may be a selected subgroup of the population, chosen because they satisfy specified eligibility criteria or because they are expected to be more cooperative and compliant with trial procedures. Such subgroups are often at lower risk of the outcome of interest. Second, trial enrolment is often accompanied by information, counselling or education that may result in safer behaviour resulting in lower incidence of the outcome. This is an important issue in trials of HIV preventive interventions for example. Third, where cohorts are followed up for the incidence of an outcome, the incidence rate is often found to decrease over time. This may occur, for example, when individuals most at risk experience the outcome early during follow-up, leaving behind a relatively low-risk cohort continuing under follow-up. By keeping incidence rates under regular review, a DMC may be able to give helpful advice on the need for recruitment or follow-up to be extended.

In a CRT, the DMC will in addition wish to see data on the *between-cluster variability* or *intracluster correlation* of the main study outcomes as these become available. As we have seen in Chapter 7, these parameters are of critical importance in determining sample size requirements for a CRT, but are often based on guess-work or limited prior data. As soon as reliable empirical estimates of these parameters are available, it is important to review them to determine whether the planned sample size is adequate and whether any adjustment to the study design is called for.

14.2.6 Assessing Comparability of Treatment Arms

An important objective of the DMC is to help ensure the *validity* and *credibility* of the trial results. In a CRT, particularly one with a relatively small number of clusters, this will depend to a large extent on the *balance* between the treatment arms. In previous chapters, we have discussed a number of design strategies that can be used to improve balance. Depending on the success of these strategies, however, it may still be necessary to *adjust* for any imbalances in the analysis. DMCs may wish to examine data on baseline comparability so that they can advise the investigators on whether such adjustments are necessary.

14.2.7 Approving the Analytical Plan

As we have seen, the options available to investigators for the analysis of CRTs are more varied than standard methods for the analysis of clinical trials, and alternative methods have different advantages and disadvantages. Because of the variety of methods available, investigators may be accused by a critical readership of trying different statistical methods and selectively choosing a method for publication that best fits their interests.

For this reason, it may be considered good practice for the investigators to present their proposed analytical plan for comment and approval by the DMC. The analytical plan may include details of which variables are to be adjusted for, and this may be informed by the baseline comparisons discussed in the previous section.

If the analytical plan is reviewed and approved prior to the end of the trial, and before data are unblinded or analysed by treatment arm, the investigators are protected against any allegation of selective choice of methods. Furthermore, the DMC may be able to give helpful advice on the analysis and presentation of the data, and preparing the analytical plan well in advance of the final analysis also helps to avoid unnecessary delays in the presentation and publication of the trial findings.

14.2.8 Presentation of Data to the DMC

The frequency and format of periodic reports to the DMC are usually agreed through discussion between the Chair of the DMC and the investigators. The reader is referred to the textbook by Ellenberg et al. (2003) for a useful discussion of the contents of DMC reports.

In most cases, DMCs request to see the accumulating data on efficacy endpoints, adverse events and other variables broken down by treatment arm. This is generally an appropriate request, since the DMC is the main group charged with protecting the interests of the study participants and this responsibility is usually discharged most effectively if the committee has full access to all data that might inform their decisions about trial continuation or modification. In contrast, it is usually considered preferable for the study investigators to remain blind to the treatment arm when analysing or inspecting data on study endpoints prior to completion of the trial. This can usually be achieved even if the trial is not double-blind or placebo-controlled.

A particular issue in the case of a CRT is that the DMC is likely to request data tabulated or analysed by study cluster. The data need to be organised in this way so that any statistical analyses can take appropriate account of between-cluster variation, and so that the DMC can check that the assumed estimate of k or ρ in the study protocol is accurate. In addition, these data can help the DMC to monitor whether there are any clusters in which study procedures are not being carried out with due diligence. Care must be taken when preparing the tables for the DMC that investigators are not *unblinded inadvertently*. For example, the tables may show the treatment arms labelled A and B, rather than Intervention and Control, but if the number of clusters differs between arms, or if sample sizes differ between clusters and are shown in the table, investigators may be able to recognise which is the intervention arm. To avoid this, it may be preferable for the DMC tables to be prepared by an independent statistician who is not a member of the study team, and to avoid the investigators seeing tables in which outcome data are shown by treatment arm even if these are labelled arbitrarily.

14.3 Interim Analyses

14.3.1 Introduction

As we have seen, in addition to their responsibilities for monitoring trial progress and adverse events, DMCs often carry out one or more *interim analyses* of efficacy against the outcomes of interest. The main aim of an interim analysis is to guide a recommendation regarding the continuation or early termination of the trial. Early termination might be called for if there is already convincing evidence that the intervention is beneficial, that it is harmful or that a benefit large enough to be of clinical or public health value can be ruled out. Early termination might also be recommended on the grounds of *futility* if the accumulating data indicate that if the trial were to continue as planned there would be little chance of demonstrating efficacy or obtaining an adequate measure of the intervention effect.

It is well known that if the accumulating data from a trial are analysed repeatedly, and if a standard significance test of the null hypothesis of no intervention effect is carried out on each occasion, then the probability of obtaining at least one "significant" result may considerably exceed the nominal size of the test. When examining the results of interim analyses, DMCs need to take this into account and, as we shall see, they may do this either informally or by using specially derived *stopping rules* that allow for the repeated examination of the data. For similar reasons, it is common when using a formal stopping rule to base the analysis on a single *primary outcome variable*, since repeated analysis of multiple endpoints will again increase the probability of detecting spurious effects. Despite this, DMCs will usually wish to take account of data on other outcomes, in combination with the results for the primary outcome, in reaching their final recommendation.

There is a substantial literature on statistical methods for interim analysis in clinical trials, but our main emphasis will be on the special requirements for CRTs. This is an area which has received relatively little attention and where further research is called for.

14.3.2 Timing of Interim Analyses

Where a DMC resolves that it is appropriate to carry out interim analyses, it must decide how many should be conducted and when they should take place.

Sometimes, the study design means that there is little choice in this. For example, if a CRT involves 2 years of follow-up with a baseline survey followed by an interim survey after 1 year and a final survey after 2 years, an interim analysis after 1 year may be the only realistic choice. In other trials, particularly if endpoints are measured continuously over time, there may be a wider range of choices open to the DMC.

A general recommendation in individually randomised trials is that it is seldom helpful to plan for more than two or three interim analyses in addition to the final analysis. In CRTs, because of the role of between-cluster variability, the additional statistical information provided as the follow-up time increases is less than in an individually randomised trial. We conclude that the case for limiting the number of interim analyses is even stronger for a CRT.

The timing of interim analyses also needs to be considered. A common choice is to carry out analyses at equal intervals of *calendar time*. For example in a trial extending over 3 years, interim analyses might be carried out at the end of the first and second years. This is logistically convenient, helping to spread out the data management tasks involved in preparing for an interim analysis, and provides a regular schedule for DMC meetings feeding into annual reports to the funding agency and ethical or regulatory boards. However, equal spacing in calendar time may not provide equal amounts of information between consecutive analyses. For this reason, some trials schedule interim analyses so that the amounts of incremental information provided at each analysis are roughly equal.

Example 14.3

Suppose 1000 subjects are to be recruited over 1 year, and each subject is to be followed for 2 years. In addition, suppose that the primary endpoint of interest is recorded continuously over time and that the rate of this endpoint can be assumed roughly constant.

For such an endpoint, the amount of *information* can be represented by the reciprocal of the variance of the estimated intervention effect. If we take the log(rate ratio) as our effect measure, it may be shown that the information is proportional to the total number of *events* observed.

The numbers of person-years of observation during the 3 years of the above trial (ignoring losses to follow-up and assuming that the endpoint is rare) are 500, 1000 and 500, respectively. Thus, if three interim analyses were to be carried out, equal incremental information would be provided if these were scheduled for 12 months, 18 months and 24 months, whereas equal spacing in calendar time would imply interim analyses at 9 months, 18 months and 27 months.

For CRTs, the situation is more complex because, as noted above, the variance of the effect estimate is influenced by the between-cluster variability as well as the numbers of observed events. Because of this phenomenon, the *incremental* information provided by the second 100 events recorded in a CRT is less than the information provided by the first 100 events. If interim analyses were to be carried out with equal spacing in terms of incremental information, this would imply more frequent interim analyses at the start of the trial. However, this might increase the probability of premature termination, which needs to be carefully guarded against for reasons set out in Section 14.3.4.

14.3.3 Stopping Rules

We have seen that it is important to take into account the increased probability of obtaining a false-positive statistically significant result due to repeated testing of the accruing data. In practice, DMCs approach this in different ways.

In some cases, DMCs take the view that their recommendation should be based on careful consideration of all the data available to them, including data on adverse events and on a range of endpoints of interest. They may consider that the overall pattern of results, including the consistency of any effects, is more important than a single test based on a specified primary endpoint, and may therefore choose not to specify any formal stopping rule. Even in this case, however, it is important that the DMC exercises due caution in interpreting the results of any significance tests at interim analysis, especially if multiple endpoints are analysed.

Other DMCs may adopt a formal stopping rule which is not based on any specific statistical operating characteristics. For example, in a trial with a single interim analysis a DMC, noting the possible dangers of terminating a trial prematurely (see Section 14.3.4), might determine that early termination will only be considered if the effect on the primary endpoint is significant at a stringent level, say $p < 0.001$ or $p < 0.01$.

Finally, it is increasingly common for DMCs to adopt a formal stopping rule that has been developed to satisfy specific statistical requirements. Such stopping rules are often designed to avoid termination at an early stage of follow-up and to ensure that, if the trial proceeds to completion as planned, any correction to the final analysis to take account of the repeated significance testing is negligible and can be ignored.

A number of such stopping rules, based on *group sequential tests*, are available and the reader is referred to standard texts for full details (Ellenberg et al. 2003; Jennison and Turnbull 1999; Proschan et al. 2006). The most commonly used is the O'Brien–Fleming (OBF) rule. This specifies boundary values b_t ($t = 1, 2, \ldots, T$) which are used to assess the test statistic on up to T occasions ($T - 1$ interim analyses and one final analysis). The OBF rule provides very stringent requirements for stopping at early analyses, and less stringent requirements at later analyses.

Computer software is available to provide the required OBF boundary values for a test statistic that can be assumed to follow the standard normal distribution under the null hypothesis. The user needs to specify, in advance, the proposed number of interim analyses as well as the timing of these analyses. The latter is specified in terms of the proportion of *information* that is available at the time of each analysis. As we have seen, the *information* is defined as the reciprocal of the variance of the effect estimate of interest.

In order to arrive at suitable boundary values for a CRT, we need to estimate the *information fraction* (the proportion of information available at each planned interim analysis) taking into account the effect of between-cluster variability. We provide approximate formulae that can be used to estimate information fractions for event rates, proportions and means, assuming that we have an estimate of the between-cluster coefficient of variation, k. These formulae assume a simple unmatched CRT with equal numbers of clusters in the two treatment arms (c in each arm).

14.3.3.1 Event Rates

Let e_1 and e_0 be the expected numbers of events occurring in the intervention and control arms at or before a specified time-point for an interim analysis. Then the variance of the effect estimate, assumed here to be the log(rate ratio), is given by:

$$Var(\log RR) = Var(\log \bar{r}_1) + Var(\log \bar{r}_0) \approx \left(\frac{1}{e_1} + \frac{1}{e_0}\right) + \frac{2k^2}{c} \qquad (14.1)$$

By obtaining the information as the reciprocal of this expression, the information accrued at different time points relative to the total information at the end of the trial can be estimated.

Setting $k=0$ we note that, for an individually randomised trial or in the absence of clustering, the information increases in proportion to the total number of observed events. As a result of between-cluster variation, however, the amount of additional information provided by increasing the number of events is reduced because the second term in Equation 14.1 remains constant.

14.3.3.2 Proportions

Let e_1 and e_0 be the expected numbers of individuals with the (binary) outcome of interest in the intervention and control arms, respectively. Then the variance of the effect estimate, assumed here to be the log(risk ratio), is given by:

$$Var(\log RR) = Var(\log \bar{p}_1) + Var(\log \bar{p}_0) \approx \frac{1-\pi_1}{e_1} + \frac{1-\pi_0}{e_0} + \frac{2k^2}{c} \qquad (14.2)$$

where π_1 and π_0 are the true proportions with the outcome in the two treatment arms.

Note that for rare outcomes, this is identical to Equation 14.1. As before, the information, obtained as the reciprocal of the variance, increases in proportion to the number of individuals with the outcome of interest if there is no clustering. As a result of between-cluster variation, the information provided by additional observations is reduced because the final term in Equation 14.2 remains constant.

14.3.3.3 Means

Let μ_1 and μ_0 be the true means, and σ_{W1} and σ_{W0} be the (within-cluster) standard deviations of the quantitative outcome of interest in the intervention and control arms, respectively. Then the variance of the effect estimate, assumed here to be the mean difference, is given by:

$$Var(\bar{x}_1 - \bar{x}_0) \approx \frac{\sigma_{W1}^2}{n_1} + \frac{\sigma_{W0}^2}{n_0} + \frac{k^2}{c}\left(\mu_1^2 + \mu_0^2\right) \qquad (14.3)$$

where n_1 and n_0 are the *total* numbers of observations in the two treatment arms.

In the absence of clustering, the information, obtained as the reciprocal of the variance, increases in proportion to the total number of observations. As a result of between-cluster variation, the information provided by additional observations is reduced because the final term in Equation 14.3 remains constant.

Example 14.4

Consider an unmatched CRT with six clusters per treatment arm and an assumed between-cluster coefficient of variation of $k=0.25$. The primary analysis is to be based on comparison of person-year event rates of a specified outcome. The expected numbers of events in the two treatment arms at the end of the trial are 100 and 80 corresponding to a rate ratio of 0.8. It is planned to carry out three interim analyses, and these are to be equally spaced in terms of total numbers of events observed. Thus, the four analyses (three interim and one final) will be conducted after 45, 90, 135 and 180 events have been observed.

Based on Equation 14.1, Table 14.1 shows estimated values of the variance, and hence the information and information fraction, at each interim analysis. These are shown for $k=0.25$, and also for $k=0$ for comparison.

Note that, in the absence of clustering, the amount of information increases in direct proportion to the number of observed events. As a result of between-cluster variation, the overall amount of information provided by the 180 observed events is reduced from 44.4 to 23.1, and this corresponds to a *design effect* of 44.4/23.1 or 1.93. Moreover, the information no longer increases in proportion to the number of events. In fact, the first 50% of observed events provide 66% of the available information. This is because increasing the person-years of observation does not reduce the component of variance in the effect measure due to between-cluster variation, although it will provide a more precise estimate of k.

At the design stage of this CRT, these estimates of the information fraction at each interim analysis could be used to obtain the appropriate OBF boundaries as discussed.

A limitation of the above approach, which does not apply to individually randomised trials, is that it requires an estimate of k before the trial commences. While we have seen that this is necessary for sample size calculations, we have

TABLE 14.1

Estimated Variance and Information at Three Interim Analyses and Final Analysis in a CRT with Six Clusters per Arm and 180 Total Expected Events, for Two Values of k

Proportion of Total Events	$k=0$			$k=0.25$		
	Variance	Information	Proportion of Total	Variance	Information	Proportion of Total
25%	0.090	11.1	25%	0.111	9.0	39%
50%	0.045	22.2	50%	0.066	15.2	66%
75%	0.030	33.3	75%	0.051	19.7	85%
100%*	0.022	44.4	100%	0.043	23.1	100%

*Final analysis.

also noted that accurate estimates of k are seldom available. This may mean that the boundaries used for interim stopping rules are inappropriate.

An alternative approach is to use the *alpha-spending* functions proposed by Lan and DeMets (1983). This approach avoids having to specify the number or spacing of interim analyses in advance. The test boundaries are computed in such a way that the available *alpha* is shared out between the various analyses (interim and final) while preserving the overall probability of a type 1 error.

Use of the Lan–DeMets (LDM) alpha-spending function requires an estimate of the information fraction at each analysis, and these estimates can be obtained as explained above. At the first interim analysis, the LDM boundary can be computed from an information fraction based on the value of k estimated from initial observations on the study clusters. This value of k is likely to be very inaccurate, and so at the next interim analysis the computations can be updated based on the additional data collected in order to arrive at a suitable LDM boundary for the second analysis, and so on. Software for implementation of the LDM approach is available from http://www.biostat.wisc.edu/landemets.

14.3.4 Disadvantages of Premature Stopping

While it is clearly important for a trial to be terminated early if there are compelling reasons to do so, the disadvantages of premature stopping need to be considered carefully. First, early findings are based on small amounts of data, and it is quite common to see what appear to be impressive trends that disappear or are much attenuated as more data are accrued. Statistical significance tests can of course be used to assess whether trends are stronger than would be expected to occur by chance. However, DMCs usually examine data on multiple endpoints and this increases the chance of false-positive findings even if allowance is made for repeated testing over time using the methods of the last section. The *power* to detect genuine effects at an early analysis is generally low, and this increases the likelihood that observed significant effects are due to chance. Furthermore, the *precision* of effect estimates is likely to be very low if a trial is terminated at an early stage, reducing the usefulness of the results for policy making. Finally, rare adverse events are unlikely to be detected if the period of follow-up is too short.

The above considerations apply equally to individually randomised trials and CRTs, but there are additional reasons to be cautious about premature stopping of CRTs.

First, stopping at an early stage due to *futility* or lack of effect may not be advisable. This is especially the case for behavioural programmes and other complex interventions, where effects may take some time to develop. For example, implementers may take some time to become familiar with the intervention methods, or it may take some time for community members to react to health education messages or for community norms to change. In the case of interventions against infectious diseases, we have seen that *indirect effects* of the intervention may sometimes be very important and these often accumulate over time. Early termination would risk missing the detection of a potentially effective intervention.

Early stopping for *efficacy* may also be problematic. In some cases, interventions may have a strong initial effect when implementers are newly trained, supervision is at its most intensive and the attention of the community is engaged by a novel activity. It is possible, however, that the immediate benefit soon wanes as implementers are distracted by other tasks, supervision becomes less intensive and community interest declines.

Example 14.5

We return to the trial of an adolescent sexual health intervention in Mwanza, Tanzania, previously discussed in Example 12.3 (Ross et al. 2007). The main component of this intervention was a health education programme delivered to students in the last 3 years of primary school with a focus on promoting safer sexual behaviour. In this trial, a cohort of around 9000 students was followed up for 3 years with an interim survey after 18 months.

Early termination of this trial for *futility* would be inappropriate for several reasons. First, the school-based programme used interactive teaching methods that were quite novel when compared with usual practice in primary schools in rural Tanzania. Selected teachers from each school were trained to deliver these methods, but it might be expected that they would take time to become familiar with the methods and materials. The quality of delivery of the intervention might therefore increase over time, particularly if refresher training and supervision were sustained. Second, patterns of sexual behaviour are known to be influenced by peer pressure as well as the cultural context and norms in the wider community. These are likely to take time to change, and so one might expect an effective intervention to show increasing evidence of impact over time. Third, the primary endpoints in this trial were the incidence of HIV infection and the prevalence of HSV2 infection. Because an individual's infection risk depends on the prevalence of infection among their sexual partners, there may be important *indirect effects* of the intervention, and these may accumulate over time. A particular reason that this may be of importance in this trial is that the male sexual partners of young women in the trial communities are on average several years older than the women themselves. During the first years of follow-up, these partners may be too old to have received the school-based programme, and it may therefore be several years before the full impact of the intervention can be observed.

Early termination for *efficacy* would also be questionable in this trial. Effects of health education interventions are often strongest soon after the intervention begins, when delivery may be optimal and before message fatigue sets in. A particular concern in the Tanzanian trial is that any effect of the educational intervention might wear off when students leave school, forget the programme messages and become subject to the influences and pressures of the wider community as they take on their new role as young adults.

15

Reporting and Interpretation

15.1 Introduction

However well a cluster randomised trial is designed and implemented, its results are likely to have little effect on health policy and practice unless the trial is adequately reported. The main emphasis of this book has been on trials of health-related interventions, and these are usually published in peer-reviewed medical journals. In this chapter, we focus mainly on the reporting of CRTs in such journals.

As we have seen, CRTs are often large studies involving the investment of substantial financial, logistical and human resources. There is perhaps a particular onus on CRT investigators to ensure that the reporting of such trials is carried out to the highest standards, to maximise the chances that the findings are interpreted correctly and the appropriate lessons drawn for future health policy.

Issues in the reporting of CRTs are discussed in Section 15.2. The CONSORT statement provides guidelines for the reporting of randomised trials, and we begin by presenting the extended CONSORT statement which adapts these guidelines for use with CRTs. We also review the possible role of publication bias. Reporting of methods and results are then considered in turn.

The interpretation of CRTs is considered in Section 15.3. Interpretation of individually randomised clinical trials is often relatively straightforward providing they are adequately powered and implemented. However, CRTs introduce additional complexities that may render their interpretation much more problematic. Finally, we discuss the incorporation of evidence from CRTs in meta-analyses and systematic reviews.

15.2 Reporting of Cluster Randomised Trials

15.2.1 Overview

Randomised trials are considered to be the gold standard for evaluating the effects of health interventions, thus contributing the highest grade of evidence for developing health policy and defining optimal treatments and preventive measures. They can only fulfil this role properly, however, if they are reported fully and accurately, and there is clear evidence that inadequate reporting of trials is associated with biased estimates of treatment effects.

Noting that trial reports often did not meet the highest standards, the editors of leading medical journals sponsored the publication of the Consolidation of Standards for Reporting of Trials (CONSORT) statement in 1996 (Begg et al. 1996). This provides an evidence-based checklist for investigators preparing a trial report and in particular stipulates the provision of a flow diagram showing the progress of participants through the various stages of a trial from screening to final follow-up.

15.2.1.1 Extended CONSORT Statement

The original CONSORT guidelines were designed for use with individually randomised trials, and did not consider the special features of CRTs that need to be addressed when reporting such trials (Elbourne and Campbell 2001). Subsequently, an extended statement was published that provided guidelines adapted for use with CRTs (Campbell, Elbourne, and Altman for the CONSORT Group 2004). All reports of CRTs submitted to the sponsoring journals must comply with these extended guidelines.

The adapted checklist is shown in Table 15.1. For each topic, additions to the standard CONSORT list are shown in italics. In some cases, the adaptations are obvious. Other points are discussed in more detail in the sections that follow.

An important point is that the title or abstract of the report should clearly identify the study as a cluster randomised trial. This ensures that the study is indexed as a CRT in the major catalogues, and that its design can be identified accurately during systematic reviews and literature searches. In addition, it is important that the main features of a study are clear from the abstract, since many readers do not study the main text. The form of randomisation is a fundamental aspect of the study design that should be stated clearly in the abstract.

15.2.1.2 Publication Bias

In deciding whether a health intervention is beneficial, it is important that we take into consideration the evidence from all relevant studies. Unfortunately, it has been recognised for some time that trials with negative findings are less likely to be reported and, even if they are reported, they may be published in journals that are less accessible in a search of the literature. The consequence is that systematic reviews of published trials in the area may conclude that an intervention is more effective than it really is, a phenomenon known as *publication bias*.

There are two main strategies to avoid this. First, every randomised trial should be registered, when it commences, in one of the recognised clinical

TABLE 15.1

Checklist of Items to Include When Reporting a Cluster Randomised Trial: Adaptations from Standard Guidelines Shown in Italics

Paper Section and Logic:	Item	Descriptor
Title and abstract		
Design	1*	How participants were allocated to interventions (e.g., random allocation, randomised, or randomly assigned), *specifying that allocation was based on clusters*
Introduction		
Background	2*	Scientific background and explanation of rationale, *including the rationale for using a cluster design*
Methods		
Participants	3*	Eligibility criteria for participants *and clusters* and the settings and locations where the data were collected
Interventions	4*	Precise details of the interventions intended for each group, *whether they pertain to the individual level, the cluster level, or both, and how and when they were actually administered*
Objectives	5*	Specific objectives and hypotheses *and whether they pertain to the individual level, the cluster level, or both*
Outcomes	6*	Report clearly defined primary and secondary outcome measures, *whether they pertain to the individual level, the cluster level, or both, and, when applicable,* any methods used to enhance the quality of measurements (e.g., multiple observations, training of assessors)
Sample size	7*	How *total* sample size was determined *(including method of calculation, number of clusters, cluster size, a coefficient of intracluster correlation (ICC or k), and an indication of its uncertainty)* and, when applicable, explanation of any interim analyses and stopping rules
Randomisation:		
Sequence generation	8*	Method used to generate the random allocation sequence, including details of any restriction (e.g., blocking, stratification, *matching*)
Allocation concealment	9*	Method used to implement the random allocation sequence, *specifying that allocation was based on clusters rather than individuals* and clarifying whether the sequence was concealed until interventions were assigned
Implementation	10	Who generated the allocation sequence, who enrolled participants, and who assigned participants to their groups

(continued)

TABLE 15.1 (Continued)

Paper Section and Logic:	Item	Descriptor
Blinding (masking)	11	Whether participants, those administering the interventions, and those assessing the outcomes were blinded to group assignment. If done, how the success of blinding was evaluated
Statistical methods	12*	Statistical methods used to compare groups for primary outcome(s) *indicating how clustering was taken into account*, methods for additional analyses, such as subgroup analyses and adjusted analyses
Results		
Participant flow	13*	Flow of *clusters and* individual participants through each stage (a diagram is strongly recommended). Specifically, for each group report the numbers of *clusters and* participants randomly assigned, receiving intended treatment, completing the study protocol, and analysed for the primary outcome. Describe protocol deviations from study as planned, together with reasons
Recruitment	14	Dates defining time periods of recruitment and follow up
Baseline data	15*	Baseline information for each group *for the individual and cluster levels as applicable*
Numbers analysed	16*	Number of *clusters and* participants (denominator) in each group included in each analysis and whether the analysis was by intention to treat. State the results in absolute numbers when feasible (e.g., 10/20 not 50%)
Outcomes and estimation	17*	For each primary and secondary outcome, a summary of results for each group *for the individual or cluster level as applicable*, and the estimated effect size and its precision (e.g., 95% CI) *and a coefficient of intrauster correlation (ICC or k) for each primary outcome.*
Ancillary analyses	18	Address multiplicity by reporting any other analyses performed, including subgroup analyses and adjusted analyses, indicating those prespecified and those exploratory
Adverse events	19	All important adverse events or side effects in each intervention group
Discussion		
Interpretation	20	Interpretation of the results, taking into account study hypotheses, sources of potential bias or imprecision and the dangers associated with multiplicity of analyses and outcomes.
Generalisability	21*	Generalisability (external validity) *to individuals and/or clusters (as relevant)* of the trial findings
Overall evidence	22	General interpretation of the results in the context of current evidence

Source: Reproduced from Campbell, M.K., Elbourne, D.R., and Altman, D.G. for the Consort Group. CONSORT statement: Extension to cluster randomized trials. *BMJ* 2004, 328, 702–8.

*Addition to CONSORT guidelines 2001.

trials registers. The World Health Organisation administers the International Clinical Trials Registry Platform (ICTRP: http://www.who.int/ictrp), which brings together a number of primary trials registers. Registering a trial with one of these ICTRP registers ensures that when systematic reviews are carried out, the reviewers are able to identify all relevant trials. As with the CONSORT guidelines, major medical journals as well as funding agencies now insist that trials are registered in this way.

Second, well-powered trials are more likely to be published than small trials that are inadequately powered, especially if they are unable to show an effect. This is because the confidence interval for the intervention effect in a small trial is likely to be very wide, so that a non-significant result cannot rule out a substantial and clinically important effect. Although such trials may not be conclusive when taken alone, it is important that their results are included when evidence is combined across all studies. If trials are adequately powered, this helps to ensure that they are published.

CRTs are often large and highly visible studies, and so it is perhaps less likely that they will remain unpublished if their findings are negative. Nevertheless, investigators would be well advised to follow the basic principles outlined above.

15.2.2 Reporting of Methods

15.2.2.1 Rationale for Cluster Randomisation

The CONSORT guidelines call for a justification to be provided for the use of a cluster randomised design. They argue that individual randomisation generally provides greater power and precision for the same total sample size, and that the rationale for cluster randomisation therefore needs to be carefully explained.

In some cases, for example in trials of community-level interventions, the rationale for cluster randomisation is so clear that it hardly needs stating. In other cases, and particularly where either design could potentially be used, it is helpful to give a clear explanation of the reasons for randomising by cluster. As we have seen in Chapter 3, there may be several reasons for this choice, especially in trials of interventions against infectious diseases.

15.2.2.2 Description of Clusters and Interventions

In an individually randomised trial, it is usual to describe the eligibility criteria for trial enrolment. This is clearly important when considering the generalisability of trial results.

In a CRT, it is *clusters* that are randomly allocated to the treatment arms under study. The trial results refer to the specific set of clusters that are studied, in the same way that the results of an individually randomised clinical trial refer to the sample of enrolled patients. It is therefore important that characteristics of the clusters are carefully described in reporting a CRT.

This should include a clear definition of a "cluster" and an explanation of how the specific study clusters were selected.

In some CRTs, all individuals within the selected clusters are automatically enrolled. In others, there may be additional eligibility criteria for individuals to be enrolled. We may also choose to study a sample of individuals within each cluster, rather than the entire cluster. It is therefore important to describe eligibility criteria and sampling methods at both cluster and individual levels.

A clear description of the intervention under study is also important if the results of the trial are to be put into practice in other settings. CRTs are sometimes used to evaluate the effects of *complex interventions*, which often comprise a package of measures that may be applied at either the cluster level or individual level or both. The description of such interventions may clearly be far more involved than the description of an experimental treatment in a clinical trial. This can be quite challenging given the space constraints of medical journals. Two possible strategies are to publish the details of the intervention in a separate paper and to present only a brief outline in the main results paper, referring the reader to the design paper for more information; or to describe the intervention in an online appendix to the main paper.

Example 15.1

We return to the trial of the *MEMA kwa Vijana* adolescent sexual health intervention, first described in Example 2.4 (Ross et al. 2007). This trial was carried out in 20 rural study communities in Mwanza Region, Tanzania. Each cluster in this trial consisted of around five to six villages, five to six primary schools and one or two health units, and corresponded roughly to an administrative area known as a "ward". For the impact evaluation, all students aged 14 years and over attending primary schools within these clusters were eligible for enrollment.

The size of these clusters was chosen to produce a cohort of around 500 students per cluster. They were not randomly sampled from a larger set of eligible clusters, but purposively selected using a map of the region, taking into account the need to avoid contamination by arranging for adequate spacing of clusters, and buffer zones between neighbouring clusters.

The *MEMA kwa Vijana* programme is a complex intervention involving four main components: school-based sexual health education, youth-friendly health services for sexual and reproductive health, community-based youth condom promotion and distribution, and supportive community activities. A full description of each of these components would be very lengthy. For example, the school-based education programme was teacher-led and peer-assisted, covered a wide range of topics and used role-play, drama and interactive teaching methods.

In an attempt to provide sufficient detail, the designs of the intervention and of the trial were published in two separate journal papers prior to publication of the main study results (Hayes et al. 2005; Obasi et al. 2006).

15.2.2.3 Sample Size

It is usual when reporting the results of a trial to describe the assumptions used in selecting the sample size. This helps the reader to evaluate whether the study was adequately powered, and will indicate what, at the outset, was important to the investigators and how this may have changed over time. In addition, examination of the differences between assumptions and realised data can help others who are planning similar studies, or studies with similar endpoints.

As we have see in Chapter 7, sample size calculations in CRTs need to take account of between-cluster variability. It is therefore important when reporting a CRT to set out the assumptions regarding the intracluster correlation coefficient (ρ) or between-cluster coefficient of variation (k) on which the sample size calculations were based, together with a justification for the values used, whether this is based on empirical estimates or otherwise.

In some CRTs, only a sample of individuals within each cluster is studied. In this case, a justification should be given for the number of individuals sampled per cluster as well as the number of clusters to be studied.

15.2.2.4 Matching, Stratification and Randomisation

We have seen that randomisation cannot always be relied on to ensure close similarity of treatment arms in CRTs, because such trials often involve a relatively small number of clusters. A number of design strategies can be used in an effort to improve the balance between treatment arms, and these include matching, stratification and restricted randomisation. Matched or stratified designs may also be chosen to reduce between-cluster variability in the main outcomes of interest.

These aspects of the design of a CRT need to be described carefully when the trial is reported. For matched or stratified trials, the trial report should define the matching factors and explain what assumptions were made about the effect of matching on between-cluster variability. If restricted randomisation was used, the criteria for balance should be stated. It may also be helpful to explore the validity of the restricted randomisation scheme, as discussed in Section 6.2.

15.2.2.5 Blinding and Allocation Concealment

As in individually randomised trials, blinding and allocation concealment should be adopted wherever possible to reduce selection bias as well as bias in the ascertainment or reporting of outcomes or bias resulting from differences in behaviours if treatment allocations are known.

Blinding during the trial may or may not be possible depending on the nature of the intervention. In the trial of vitamin A supplementation in Northern Ghana, first discussed in Example 3.4, it was possible to maintain blindness by giving a placebo supplement in the control clusters (Ghana VAST Study Team 1993). In the *MEMA kwa Vijana* trial discussed above in Example 15.1, it was clearly not possible to blind participants to the treatment allocation given the nature of this intervention involving intensive school-based sexual health education (Obasi et al. 2006). Even when full blinding is not possible, however, it may be feasible to blind certain individuals, for example field workers administering study questionnaires or laboratory personnel carrying out diagnostic tests.

In CRTs, allocation to treatment arms is carried out at cluster level. While in individually randomised trials, individuals are sometimes allocated to treatment arms sequentially, it is more common in CRTs for cluster allocation to be carried out at one time at the start of the trial, and it should be possible to ensure allocation concealment. A serious consideration in some CRTs, however, is that individuals within clusters may be enrolled in the trial subsequent to cluster allocation and, if they are aware of the treatment allocation of their cluster, this may influence their decision to enrol, leading to possible selection bias.

Example 15.2

A feasibility study was carried out in preparation for a randomised trial of different treatments for back pain in primary care settings in the U.K. (Farrin et al. 2005). In this feasibility study, known as the Back pain, Exercise, Active management and Manipulation (U.K. BEAM) study, 26 general practices were randomly allocated to two arms providing either active or traditional management for patients with back pain. The characteristics of the practices, including the numbers of registered patients, were found to be broadly similar in the two treatment arms.

Following randomisation, the target was to enrol approximately 120 patients presenting with back pain in each treatment arm. In the event, 165 patients were enrolled in the 13 practices in the active management arm, but only 66 in the 13 practices in the traditional management arm. There were also found to be systematic differences in the characteristics of the patients enrolled in the two arms, the cases in the active management arm being less severe, on average, than in the traditional management arm.

The investigators concluded that because enrolment of patients was carried out following randomisation, when the treatment allocation was known both to patients and to practitioners, eligible patients in the active management practices were more likely to be identified and enrolled than in the traditional management practices. The resulting selection bias would likely distort the results of the trial. As a result, the investigators modified the proposed trial design to avoid randomisation by practice.

Measures can sometimes be taken to avoid selection bias in such trials. For example, it may be possible to draw up a list of eligible patients prior to randomisation and allocation. Or, if this is not possible, an independent clinician could be designated to identify suitable patients in practices in both arms of the trial. However, there is still the potential for selection bias if patients are asked for individual informed consent to enrol in the trial knowing their treatment allocation.

Depending on the particular context of the trial, any measures to ensure blinding or allocation concealment, or to avoid the type of selection bias discussed above, should be clearly described in the trial report.

15.2.2.6 Definition of Primary Endpoints

In most CRTs, data are collected on a range of different endpoints. If intervention effects on all these endpoints are analysed and presented, it is likely that some statistically significant effects will be obtained just by chance. While statistical procedures are available which allow for this problem of repeated testing, these generally require the use of more stringent criteria to declare differences significant, thus reducing the power of the trial to detect effects on key outcomes.

As in individually randomised trials, therefore, it is advisable to define one, or at most two or three, *primary endpoints* in advance of the trial. The argument is that significant effects on pre-defined primary endpoints would be given more weight than isolated significant effects when a large number of endpoints are analysed. The primary and secondary endpoints should be set out in the analytical plan, which should be finalised before the results of the trial are analysed. They should also be clearly defined in the trial report so that readers have some basis on which to assess the strength of evidence for intervention effects on different endpoints.

15.2.2.7 Statistical Methods

A clear description of statistical methods is an essential component of the published report of any randomised trial.

We have seen in Chapters 9 through 12 that a much wider range of statistical methods may be applied to CRTs than would generally be used for the analysis of individually randomised trials. We have reviewed methods based on cluster summaries as well as more sophisticated regression methods that can be applied to individual level data. Each of these methods has its advantages and disadvantages. There are two important consequences of this. First, because the analysis of CRTs is less standardised than for simple clinical trials, it is important that the methods used are set out clearly. Second, the wide variety of available methods may lead to the suspicion that investigators have tried multiple approaches until they have obtained the most favourable result. If investigators can report that the analytical methods were specified in advance, in an approved analytical plan, this helps to protect them against such accusations.

A special feature of CRTs is that there may be important baseline imbalances between the treatment arms, even if design strategies have been used to minimise these. Adjusted analyses are therefore more common in CRTs than in individually randomised trials, in which randomisation of large numbers of individuals can usually be relied upon to ensure adequate balance. As with the choice of statistical methods, the adjustments to be carried out should be decided before the main trial results are analysed. Since this may depend on baseline observations that are sometimes carried out after randomisation, it may not be possible for such adjustments to be pre-specified in the trial protocol. However, it should be possible to specify them in the analytical plan which can be finalised when baseline observations are complete but before results for the main endpoints are analysed.

15.2.3 Reporting of Results

15.2.3.1 Flow Diagram

An important component of the report of any randomised trial is a flow diagram showing the numbers of participants who are eligible, the numbers randomised to the different treatment arms, the numbers lost to follow-up or excluded at each stage of the trial, and the numbers analysed for the main trial endpoints. Providing such a flow diagram is a key requirement of the CONSORT guidelines.

The extended CONSORT guidelines also require such flow diagrams to be reported for CRTs. An important modification for CRTs is that both the number of clusters and the number of individual participants should be reported at each stage. This provides useful information on the number of individuals enrolled per cluster, which may be relevant to the assessment of selection bias due to differential recruitment in the intervention and control arms as discussed in Section 15.2.2. It also shows clearly whether any clusters were removed from the trial or lost to follow-up, and this is again of importance in assessing selection bias and the generalisability of trial findings.

The extended CONSORT guidelines acknowledge that the exact format of the flow diagram should be adapted to the particular trial design. As an example, Figure 15.1 shows the published flow diagram for the *MEMA kwa Vijana* trial in which 20 rural communities in Tanzania were randomly allocated to an adolescent sexual health intervention or a control condition (Ross et al. 2007). In this trial, as in many CRTs, all 20 trial communities were successfully followed up to the end of the trial. The diagram also provides useful information on the variation of cluster size and reasons for exclusions and losses to follow-up, and shows that follow-up rates were similar in the two treatment arms.

15.2.3.2 Baseline Comparisons

The first table in a published trial report usually presents baseline characteristics of individuals in the different treatment arms, and shows whether the randomisation has been effective in achieving comparable treatment groups. This is even more important when reporting a CRT, because comparability is not guaranteed when relatively small numbers of clusters are randomised.

In CRTs it may be helpful to present data on the baseline characteristics of both clusters and individuals. For individuals, baseline comparisons can be based on either cluster summaries or individual-level data. For example, a binary variable could be presented by displaying the mean of the cluster-level proportions in each treatment arm, or the overall proportion for all individuals in that arm. If cluster sizes are similar, the two results will be very similar and it is probably more straightforward to show the individual-level data since then the raw numbers that make up the proportion can also be displayed.

Whichever approach is taken, it is not appropriate to carry out significance tests for differences between arms, with or without adjustment for clustering.

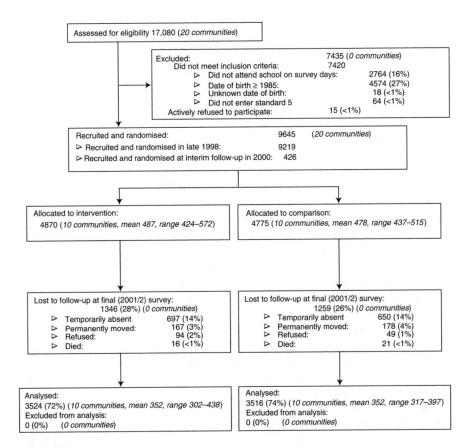

FIGURE 15.1
Flow diagram for the *MEMA kwa Vijana* trial of an adolescent sexual health intervention in rural Tanzania. (From Ross, D.A., Changlaucha, J., Obasi, A.I.N., et al. Biological and Behavioral impact of an adolescent sexual health intervention in Tanzania: A community-randomized trial. *AIDS* 2007, 21, 1943–55. With permission.)

This is because, if randomisation has been used to allocate clusters to treatment arms, any differences between those arms must necessarily be attributable to chance and so the null hypothesis is known to be true. Instead of carrying out tests, the data can be examined to evaluate whether there are *important* differences between treatment arms. To do this, we need to examine the size of any imbalances and to consider which baseline variables are likely to be important determinants of the primary outcomes. As discussed previously, these considerations should guide decisions on whether analyses of trial endpoints need to be adjusted for any imbalances.

15.2.3.3 Analysis of Endpoints

The most important tables in a CRT report are those showing the estimated effects of the intervention on the main endpoints of interest. As discussed previously, the report should state clearly which endpoints were pre-specified *primary endpoints* and which were *secondary endpoints*. The tables should show estimated intervention effects together with confidence intervals, obtained using appropriate methods of statistical analysis that take account of between-cluster variability, as explained in Chapters 9 through 12. If adjustment is required for baseline imbalances, it is generally helpful to show both unadjusted and adjusted estimates of effect, so that the reader can assess the effect of the adjustment.

In presenting data on endpoints in CRTs, it is important to provide clear information on the denominators used for each analysis, indicating where there were missing data for either clusters or individuals.

In most CRTs, the primary analysis is based on the *intention-to-treat* principle, so that all clusters, and individuals within these clusters, are analysed according to the treatment to which the cluster was randomised. The objective of most CRTs is to estimate the population-level effect of assigning whole communities or clusters to a particular intervention. The measured effect captures indirect effects of the intervention (as discussed in Chapter 3) but will also be influenced by the level of adherence to the intervention. Depending on the level of adherence, the effect measure may therefore be regarded as an estimate of the *effectiveness* of the intervention rather than its *efficacy*.

If some clusters do not receive the intervention they were assigned, further *on-treatment* analyses can be carried out in which clusters are analysed according to the intervention they actually received, or *per-protocol* analyses in which clusters not receiving the correct intervention are excluded. These would usually be regarded as secondary analyses, however, since the randomisation is violated when clusters are allowed to switch groups, and the treatment arms may no longer be comparable, thus introducing selection bias.

Similarly problematic are analyses which try to take account of differences in adherence among *individuals*. The analysis could be restricted to those individuals in each cluster who show a high level of adherence to the intervention. However, such good adherers are a selected subgroup of the population, and so valid comparisons can only be made if these individuals can be compared with similar individuals in the control arm. This is only likely to be possible in a placebo-controlled trial, and even then there may be differences in selection effects, for example if adverse effects (or other effects) lead to different selection pressures in the two treatment arms.

15.2.3.4 Subgroup Analyses

Effect measures may also be reported in specific subgroups of clusters or individuals within clusters.

At the cluster level we might, for example, wish to look at the effect of a community-level intervention separately in rural and urban communities; in communities varying in the transmission intensity of an infectious disease; or in large and small medical practices. Unless there are large numbers of clusters in a CRT, however, there will often be insufficient power or precision to estimate intervention effects in such subgroups.

More commonly, we may wish to look at intervention effects across all clusters but in specific subgroups of individuals, for example according to age, sex or other baseline characteristics, or according to adherence.

As in individually randomised trials, differences in effect between subgroups should be interpreted with caution. Significance tests for interaction (effect modification) could be carried out to assess whether these differences could easily have occurred by chance.

In addition, there are many potential subgroup analyses that could be carried out, with the problem of repeated significance testing, and more weight should be given to subgroup analyses that were pre-specified in the analytical plan.

15.2.3.5 Contamination

Cluster randomisation is often selected to avoid the contamination that could occur if individuals in close proximity, for example in the same community, institution or medical practice, were assigned different treatments. Contamination may still occur in CRTs, however. For example, this can occur if clusters are geographically close, or through migration or travel of individuals between different clusters. If there is a large amount of contamination, this might dilute the measured effect of the intervention. Where possible, investigators should therefore aim to collect data to gauge the extent of any contamination.

Example 15.3

In the STD treatment trial in Mwanza, first presented in Example 1.1, the 12 trial communities were specifically chosen to be geographically distant so as to mini-mise the likelihood that patients with STDs would travel to other trial communities to receive treatment (Grosskurth et al. 1995; Hayes et al. 1995). However, the investigators used clinic records, which included information on patients' places of residence, to count the number of STD patients who came from other trial communities either in the same or opposite treatment arm. The proportion of such patients was very small, suggesting that there would have been little dilution of effect due to contamination in this trial.

15.2.3.6 Estimates of Between-cluster Variability

An important problem when designing CRTs is that sample size calculations require estimates of the intracluster correlation coefficient (ρ) or between-cluster coefficient of variation (k), and empirical values of these coefficients are often unavailable for the chosen study population. The extended CONSORT guidelines therefore recommend that when CRTs are published, the observed values of ρ or k should be reported. Investigators planning new trials can then draw on the accumulating evidence on appropriate values of these coefficients for different endpoints and different types of study population. It may be helpful to report these values for secondary as well as primary endpoints. This information could be given in an online appendix if there is insufficient space in the main paper.

While values recorded in previous CRTs may be useful for trial planning, caution is needed in using such values, for two main reasons. First, except in the largest trials, estimates of ρ or k are usually imprecise, since they rely on the empirical variance of the outcome of interest between clusters. Ideally, therefore, estimates of ρ or k should be accompanied by confidence intervals, but the difficulty of doing so generally precludes this level of reporting. Second, even if a precise estimate is available from a previous trial, we must remember that this applies to the specific clusters studied in that trial. It may or may not be appropriate to assume that a similar value would apply in a different geographical location. Not only do health outcomes tend to vary between populations, but the degree of *heterogeneity* in such measures may also show considerable variation.

By systematically reporting such values, however, we can hope to build an evidence base that will help us develop a clearer understanding of the size and variation of ρ and k in different settings.

15.3 Interpretation and Generalisability

15.3.1 Interpretation

In the published report of a CRT, the investigators' interpretation of the trial results would usually be set out in the Discussion section. As in the report of any trial, the authors will wish to discuss the limitations of the study and the bias that may result from these, including the likely direction and magnitude of any such bias.

As discussed previously, the main focus should be on the primary endpoints. While effects on secondary endpoints, or in particular subgroups, can be reported and discussed, the interpretation of these should be much more cautious. There is usually a large number of potential secondary analyses, including subgroup analyses. Given the repeated significance testing that this involves, and the low power of many trials to detect such effects, we can assume that many, or even most, of the significant effects obtained are due to chance. Such findings may, however, guide future research and may lead to confirmatory tests in further trials, especially if there is a strong biological rationale or supporting evidence from other studies.

Whether or not the primary endpoints show a significant impact, more attention should be paid to the confidence interval than the point estimate of effect or significance level. The confidence interval is the most useful summary of the range of plausible values for the intervention effect, and this should form the main basis for the discussion of the clinical or public health relevance of the findings. This is particularly important when a non-significant effect is reported. While this means that any effect may be due to chance, the confidence interval tells us whether the data are consistent with an important positive or negative effect. If the confidence interval includes substantial positive effects, it would be wrong to use a non-significant result to rule out implementation of an intervention. Further research would be needed to obtain a more precise effect estimate and to clearly establish whether the intervention is of value.

15.3.2 Generalisability

In interpreting the results of any randomised trial, the investigators need to consider and discuss the generalisability of the results. The generalisability of results of CRTs has been discussed in some detail in Section 3.4.4, and we will only review the main points here.

The results of a CRT tell us, within a specified margin of error, the estimated effect of the intervention within the specific study population and as implemented during the trial. The effects seen if the intervention is introduced in a different population or under different conditions may not be the same for several reasons.

- The quality and intensity of intervention are often less when implemented routinely than in a carefully controlled and well-resourced randomised trial. Moreover, the quality of implementation may vary over time. Trends in effect over time may be positive, if it takes time for implementers or the population to become familiar with the intervention, or negative, if initial enthusiasm for the intervention is difficult to sustain.
- Effects may vary because of differences in the characteristics of individuals in different populations. These might, for example, include differences in literacy, health or nutritional status, genetic factors, socioeconomic conditions or cultural factors.
- Effects may vary because the implementation of the intervention differs between populations. For example, the effects of a school-based intervention may depend on the characteristics of the school system, the age-range of the students, the training and skills of the teachers, and many other factors. In some cases, intervention materials have to be adapted to the local context, perhaps involving translation into local languages, and such adaptations may influence intervention effects.
- In trials of interventions against infectious diseases, effects may vary according to the epidemiological characteristics of the infection in specific populations. This was illustrated in Example 3.14, which discussed the differing effects of STD treatment interventions on HIV transmission in three CRTs in East Africa. These differences may be due to differences in the prevalence of STDs and the maturity of the HIV epidemic in different settings (Korenromp et al. 2005).

Some of these factors also limit the generalisability of clinical trials of drug treatments. However, the interventions tested in CRTs are often complex interventions that operate on the health endpoints of primary interest through an elaborate web of cause and effect. Sometimes these interventions depend for their effects on changes in behaviours that may be strongly influenced by social, cultural and economic factors. It is therefore perhaps not surprising that CRTs sometimes seem to show less consistent effects than simple clinical trials.

15.3.3 Systematic Reviews

With the increasing emphasis on evidence-based health-care, an important objective is to base policy decisions on the cumulative evidence from all relevant research studies. Despite their limitations, randomised trials are still regarded as the gold standard for evaluating the effects of health interventions, and play a central role in systematic reviews and meta-analyses carried out to summarise the evidence on specific interventions.

In the past, the major emphasis has been on summarising the evidence on the effects of treatments and other interventions aimed at individuals, and meta-analyses have been based mostly on the results of individually randomised trials. More recently, there has been increasing interest in reviewing the effects of more complex interventions that are applied and evaluated more naturally at population or cluster level. We can therefore expect that systematic reviews and meta-analyses will increasingly make use of data from CRTs. In general, the principles of systematic reviews are similar for CRTs and individually randomised trials. Two points, however, deserve special emphasis.

First, meta-analysts sometimes obtain the primary data from component trials and reanalyse the individual-level data. This is done partly to ensure standardisation of methods of analysis across trials. This is likely to be more problematic for CRTs, where different methods of analysis may be needed for different trials and where adjustments for baseline values are also likely to vary across studies. While a fully standardised analysis may not be feasible, however, it is still possible to combine the evidence from different trials providing that a valid effect estimate and measure of precision are available for each trial. This approach can also be used to combine data from individually randomised trials and CRTs, where both types of study design have been used. In using data from published reports of CRTs, however, authors of systematic reviews need to check carefully that analyses have accounted properly for between-cluster variability, otherwise CRTs with large overall sample sizes may inappropriately dominate the meta-analysis. If clustering has not been accounted for, it may be possible to use external estimates of k or ρ, where these are available, to adjust published estimates for inclusion in a meta-analysis (Donner and Klar 2002; White and Thomas 2005).

Second, meta-analysis can be done using either fixed effects or random effects approaches. As discussed above, we would often expect the effects seen in CRTs to show heterogeneity between trials and study populations. For this reason, random effects meta-analysis is often likely to be the method of choice.

As familiarity with the CRT design increases, and knowledge of the best methods of design and analysis continues to develop, we hope that the next few years will see a continuing improvement in the methodological quality of such trials. If used appropriately, CRTs have the potential to make an important contribution to the development of evidence-based health, educational and social interventions in the years ahead.

References

Adams, G., M. C. Gulliford, O. C. Okoumunne, et al. 2004. Patterns of intra-cluster correlation from primary care research to inform study design and analysis. *Journal of Clinical Epidemiology* 57: 785–94.

Anderson, R. M., and R. M. May. 1991. *Infectious diseases of humans: Dynamics and control.* Oxford: Oxford University Press.

Auvert, B., D. Taljaard, E. Lagarde, et al. 2005. Randomized, controlled intervention trial of male circumcision for reduction of HIV infection risk: The ANRS 1265 trial. *PLoS Medicine* 2 (11): e298.

Ayles, H. M., C. Sismanidis, N. Beyers, R. J. Hayes, and P. Godfrey-Faussett. 2008. ZAMSTAR, the Zambia South Africa TB and HIV Reduction Study: Design of a 2x2 factorial community randomized trial. *Trials* 9: 63.

Bailey, R. 1983. Restricted randomization. *Biometrika* 70: 183–98.

Bailey, R. A. 1987. Restricted randomization: A practical example. *Journal of the American Statistical Association* 82: 712–19.

Begg, C., M. Cho, S. Eastwood, et al. 1996. Improving the quality of reporting of randomized controlled trials. The CONSORT statement. *Journal of the American Medical Association* 276: 637–39.

Bellamy, S. L., R. Gibberd, L. Hancock, et al. 2000. Analysis of dichotomous outcome data for community intervention studies. *Statistical Methods in Medical Research* 9: 135–59.

Berry, D. A., and S. G. Eick. 1995. Adaptive assignment versus balanced randomization in clinical trials: A decision analysis. *Statistics in Medicine* 14: 231–46.

Binka, F. N., A. Kubaje, M. Adjuik, et al. 1996. Impact of permethrin impregnated bednets on child mortality in Kassena-Nankana district, Ghana: A randomized controlled trial. *Tropical Medicine and International Health* 1: 147–54.

Borm, G. F., R. J. F. Melis, S. Teerenstra, and P. G. Peer. 2005. Pseudo cluster randomization: A treatment allocation method to minimize contamination and selection bias. *Statistics in Medicine* 24: 3535–47.

Campbell, M. K., D. R. Elbourne, and D. G. Altman for the CONSORT Group. 2004. CONSORT statement: Extension to cluster randomised trials. *British Medical Journal* 328: 702–8.

Cheung, Y. B., D. Jeffries, A. Thomson, and P. Milligan. 2008. A simple approach to test for interaction between intervention and an individual-level variable in community randomized trials. *Tropical Medicine and International Health* 13: 247–55.

COMMIT Research Group. 1995a. Community Intervention Trial for Smoking Cessation (COMMIT): I. Cohort results from a four-year community intervention. *American Journal of Public Health* 85: 183–92.

COMMIT Research Group. 1995b. Community Intervention Trial for Smoking Cessation (COMMIT): II. Changes in adult cigarette smoking prevalence. *American Journal of Public Health* 85: 193–200.

Council for International Organizations of Medical Sciences (CIOMS) in collaboration with the World Health Organization (WHO). 2002. *International ethical guidelines for biomedical research involving human subjects.* Geneva: CIOMS.

D'Alessandro, U., B. O. Olaleye, W. McGuire, et al. 1995. Mortality and morbidity from malaria in Gambian children after introduction of an impregnated bednet programme. *Lancet* 345: 479–83.

Diehr, P., D. C. Martin, T. Koepsell, and A. Cheadle. 1995. Breaking the matches in a paired *t*-test for community interventions when the number of pairs is small. *Statistics in Medicine* 14: 1491–1504.

Donner, A., N. Birkett, and C. Buck. 1981. Randomization by cluster: Sample size requirements and analysis. *American Journal of Epidemiology* 114: 906–14.

Donner, A., K. S. Brown, and P. Brasher. 1990. A methodological review of non-therapeutic intervention trials employing cluster randomization, 1979–1989. *International Journal of Epidemiology* 19: 795–800.

Donner, A., and N. Klar. 2000. *Design and analysis of cluster randomization trials in health research*. London: Arnold.

———. 2002. Issues in the meta-analysis of cluster randomized trials. *Statistics in Medicine* 21: 2971–80.

Elbourne, D. R., and M. K. Campbell. 2001. Extending the CONSORT statement to cluster randomized trials: For discussion. *Statistics in Medicine* 20: 489–96.

Ellenberg, S. S., T. R. Fleming, and D. L. DeMets. 2003. *Data monitoring committees in clinical trials: A practical perspective*. Chichester, UK: Wiley.

Farrin, A., I. Russell, D. Torgerson, et al. 2005. Differential recruitment in a cluster randomized trial in primary care: The experience of the UK Back pain, Exercise, Active management and Manipulation (UK BEAM) feasibility study. *Clinical Trials* 2: 119–24.

Feder, G., C. Griffiths, S. Eldridge, and M. Spence. 1999. Effect of postal prompts to patients and general practitioners on the quality of primary care after a coronary event (POST): Randomised controlled trial. *British Medical Journal* 318: 1522–26.

Gambia Hepatitis Study Group. 1987. The Gambia hepatitis intervention study. *Cancer Research* 47: 5782–87.

Gessner, B. D., A. Sutanto, M. Linehan, et al. 2005. Incidences of vaccine-preventable *Haemophilus influenzae* type b pneumonia and meningitis in Indonesian children: Hamlet-randomised vaccine-probe trial. *Lancet* 365: 43–52.

Ghana VAST Study Team. 1993. Vitamin A supplementation in northern Ghana: Effects on clinic attendances, hospital admissions, and child mortality. *Lancet* 342: 7–12.

Grosskurth, H., F. Mosha, J. Todd, et al. 1995. Impact of improved treatment of sexually transmitted diseases on HIV infection in rural Tanzania: Randomised controlled trial. *Lancet* 346: 530–36.

Habluetzel, A., D. A. Diallo, F. Esposito, et al. 1997. Do insecticide-treated curtains reduce all-cause child mortality in Burkina Faso? *Tropical Medicine and International Health* 2: 855–62.

Halloran, M. E., I. M. Longini Jr, and C. J. Struchiner. 1999. Design and interpretation of vaccine field studies. *Epidemiological Reviews* 21: 73–88.

Halloran, M. E., and C. J. Struchiner. 1991. Study designs for dependent happenings. *Epidemiology* 2: 331–38.

Hargrove, J. W., J. H. Humphrey, K. Mutasa, et al. 2008. Improved HIV-1 incidence estimates using the BED capture enzyme immunoassay. *AIDS* 22: 511–18.

Hayes, R. J., and S. Bennett. 1999. Simple sample size calculation for cluster-randomized trials. *International Journal of Epidemiology* 28: 319–26.

Hayes, R. J., J. Changalucha, D. A. Ross, et al. 2005. The MEMA kwa Vijana Project: Design of a community randomised trial of an innovative adolescent sexual health intervention in rural Tanzania. *Contemporary Clinical Trials* 26: 430–42.

Hayes, R., F. Mosha, A. Nicoll, et al. 1995. A community trial of the impact of improved sexually transmitted disease treatment on the HIV epidemic in rural Tanzania: 1. Design. *AIDS* 9: 919–26.

Hughes, J. P. 2005. Using baseline data to design a group randomized trial. *Statistics in Medicine* 24: 1983–94.

Hussey, M. A., and J. P. Hughes. 2007. Design and analysis of stepped wedge cluster randomized trials. *Contemporary Clinical Trials* 28: 182–91.

International Conference on Harmonisation of Technical Requirements for Registration of Pharmaceuticals for Human Use. 1996. *ICH harmonised tripartite guidelines: Guideline for good clinical practice E6(R1)*. ICH.

Jennison, C., and B. W. Turnbull. 1999. *Group sequential methods with applications to clinical trials*. Boca Raton: Chapman and Hall.

Kamali, A., M. Quigley, J. Nakiyingi, et al. 2003. Syndromic management of sexually-transmitted infections and behaviour change interventions on transmission of HIV-1 in rural Uganda: A community randomised trial. *Lancet* 361: 645–52.

Kish, L. 1965. *Survey sampling*. New York: John Wiley.

Klar, N., and Donner, A. The merits of matching in community intervention trials: A cautionary tale. *Statistics in Medicine* 1997, 16: 1753–64.

Korenromp, E. L., R. G. White, K. K. Orroth, et al. 2005. Determinants of the impact of sexually transmitted infection treatment on prevention of HIV infection: A synthesis of evidence from the Mwanza, Rakai and Masaka intervention trials. *Journal of Infectious Diseases* 191 (suppl. 1): S168–75.

Lan, K. K. G., and D. L. DeMets. 1983. Discrete sequential boundaries for clinical trials. *Biometrika* 70: 659–63.

Littenberg, B., and C. D. MacLean. 2006. Intra-cluster correlation coefficients in adults with diabetes in primary care practices: The Vermont diabetes information system field survey. *BMC Medical Research Methodology* 6: 20.

Longini, I. M. Jr, K. Sagatelian, W. N. Rida, and M. E. Halloran. 1998. Optimal vaccine trial design when estimating vaccine efficacy for susceptibility and infectiousness from multiple populations. *Statistics in Medicine* 17: 1121–36.

McDougal, J. S., C. D. Pilcher, B. S. Parekh, et al. 2005. Surveillance for HIV-1 incidence using tests for recent infection in resource-constrained countries. *AIDS* 19: S25–S30.

Medical Research Council. 2002. *Cluster randomised trials: Methodological and ethical considerations*. London: MRC.

Moulton, L. H. 2004. Covariate-based constrained randomization of group-randomized trials. *Clinical Trials* 1: 297–305.

Moulton, L. H., J. E. Golub, B. Durovni, et al. 2007. Statistical design of THRio: A phased implementation clinic-randomized study of a tuberculosis preventive therapy intervention. *Clinical Trials* 4: 190–99.

Moulton, L. H., K. L. O'Brien, R. Kohberger, et al. 2001. Design of a group-randomized *Streptococcus pneumoniae* vaccine trial. *Controlled Clinical Trials* 22: 438–52.

Moulton, L. H., K. L. O'Brien, R. Reid, R. Weatherholtz, and M. Santosham. 2006. Evaluation of the indirect effects of a pneumococcal vaccine in a community-randomized study. *Journal of Biopharmaceutical Statistics* 16: 453–62.

Moulton, L. H., and S. L. Zeger. 1989. Analyzing repeated measures on generalized linear models via the bootstrap. *Biometrics* 45: 381–94.

Nagot, N., A. Ouedraogo, V. Foulongne, et al. 2007. Reduction of HIV-1 RNA levels with therapy to suppress Herpes simplex virus. *New England Journal of Medicine* 356: 790–99.

Nevill, C. G., E. S. Some, V. O. Mung'ala, et al. 1996. Insecticide-treated bednets reduce mortality and severe morbidity from malaria among children on the Kenyan coast. *Tropical Medicine and International Health* 1: 139–46.

Obasi, A. I., R. Balira, J. Todd, et al. 2001. Prevalence of HIV and *Chlamydia trachomatis* infection in 15–19-year olds in rural Tanzania. *Tropical Medicine and International Health* 6: 517–25.

Obasi, A. I., B. Cleophas, D. A. Ross, et al. 2006. Rationale and design of the *MEMA kwa Vijana* adolescent sexual and reproductive health intervention in Mwanza Region, Tanzania. *AIDS Care* 18: 311–22.

O'Brien, K. L., L. H. Moulton, R. Reid, et al. 2003. Efficacy and safety of seven-valent conjugate pneumococcal vaccine in American Indian children: Group randomised trial. *Lancet* 362: 355–61.

Orroth, K. K., E. L. Korenromp, R. G. White, et al. 2003. Higher risk behaviour and rates of sexually transmitted diseases in Mwanza compared to Uganda may help explain HIV prevention trial outcomes. *AIDS* 17: 2653–60.

Pan, W., and M. M. Wall. 2002. Small-sample adjustments in using the sandwich variance estimator in generalized estimating equations. *Statistics in Medicine* 21: 1429–41.

Pocock, S. J., and R. Simon. 1975. Sequential treatment assignment with balancing for prognostic factors in the controlled clinical trial. *Biometrics* 31: 103–15.

Proschan, M. A., K. K. G. Lan, and J. T. Wittes. 2006. *Statistical monitoring of clinical trials: A unified approach.* New York: Springer.

Raab, G. M., and I. Butcher. 2001. Balance in cluster randomized trials. *Statistics in Medicine* 20: 351–65.

Rose, G. 1992. *The strategy of preventive medicine.* Oxford: Oxford University Press.

Ross, D. A., J. Changalucha, A. I. N. Obasi, et al. 2007. Biological and behavioural impact of an adolescent sexual health intervention in Tanzania: A community-randomized trial. *AIDS* 21: 1943–55.

Signorini, D. F., O. Leung, R. J. Simes, et al. 1993. Dynamic balanced randomization for clinical trials. *Statistics in Medicine* 12: 2343–50.

Simpson, J. M., N. Klar, and A. Donner. 1995. Accounting for cluster randomization: A review of primary prevention trials, 1990 through 1993. *American Journal of Public Health* 85: 1378–82.

Sismanidis, C., L. Moulton, H. Ayles, et al. 2008. Restricted randomization of Zamstar: A 2x2 factorial cluster randomized trial. *Clinical Trials* 2008, 5: 316–27.

Thiam, S., A. M. LeFevre, and F. Hane, et al. 2007. Effectiveness of a strategy to improve adherence to tuberculosis treatment in a resource-poor setting: A cluster randomized controlled trial. *Journal of the American Medical Association* 297: 380–86.

Todd, J., L. Carpenter, and L. Xianbin, et al. 2003. The effects of alternative studyt designs on the power of community randomized trials: Evidence from three studies of human immunodeficiency virus prevention in East Africa. *International Journal of Epidemiology* 32: 755–62.

Torgerson, D. J. 2001. Contamination in trials: Is cluster randomisation the answer? *British Medical Journal* 322: 355–57.

Turner, R. M., S. G. Thompson, and D. J. Spiegelhalter. 2005. Prior distributions for the intracluster correlation coefficient, based on multiple previous estimates, and their application in cluster randomized trials. *Clinical Trials* 2: 108–18.

UNAIDS/WHO. 2007. *Ethical considerations in biomedical HIV prevention trials.* Geneva: UNAIDS.

Wawer, M. J., R. H. Gray, N. K. Sewankambo, et al. 1998. A randomized, community trial of sexually transmitted disease control for AIDS prevention, Rakai, Uganda. *AIDS* 12: 1211–25.

Wawer, M. J., N. K. Sewankambo, D. Serwadda, et al. 1999. Control of sexually transmitted diseases for AIDS prevention in Uganda: A randomised community trial. *Lancet* 353: 525–35.

White, I. R., and J. Thomas. 2005. Standardized mean differences in individually-randomized and cluster-randomized trials, with applications to meta-analysis. *Clinical Trials* 2: 141–51.

White, R. G., K. K. Orroth, E. L. Korenromp, et al. 2004. Can population differences explain the contrasting results of the Mwanza, Rakai, and Masaka HIV/sexually transmitted disease intervention trials? A modeling study. *Journal of Acquired Immune Deficiency Syndromes* 37: 1500–13.

Wight, D., G. M. Raab, M. Henderson, et al. 2002. Limits of teacher delivered sex education: Interim behavioural outcomes from randomised trial. *British Medical Journal* 324: 1430–35.

Zeger, S., and Liang, K. -Y. 1986. Longitudinal data analysis for discrete and continuous outcomes. *Biometrics* 42: 121–30.

Zelen, M. 1979. A new design for randomized clinical trials. *New England Journal of Medicine* 300: 1242–45.

Zelen, M. 1990. Randomized consent designs for clinical trials: An update. *Statistics in Medicine* 9: 645–56.

Index